Snowshoe & Lancet

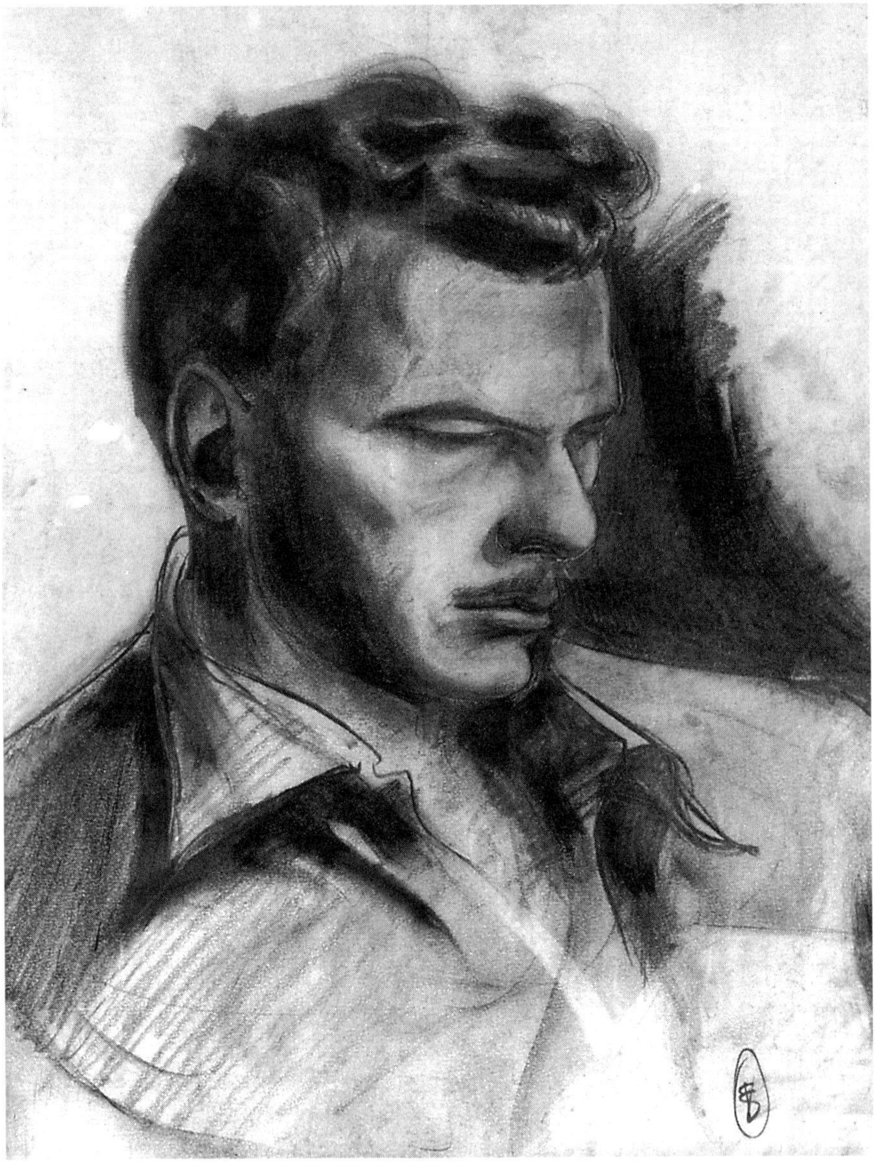

Charcoal portrait of RSE by Ted Drover.

Snowshoe & Lancet

Memoirs of a Frontier Newfoundland Doctor

1937–1948

ROBERT SKIDMORE ECKE, M.D.

Foreword by Gary Saunders

PETER E. RANDALL PUBLISHER
Portsmouth, New Hampshire · 2000

Published in the United States of America

Design; Tom Allen, Pear Graphic Design

Peter E. Randall Publisher
Box 4726, Portsmouth, NH 03802

Distributed by University Press of New England
Hanover and London

Library of Congress Cataloging-in-Publiction Data

Ecke, Robert Skidmore, 1909-
Snowshoe & lancet : memoirs of a frontier Newfoundland doctor, 1937-1948 / Robert Skidmore Ecke
p. ; cm.
ISBN 0914339-85-0 (alk. paper)
1. Physicians--Newfoundland--Biography. 2. Missions, Medical--Newfoundland--Biography. I. Title: Snowshoe and lancet. II. Title.
[DNLM: 1. Ecke, Robert Skidmore, 1909- 2. Physicians--Personal Narratives. WZ 100
E189 2000
R722.32.E27 A3 2000
610'.92--dc21
[B]

00-035305

In sweet remembrance
Of forty-seven years of friendship
1949-1996

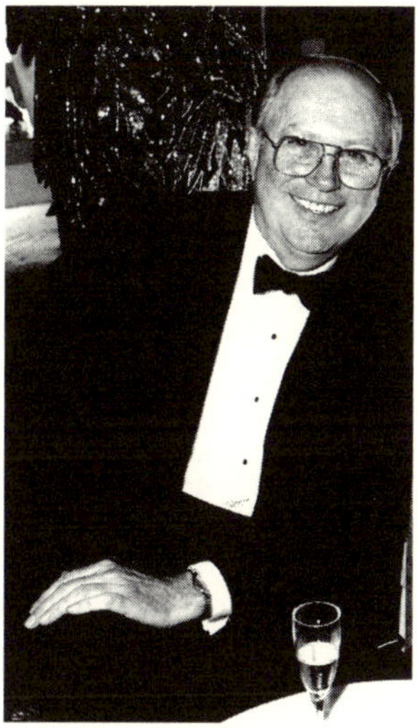

Robert Willard Olson

FOREWORD

They called him Dr. Hackie, those 1930s Newfoundlanders in their West Country dialect, and he, a Yankee newcomer, loved it. "Hackie" wasn't a nickname, nor a pun on his profession; it was simply how Notre Dame Bay people spoke the King's English. Actually they improved his surname, for "Ecke" seemed somehow too slight for this strapping young doctor who came roaring over the sheep paths on a motorcycle to born their babies and succour their ills.

They took to him readily, the more so since he worked with their beloved John McKee Olds, boss of Twillingate Hospital and its chief surgeon. Certainly Olds needed him. The hospital's clientele lived in a hundred coastal outports scattered across a sub-arctic archipelago, many reachable only by boat in summer and dog team in winter. A TB epidemic was raging—this was before miracle drugs—and the 60-bed hospital (soon expanded to 90-bed) overflowed with long-term patients. World War II worsened this situation by stealing all of Olds' RNs and most of his doctors, including, for a time, Robert Ecke.

But Ecke came back, twice. Between 1937 and 1948 he served the islanders seven years. He could easily have made more money (and stayed warmer) in Boston or Baltimore, but Newfoundland had got into his blood. A good thing, too, or we wouldn't have this book.

For he kept a journal. Hurriedly, after grueling hours in the OR and in Outpatients, or in the cramped and often tilting bunk of the hospital boat *Bonnie Nell* on another harrowing house call, he scribbled his impressions. He was keeping a record, yes; but he was also coming to terms with the welter of new experiences breaking over him like storm waves over an open skiff. Out of those journals came this memoir.

Like all good memoirs it is candid. The warts are here—both his and theirs. So are the killing hours, the sense of Arctic isolation, the almost compulsive partying, the hospital politics, the triumphs small and large.

Sometimes one feels the author is being too hard on himself. There are times when he's obviously exasperated with his patients. But you can tell he loves them.

Recently he confided to me that re-reading certain passages made him weep. Not from sadness or maudlin sentiment I am sure, but because they recall the many wonderful human beings, so brave and kind and funny, with whom he lived and worked. Former nursing aide Lorna Bradley Stuckless put it well when, chided by Dr. Olds for "carrying on" about her son's recovery at his hands, she retorted, "Doctor, there's such thing as tears of sadness but there's also tears of joy!"

All those people are here: crusty John Olds, long-suffering aides, nurses and doctors; well-off merchants, starving cod fishers, gruff sea-dogs, jolly poker partners, bona fide patients and whining malingerers, pregnant teenaged girls, rascally youngsters on the mend. So is the impoverished mother of several, recently amputeed, who quietly says when told she must undergo a caesarian: "All right, Doctor, do what you can to help me—but remember, life is sweet." Two disastrous fires are here too, and the wartime blackouts, and Olds' Goldbergian Inventions, and the excitement of the spring seal hunt.

Robert Ecke has a light touch, a lovely sense of humour and understatement. His word portraits are so vivid, his landscapes so painterly, that one feels transplanted to that place and time.

One of the best things about this book is the sense of a young man finding himself, of a person gradually maturing in his relationships and his profession. Twillingate Hospital did that to you. It was a school of Life. All its best graduates said so. None has said it better than Dr. Hackie—Guaranteed.

GARY SAUNDERS
Clifton, Nova Scotia, Canada
September 1999

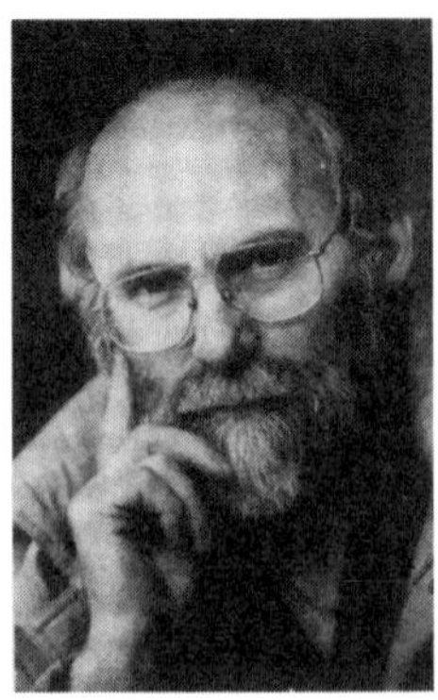

CONTENTS

INTRODUCTION

Most of this book is taken directly from my journal, beginning in 1937 and ending in 1941, when it came to pass that the winds of war wafted me away to four continents for forty-five months. I was brought home as a patient on the hospital ship *John J. Meaney,* an improbable name. It was a very stormy November crossing from Bremerhaven to Staten Island. In due course, Walter Reed Hospital released me and separated me from the service as a Lt. Colonel. My brother, Albert Dekker, of stage, screen and forum, bade me come for R&R in the San Fernando valley. I stayed on the Mojave at Rancho Yucca Loma, then in his Schindler-designed house near Hollywood. Albert was busy making movies, serving in the California legislature, and writing a muck-raking column for a local paper. He found me an amanuensis, one Milton Lubewisky, an ace typist and avowed communist. Under brotherly pressure, I dictated away for dear life using my assorted journals, notes, letters, and papers.

How and why the manuscript languished for more than half a century is a book in itself. At first, there was praise and interest. I was encouraged by people big in literary matters. Hearing some of my war stories at dinner, novelist Irving Stone said if my book was anything like the stories, I should publish. He sent me to his editor, Maxwell Perkins, editor for Hemingway, Fitzgerald and Thomas Wolfe. Dale VanEvery, a producer (*Dr. Cyclops*) and widely read author (*Bridal Journey, The Voyagers,* and five others), set up a morning appointment in his little cabin sanctuary on his one-thousand-acre spread in Santa Barbara. He sat me down and talked at length standing by the fire with my manuscript in hand. He had read it all and thought it would be published, but I must never, never let anyone change it.

Six years later, John Douglas, vice-president of CBS, sent it to his editors who threw it back in his face saying uncomplimentary things about him and me. He ruefully admitted that his department did not get along with that department. Other bits surfaced like, “This mountain of typing . . . ,” and “This self-effacing doctor is not as modest as he seems.” Viking Press assigned, and I assume paid, an editor to work with me. A month later he was seduced by an industrial giant and left without completing the project. The opus lay fallow for five decades.

My closest friend told me pointedly that constant nattering about Twillingate was boring our friends, in spades. However, several went to visit the place. One Harvard professor stayed a whole year, and a luxury cruise director took groups of his well-heeled clients. There were others. All returned raving and I don’t mean crazy.

Finally an Eliot neighbor, Deborah Perkins, interviewed me as “Curmudgeon of the Week,” for her little Eliot newsletter. She, a computer wizard, said she would like a shot at getting the now bedraggled opus published. The fat was in the fire. For the outcome, read on.

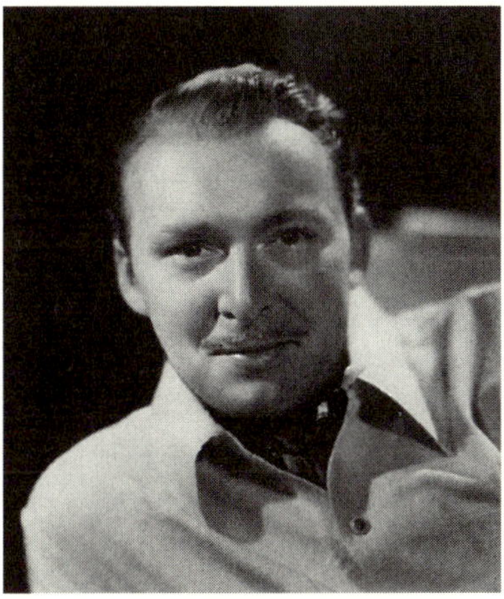

Albert Dekker
on Paramount Lot

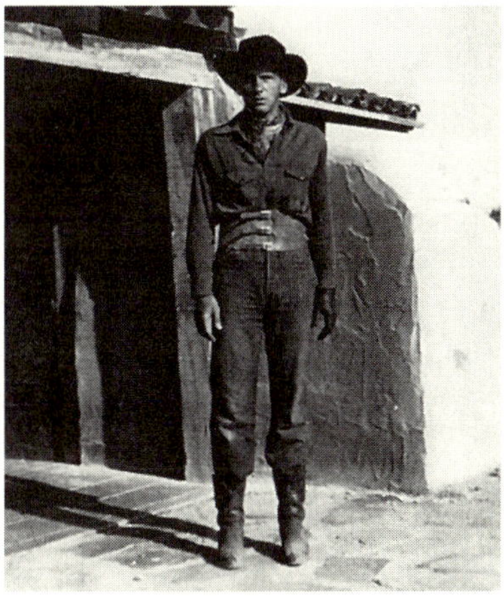

Ecke on R&R
at Rancho Yucca Loma

ACKNOWLEDGMENTS

In 1946 my brother, Albert Dekker, shamed me into getting my material into readable shape. He became a booster.

Dr. Lydia Edwards worked during World War II with Tito's partisans and so did I. She heard so much about Twillingate that she went there and became enraptured. A steady goading ensued.

John J. Murphy's eagle eye unerringly spots imperfection. He made much use of his undying passion for words in all their aspects. He gave many hours to tedious perusal.

Deborah Perkins's enthusiastic computer wizardry kept this show on the road.

Claire Blaisdell exercised her typing and proofing skills.

Vital tiresome typing and retyping was gladly performed over five decades. I am grateful to Jan Dekker, my erudite niece; Ruthie Torborg, my very dear cousin; Ellen Harris Lemire, an observing civic colleague; and Jan and Denise Sheldon, my honored gourmet associates.

CHRONOLOGY

- November 22, 1909—Born at home; Brooklyn, New York.
- Attended local public elementary school—P.S. 171.
- Was graduated from Richmond Hill High School, Queens, New York.
- Attended Bowdoin College, September, 1927 to June, 1931, was graduated with AB cum laude degree, majoring in Chemistry, with a minor in German.
- Went to Camp Winona, Denmark, Maine, for first time, in summer of 1928, as counselor.
- Summer 1929—at cottage in Randolph, N. H., White Mountains—Cold Brook Camp.
- Started as medical student at Johns Hopkins—September , 1931.
- June–September, 1934. First summer at Twillingate Hospital, as Johns Hopkins medical student; with Dick Mirick.
- September, 1934—started 4th year at Johns Hopkins, including one semester at Harvard Medical School.
- June, 1935; Received MD, Johns Hopkins.
- Summer of 1935. At Camp Winona.
- September, 1935. At Baltimore City Hospitals, Bayview—10 months.
- July, 1936. At Camp Winona.
- September, 1936. At Johns Hopkins on Poliomyelitis Fellowship, to Spring '37.
- Summer, 1937. At Camp Winona.
- Early September, 1937—Auto drive by sister Kathryn and Dot Houghton to North Sydney, Cape Breton.
- September, 1937. To Newfoundland, St. John's, to be examined for Empire Medical License, accepted; on to Twillingate as Staff doctor.
- September, 1937. Starts keeping Journal.
- Saturday, Nov. 6, 1937—Marianne arrives at Twillingate.
- Summer of 1938. At Camp Winona, with infected arm.

- September, '38. Back at Twillingate, with Dudley Sean O'Connor.
- February 7, '39. Dudley disappears.
- February 28, '39. Cottage burns.
- April–May, '39. Manhattan General Hospital. "40 days."
- June, 1939. Trip to California—3-4 weeks Hollywood.
- Summer, 1939 at Camp Winona.
- Fall, 1939—Ambulance—E.R. for Bedford Styvesant area for St. John's Hospital, Brooklyn, New York.
- June, 1940—At Wesleyville, Newfoundland, covering for Dr. Rube Waddell.
- July, 1940—Return to Twillingate, with Dudley II.
- Summer, 1940 to June 5, '41—At Twillingate.
- November, 1940—Dudley II shot.
- July, 1941—Trip to St. John's, Medical convention.
- July–August, 1941—Sister Kathryn and Dot Houghton visit Twillingate for 5 weeks.
- Fall, 1941—Continue at Twillingate.
- December 7, 1941—Pearl Harbor—Planning to take a holiday January, '42 in States, switched with Swanker for vacation. Left immediately, and en-route learned of Pearl Harbor, went to Brooklyn, NY.
- February 14, 1942—Received commission as 1st Lieutenant in U.S. Army. Sworn in by father.
- WWII.
- May–September, 1942—Quidi Vidi, Newfoundland.
- Summer, '42—official visit as Army Officer to Notre Dame Bay Hospital to alert them to possible need for medical services for U.S. military personnel.
- First assignment: to Fort Chimo, Ungava Bay, Quebec—as local Post Medical Officer at a Weather Station, then airstrip, (U.S. Army doctor with U.S. Corps of Engineers) October, '42–late 1943.
- Late 1943–1946 . Member of U.S. Army, Typhus Commission, at various places: Cairo, Egypt; Naples, Italy; other Italy; Aden; Addis Ababa; Khartoum, Sudan; four months with Yugoslav partisans; post-war: typhus consultant to SHAEF. De-mobed as Lt. Col.
- April, 1944. Father died.
- November 8, 1947–April 20, 1948—Medical Director of Notre Dame Bay Memorial Hospital, Twillingate.
- 1949–1964. CIA (no comment).

- 1964–1969. Research on adrenal cortex, Westchester County, New York, U.S.A.
- 1969–1979. Private practice Hartsdale, New York, U.S.A.
- November 2, 1970. Mother died.
- 1979—Moved to Eliot, Maine, U.S.A.

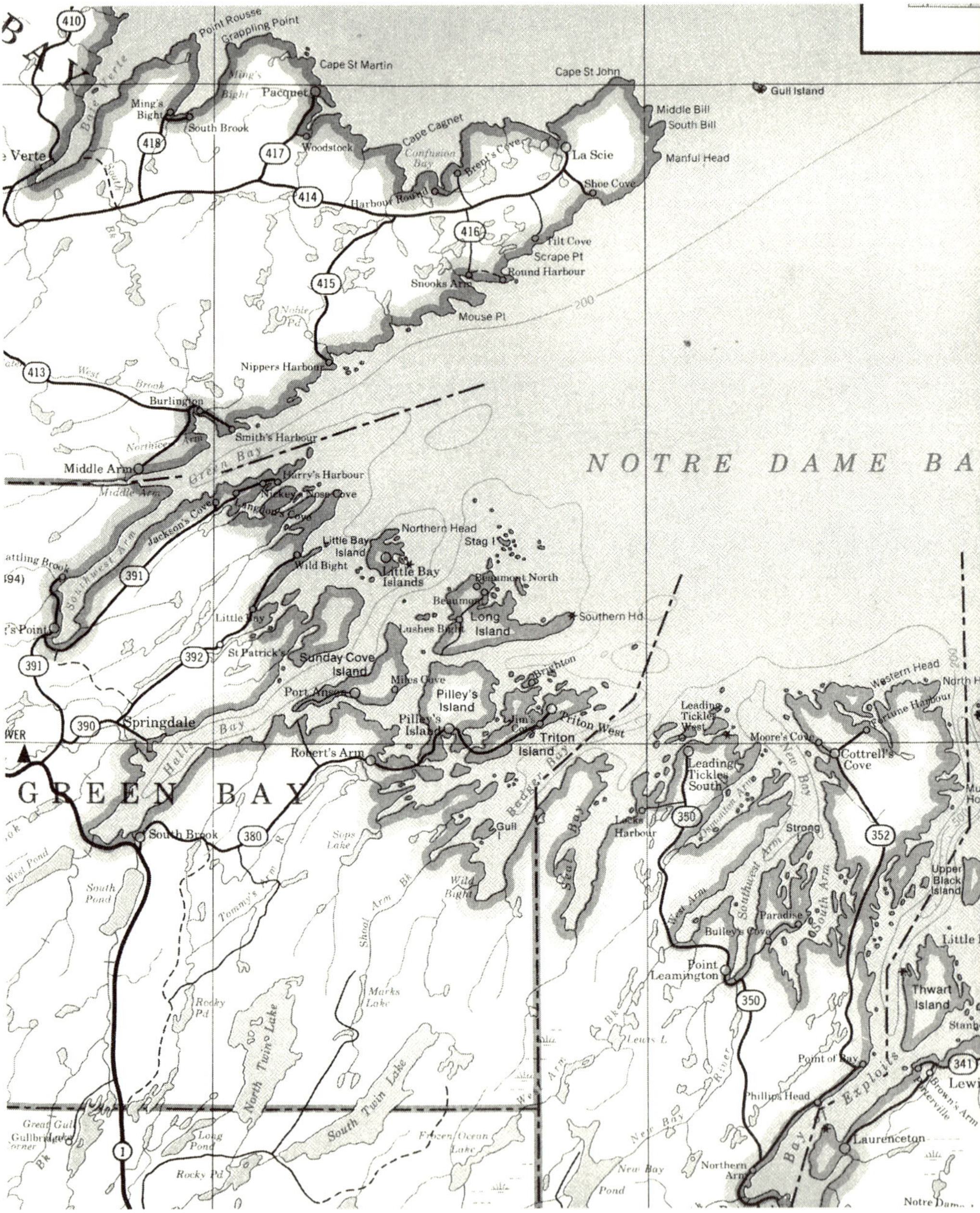

Map of Notre Dame Bay and Twillingate Island, northeast coast of Newfoundland. Used with permission, Natural Resources Canada.

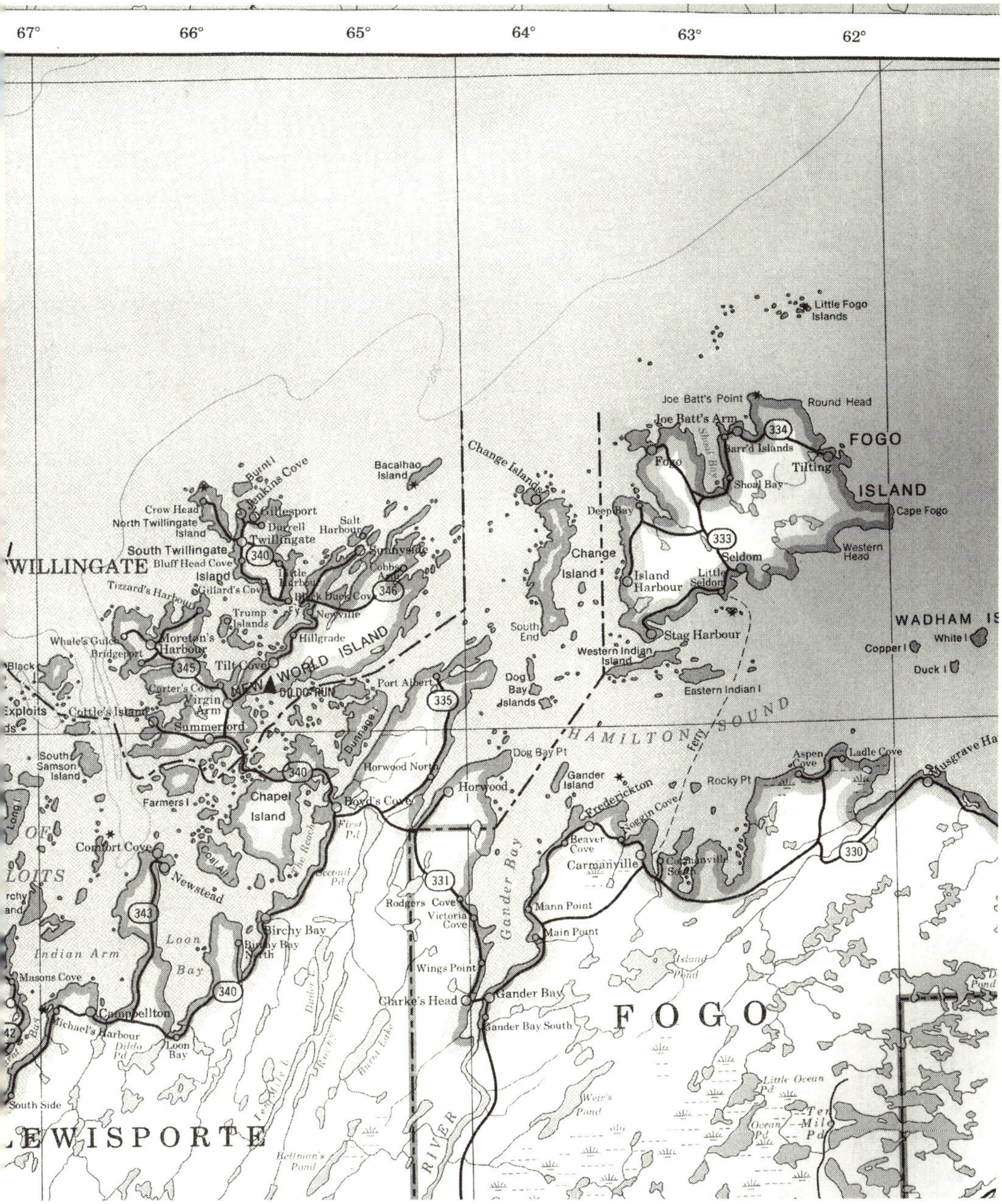

FOGO ISLAND
TWILLINGATE
NEW WORLD ISLAND
Change Islands
Change Island
HAMILTON SOUND
WADHAM IS
FOGO
LEWISPORTE
Little Fogo Islands
Joe Batt's Point
Round Head
Joe Batt's Arm
Barr'd Islands
Tilting
Shoal Bay
Cape Fogo
Seldom
Little Seldom
Western Head
Deep Bay
Island Harbour
Stag Harbour
Western Indian Island
Eastern Indian I
Copper I
White I
Duck I
Bacalhao Island
Jenkins Cove
Gillesport
Durrell
Crow Head
North Twillingate Island
South Twillingate Island
Bluff Head Cove
Gillard's Cove
Salt Harbour
Sunnyside
Cobbs Arm
Black Duck Cove
Newville
Hillgrade
Trump Islands
Moreton's Harbour
Bridgeport
Whale's Gulch
Tilt Cove
Virgin Arm
Carter's Cove
Cottle's Island
Summerford
Exploits
South Samson Island
Farmers I
Chapel Island
Port Albert
Dog Bay Islands
Dog Bay Pt
Horwood North
Horwood
Boyd's Cove
Gander Island
Frederickton
Noggin Cove
Beaver Cove
Carmanville
Carmanville South
Rocky Pt
Aspen Cove
Ladle Cove
Musgrave Harbour
Comfort Cove
Newstead
Birchy Bay
Birchy Bay North
Loon Bay
Indian Arm
Masons Cove
Campbellton
Michael's Harbour
South Side
Rodgers Cove
Victoria Cove
Wings Point
Clarke's Head
Gander Bay
Gander Bay South
Mann Point
Main Point
Island Pond
Little Ocean Pd
Ocean Pd
Ten Mile Pd
Weir's Pond
Bellman's Pond
RIVER
67°
66°
65°
64°
63°
62°

CHAPTER I

Medicine, Why Not

In 1939 I had a job in a New York hospital designed to be a citadel of private medicine. Three-story columns graced the entry, marble floors softened the suffering of the sick and impressed visitors who sought the spacious lobby. Off to one side, a broad hallway led to the ducal lair of the director-owner, who sat behind a Florentine desk in his Palazzo Venezia office with its forty-foot ceiling.

My bond called for six months as assistant resident and a year of residency. Well-meaning friends had talked me into this. "It's time," they said, "you gave up this silly wandering around among those Newfoundlanders. You've got to settle down, you know, and open an office." Now I can't walk past one of those discreet suburban offices without a shudder. I can see through that tapestry brick veneer and the iron grill downstairs doorway into the reception room with its chrome furniture and the magazines very carefully kept up-to-date by a charming receptionist. It brings back my ulcer.

This job, arranged by friends while I was a thousand miles away, was the best that could be managed with my background. Four years at Bowdoin had made it not too difficult to get into Johns Hopkins. Next, a year of surgery at Baltimore City Hospitals had led to a year of research fellowship in poliomyelitis back at Hopkins. But then I went off to Newfoundland. Two years there, it was argued, had almost irretrievably put me outside the pale of ordinary medicine.

Oh, well, I thought, the Jews had a hard time of it for 40 years. I suppose I can endure for 18 months here. Besides, I was learning from my older colleagues. As we used to gather cozily in the green room after or just before operations, I would listen to the words of wisdom: "You know,

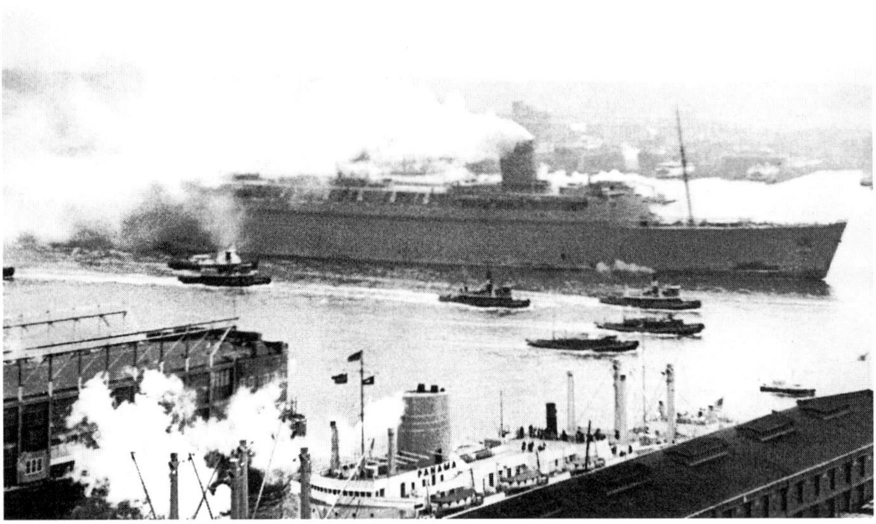

Room with a view, from the scrub room of Manhattan General, photograph by Joseph Kassheimer.

(adjusting the mask) you have got to soak these birds. If you don't charge them generously they don't think you're any good" or "we'll have to get out and find something else to do. I haven't done a mastoid in a month. This sulfa stuff will put us out of business."

A counter measure to this attitude had been provided by the architects (McKim, Meade, and White) with a window commanding a striking view of New York harbor. The ten minutes spent scrubbing for surgery are a strange, unreal ten minutes. They can seem hours long. Usually one goes into a kind of trance, leaving the mind blank and in a strangely receptive condition. Many people have visions and inspirations as they automatically wield the brush and soap in this half-dream state. It is a phase in the doctor's life neglected by propagandists. That would be the time to plant seeds or germs in the mind. Suddenly coming to, you would have something new in your thinking and not know where it came from.

Thus was I taken by the scene of the harbor ten floors below. Each morning through my cell window I would see the feathery wisps of steam from the freighters and the liners, and a moment later sense the haunting nostalgia of the deep-water whistle. Each outbound prow that cut the harbor took me further from the green room. Each tug that nudged its bigger brother into the stream separated me a little more from my bondage until at the end of 40 days and 40 nights my soul was won back to me. It was the work of but an hour to have in hand the notice that, "At his own request, Dr. R. S. Ecke is relieved from further duty." (The director of intern service was an old army man.)

Then followed a period of hectic happy preparation for the north. Skis, woolens, books were gathered; some needed supplies and instruments collected for the Twillingate Hospital, a hasty trip to California to say good-bye to my brother, farewells to my family in New York, and I was aboard the "State of Maine" Express for Brunswick, Maine, where all my journeys end and begin.

A two-day ride on the *Gull* through the Maritime Provinces of northeast Canada took me to North Sydney on Cape Breton Isle. Schedules here begin to be a little ragged. There may be days to wait for the *S.S. Caribou*—my favorite ship in the world: Newfoundland registry, best icebreaker in the North Atlantic. When the Canadian icebreakers are frozen in they get the *Caribou* to cut them out. Her 2,222 tons were Holland-built, with one of those spoon bows to rush full speed upon the pans of blue St. Lawrence ice and crush them. Captain Benjamin Tavenor skippered her and in the crew were four of his sons. I can see him now, big in all directions, walrus-mustached, quiet, playing cribbage in the saloon while we were frozen tight in the pack ice waiting ten hours for the sea to break it up. Half the crew had disappeared over the horizon, on the ice, to hunt for seal. He was very careful of his ship and had made every trip on her but one. He had been persuaded to rest ashore for once, about three years after she started this tricky one-hundred mile run between Canada and the nearest point of Newfoundland, Port aux Basques. His rest was short. In only three hours she was on the rocks and he was summoned. Tavenor made all the trips after that, even to the point of putting the helm hard over in a valiant, vain attempt to ram the German submarine who had fired a fatal torpedo. One-hundred and thirty-seven, including the captain and his sons, died in that icy water, one hundred and one were saved. The ships on that run now can't begin to replace my real love—the *Caribou*. But I am in the middle of my story.

When I am with my friends and the conversation comes around to the subject of Newfoundland (that's pretty easy to manage) certain questions are posed: Where is Newfoundland? How did you come to go there in the

2A BROOKLYN EAGLE, SUNDAY, OCT. 18, 1942

U-Boat Plowed Among Children, Women Struggling in Icy Sea

Sydney, N. S., Oct. 17 (U.P.)—Survivors of the passenger steamer Caribou, sunk in Cabot Strait Wednesday by an enemy submarine with a loss of 137 Canadians and Americans, told today how the U-boat surfaced after the sinking and plowed ruthlessly through men, women and children struggling in the icy waters.

Canadian naval rescue vessels landed 101 survivors. The bodies of 36 persons were recovered. There remained a missing list of 101, none of whom was believed to have survived.

Capt. Benjamin Tarvernor, who went down with his ship but somehow fought off the suction and popped to the surface alongside a life raft, saw the submarine after it loosed its torpedo and attempted to ram it, but the 2,222-ton Caribou's bow plunged under the waves before it could strike back.

The submarine, which had dived to avoid Captain Tarvenor's attempt to ram it, returned to the surface and threw the occupants of a lifeboat and two rafts into the water. It made no attempts to assist them but cruised about through the debris and struggling victims. Only one of 15 children aboard survived.

Navy Minister Angus MacDonald, who announced the sinking, asserted:

"If there were any Canadians who did not realize that we were up against a ruthless and remorseless enemy, there can be no such Canadians now. If anything were needed to prove the hideousness of Nazi warfare, surely this is it."

first place? Why did you like it so much? Why did you stay so long?

The first one—where is it?—ought to be easy to answer but for some reason people don't seem able to hold the country in their minds as an entity. I can spend a whole evening raving about Newfoundland only to be asked the next time I see my friend "What's the news from Alaska?" or "Have you been back to Greenland," even "I just met a man from Nova Scotia, that's where you were, isn't it?" I groan and start all over again.

As to the how and why I went there is another story. I would like to think that from the age of two, I read nothing but accounts of Newfoundland and finally saw my dream come to reality, yet search the beginnings of my life and there is no trend—no zeal for the starkness of the northern life, no consuming yen to help humanity. I grew up quite amiably in Brooklyn, USA. Throughout high school (Richmond Hill) the streets of Brooklyn and the stage of the high school dramatic club offered all the adventure I seemed to need. The summers were spent pursuing the elusive brook trout through the Poconos and the Catskills. I didn't pursue them but my father was a fanatic fly caster and the whole family had to go along like a pack in full cry, with the result that I haven't spent more than half an hour fishing in my whole life. Besides being a disciple of Isaac Walton, my father was two other things—a lawyer who knew more about real property law than anyone else in New York, and as good a colonel of infantry as we ever had in the army. My brother, sister, and mother shared this military, legal, piscatory life. The brother was always off with father on maneuvers or something equally military. He had a burning urge to be a doctor, started as a Broadway actor and wound up in the movies. The sister turned out to be a major in the Air Force. My mother retained her own sweet long-suffering identity.

After high school I developed the pleasant habit of teaching canoeing and taking out canoe trips at a Maine summer camp. This was the most valuable aspect of my pre-Newfoundland life, where I learned the joy of the life in which the important things are the basic ones: Have we food? Can we travel? Have we shelter? How is the wind? I did try to break away from this camp life. I even went so far as to get a job on a Dollar Line ship to go around the world. I looked up the ship's schedule and in what I thought was good time, presented myself at that line's office in Hoboken. I can see the Captain-of-the-Port Parker now as I announced myself. He was terse. He said, "The *President Coolidge* left a week ago." Then to his secretary, "We must remember to keep this door locked." While composing a telegram to the camp I swore I would save pennies until I could buy the Dollar Line and fix Captain-of-the-Port Parker's wagon. Unfortunately, the line went into bankruptcy before vengeance was mine.

The year my brother was born, one of my father's fellow soldiers started preaching the virtues of Bowdoin College. We packed Albert off 18 years later in Sears Roebuck corduroy and leather to brave the Maine wilds at Bowdoin. Four years later it was my turn. I was offered a scholarship to Harvard but I was steered away from the fleshpots of Boston.

The Bowdoin years went swiftly and happily. My 175 pounds were stacked six feet and that looked to people as if I ought to play end. Ends have to be kind of smart, what with catching forward passes and things so I ate steaks and baked potatoes and got up to 183 so I could play tackle. Besides that, we already had two ends. I played very faithfully and even became captain. That was in the last game of my career—with Wesleyan, where we were so far ahead that in the final minute and a half, Charlie Bowser put in the second team. The substitute for my position had a sprained elbow and was a little slow so the captaincy, as substitutions progressed, gradually devolved and as eleventh choice I became captain for the delirious ninety-second taste of power.

The Drama also attracted me. My triumph perhaps was the lead in Galsworthy's *Escape*. It will be recalled that the hero dallies with a stolen bottle of spirituous drink during the last act. At the premier I ignored the coach's directions to use a bottle of tea. A bottle of real spirits added brilliance to my performance even if I did run afoul of the boom that weighs down the curtain. No one has any concept of the works of William Shakespeare who has not heard me declaim in black tights and hired ermine, "If music be the food of love, play on."

Meanwhile I majored in chemistry and took lots of German. One of the beautiful moments of my life occurred in the physical chemistry class. The desk was decorated with molecular models. The walls held Mendelieff's periodic chart of the elements. The professor, since dead by his own hand, was expounding on the obscurities of hydrogen ion concentration. For nine seconds a rift seemed to appear in the misty clouds and a shaft of pure understanding shone. For that brief period all was clear and the mysteries of the universe and I were one. In the midst of my knowing elation the clouds closed and like O.W. Holmes, all I had left was, "It smells of ether."

College galloped toward the close. Easter vacation of my senior year, six weeks before graduation, found me undecided on my life's work. The only prospect seemed to be going to China for the Standard Oil Company. At home, my father was a little gruff about that. In fact, we didn't exchange a civil word that whole vacation. Money was not important to Dad. He didn't have much and he had no special desire to accumulate it. Nevertheless, every year for a week or two after he had paid his insurance premiums, you couldn't live with him. "Pooh," he said, "Standard Oil indeed. Look what they did to your grandfather. He and John D. started off in that business together. He worked forty years for them, invented the non-refillable oilcan and set up their plant in Cuba and what did he get out of it? They sent a lovely wreath when he died and a couple of the Pratt's came to his funeral." I didn't find out until later that father's next move had been to go to his friends among the brigands of lower Broadway and tell them not to hire me.

A day after the above interview, Dad said to me, "You have a friend in Baltimore." I nodded a tentative yes. "Why don't you go down and see him and take a look at Johns Hopkins. Here's a round trip ticket on the Pennsylvania, here's a nickel for the subway and eight cents for the Long Island Rail Road."

Meekly I accepted the gifts and set out for the heart of the old south. My friend, Ed Stafford, a fellow counselor at Camp Winona and now a

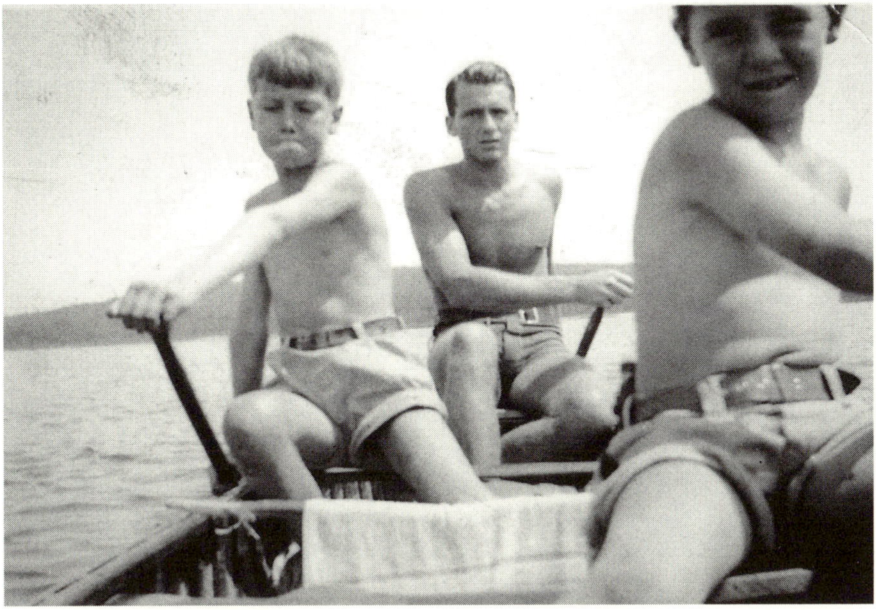

My "Chair of Canoeing." Camp Winona, Denmark, Maine..

senior at Hopkins, just happened to be at the Pithotomy Club when I called. In half an hour I was tramping Hopkins' Hallowed Halls. "I work with the dean," said my guide, "Wouldn't you like to meet him?" After a twenty-minute chat, Dr. Chesney said, "If you are thinking of applying, here's a blank and we will consider this your personal interview." I'm queer for blanks. If anyone goes to the trouble of having questions printed I feel the least I can do is answer them. In no time I was enrolled and it seemed easier to go to medical school than not.

These four years did not disappear so easily as the previous four. I broke the monotony by transferring to Harvard Medical School for the free quarter of my fourth year. This I did because I wanted to spend Christmas vacation with my friends in Maine. Living in New York, my family would have taken a dim view of my passing through the hometown on my way to some place else. Being already in Boston it didn't seem so impious to go down to Maine.

At the end of the third year, two of my close friends were planning to work for the summer at something called the Notre Dame Bay Memorial Hospital. This hospital was on the island of Twillingate in Newfoundland.

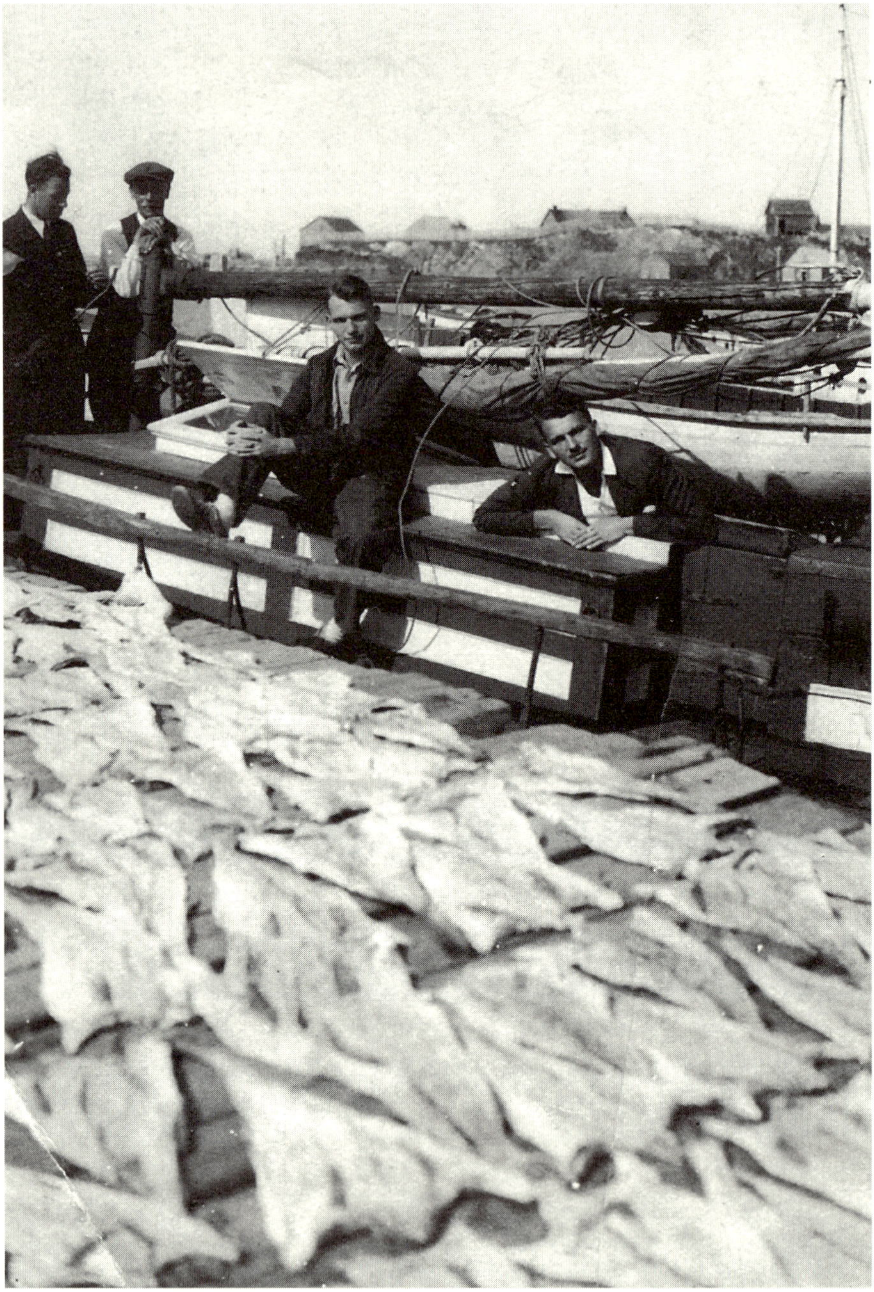

Office manager (?), Skipper Frank, Dick Mirick, and Ecke on the M.S. *Little Grace.* Drying cod! Summer 1934. Author's photograph.

The two who had been there the year before had come back with accounts of a great summer. For ten or more years, two had been going down there each summer and coming back to line up two more for the coming summer. At the last minute, one of them found he wouldn't be able to make it, and the other, Dick Mirick, asked me to take his place. I was already signed up for my usual chair of canoeing, but I was ready for a change and jumped at the chance. It was a glorious summer. The lotus was firmly planted in my digestive tract and I returned with the firm resolve to work as a doctor in Newfoundland as soon as I was qualified.

During my fourth year free quarter at Harvard, I had suffered from the illusion that I could get a surgical internship at the Massachusetts General Hospital. I neglected to apply anyplace else and late in January those appointments all went to Harvard men. In fact, if I am not mistaken, their fathers were Harvard men too and had also served on the West Service of MGH. This left me stranded until I heard from my dear friend, Charles Sommers, a medical schoolmate, that a position was open in surgery at the Baltimore City Hospitals, where he was working in Medicine. That was a profitable year professionally, but a year saddened by the death of Sommers. It was a tragic business. I watched him many a night in his oxygen tent as he bravely joked about his rising NPN and the other blood signs of increasing heart failure. I never went back there, once I was released. The year was punctuated by a slight feud with the acting chief of the surgical service. I felt that our instruction left something to be desired. I wrote him a letter comparing his regime unfavorably with that of the MGH. He called me a communist and a Bolshevik. The last three weeks, I was marking quarter days off on the calendar and the last day I got a colleague to take my calls and, seated on the floor of a taxicab, sneaked by the front door so nobody would see me.

I do confess it was a profitable year professionally. Hospital experience provides the new medical graduate with the confidence and experience that makes him useful to his patients. The system of internship is a dirty one. The intern does the work of a trained man. He has spent eight years of study before he takes the job. The work he does has to be done and no one can do it without this training. Yet, society has the insolence to accept this service without compensating the man who provides it. Older doctors were the ones responsible for the continuation of this peonage. Otherwise intelligent physicians will tell you how they worked for nothing 26 hours a day at the Gedunkus University hospital and that was what made them the great personage you are privileged to work with or for. It was good enough for them and why, pray tell, should it be changed. The experience you gain, they tell you, is worth more than anyone could pay you. This opiate suffices to keep the laboring young doctor quiet. Every operation the famous surgeon performs gives him experience (did you ever know a surgeon who wasn't famous) and yet the patient is expected to proffer the surgeon a certain recompense for his performance. It is not unknown for the famous surgeon to submerge his noble sentiments to the point of being sure of that financial and spiritual return before he dons the rubber glove. If we pay the intern, say the board of directors, we will get people who are not of noble purpose but interested only in the money. Often it is bank presidents who utter such sententious phrases.

The hospital where I interned used to pay its workers but there was a change. They built new buildings and changed the staff and decided it should be a first-rate hospital. The first move of the board was to cut out salaries for interns. That apparently was the *sine qua non* of a first-class hospital. Besides not paying its interns, I know one very very famous hospital that rather insists that you be not married. Such a division of interest is not compatible with the healing of the sick under the direction of a medical oracle with splendid financial recognition and the social *réclame* of a meat packer.

Fortunately, my family was willing to supply me with the means to purchase cigarettes and Maryland rye and make the necessary trips to Maine and New York. Well anyhow, profitable or not, paid or not, I was glad to escape from the newly built elegance of that eleemosynary institution.

A summer of canoeing made me ready for a fellowship at Johns Hopkins. A colleague of mine, Howard Howe, had been given a grant to start work there on infantile paralysis. I joined him in whitewashing ceilings and getting equipment together to establish a laboratory. We put in a good year with our 250 unfriendly monkeys. I did 200 brain operations. He stayed with the project, becoming professor in charge of the Poliomyelitis Research Center—a far cry from our little installation in the cellar of the old anatomy building. The U.S. Public Health Service wanted to commission me to continue the work at Hopkins but I had had enough of cities and streets and the madding crowd.

September of 1937 found me once more on my way to Twillingate.

CHAPTER II

Newfoundland 1937

An Introduction

(Editor's note: This chapter describes Newfoundland as it was when Dr. Ecke arrived there in the late 1930s, and sets the scene for his journal which follows. The geography remains the same although some names may have changed and some communities have now been abandoned.)

Newfoundland, roughly the size of New York State, is said to be the tenth largest island in the world forming a separate country. Contrary to the general notion, it has no connection with Canada either geographic or political, except that as Britain's senior colony, it does form part of the Empire [Ed: Newfoundland joined Canada in 1948.]

A jagged irregular island with its myriad of finger-like capes and peninsulas, it blocks the Gulf of St. Lawrence. To the westward, along the Labrador, the Strait of Belle Isle narrows to nine miles. To the southwest, the ninety-mile-wide Cabot Strait forms the other exit from the Gulf. Slicing deep into the northeast flank of Newfoundland is the cliff-shored Notre Dame Bay. It is forty miles wide at the mouth, from Cape St. John to Cape Fogo, and the "Ships-Run" is almost forty miles from the ocean to Lewisporte, the railhead, at the bottom of the bay. This bay is flecked with islands and the outermost of these is Twillingate, facing the Atlantic.

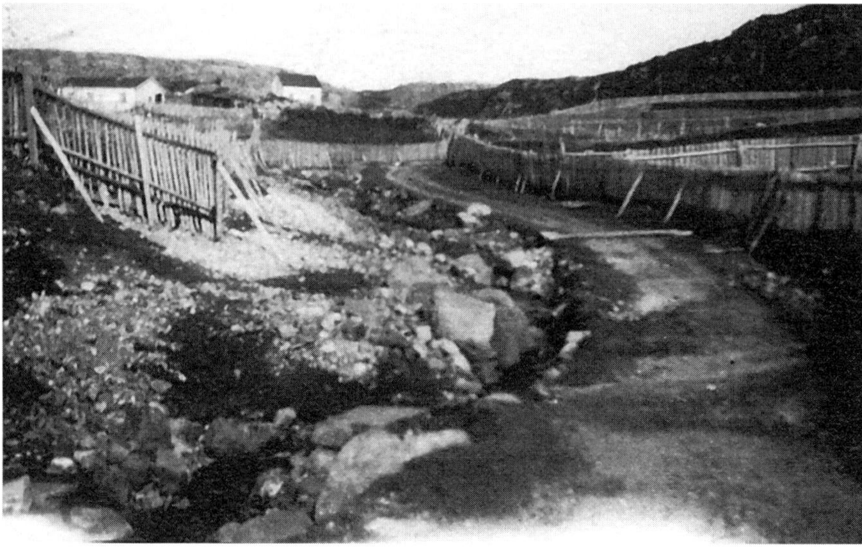

A downtown Twillingate street. Author's photograph.

Certainly to the devotees of Peary and McMillan, Twillingate cannot be called north. The north comes down on us, though. The Arctic currents from Baffin Island and Greenland and the Labrador sweep by us for four hundred miles before delivering a gleaming burden of bergs and ice-flows to the steamy bosom of the Gulf Current. That is way down near the Grand Banks where fogs are born. The isothermic line for January drops south to us from Alaska and sweeps way up north to the top of Norway and Sweden. There is no settlement of any note on this coast between us and the Pole. A scant few thousands support existence on the Labrador by trapping and catering to the thousands of fishermen who voyage hazardously "down on the Labrador," summers, in one of the great annual migrations of the world. There is much to be told of the whole families and crews who pilot their forty-ton schooners down that hungry, angry coast or pack their skiffs, spoon-fashion, on the decks of the government steamers to go to live in meager "tilts" on the rocks, to catch and make fish for a capricious market.

Twillingate, the "Metropolis of the North" and the "Pearl of Notre Dame Bay," housing but far from supporting some three thousand souls, takes the form of two islands separated at one end by a narrow passage of water (Shoal Tickle). The inlet widens between the islands to a reef-flanked mouth, leaving a good-sized harbor protected from every wind but the

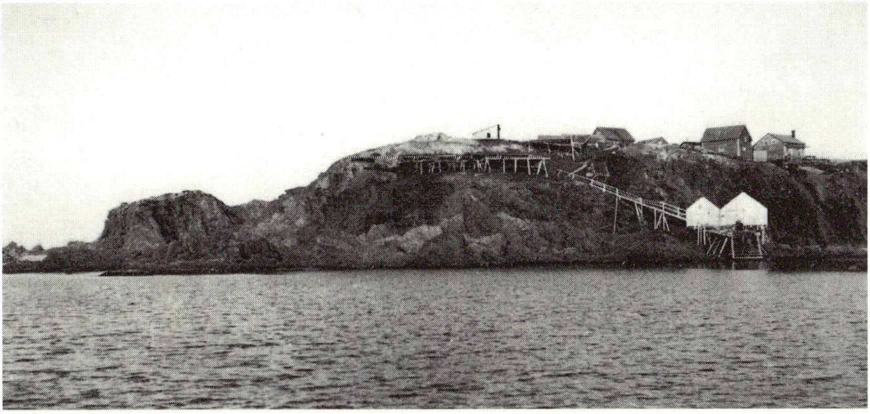

Froude's Hill at Carter's Head harbor entrance. Author's photograph.

northeast. That rages right in. In the days of brisk shipping, a northeaster could pile ten or a dozen schooners on the plentiful rocks but now it's doing well to catch a single, unwary bottom to be ground to spalls.

A cherished memory of these island dwellers was the sight three years ago, of the government wharf, two hundred feet long, her red warning lights still blinking, riding in toto down the harbor on the wings of a gale to perch high and dry on the Bedlamer Rock until the next storm broke it up.

Of the two islands, the outside one, the North Island, is the smaller. From Tickle Bridge, where it is joined to South Island, it stretches northeasterly three miles to the dramatic heights of Long Point. There the lighthouse gives warning of the sinister rocks waiting three hundred feet below. The width of this island, from Paradise to Bread and Butter Point, is only about a mile. The South Island is rather square being about four miles in length and breadth. The shores are everywhere irregular and rough. In most of the little coves and harbors there are small clusters of houses, that are all part of Twillingate but each settlement has its own name—Crow Head, Durrel's Arm, Farmer's Arm, Black Duck Cove, Gillard's Cove, Bluff Head, Tickle Point, Froude's Hill, and many more.

The network of roads is considerable; a rather good one follows the edge of the harbor and along both sides of it are strung the houses, shops, and churches which make Twillingate the important local center it is. The houses tend to be low and compact as if to get out of the wind. The weather soon mellows them to blend with the rocks on which they stand.

Almost every house has a sort of wharf or stage associated with it where boats can be tied up. On the shore end of the stage, or out on the stage itself, is a "store" where the fish and salt and gear are kept. Near the house is a "flake"—a loosely built wide platform out of the reach of dogs where the fish are spread out to dry on a thin mat of fir boughs. Each house and vegetable garden beside it is carefully and completely sealed behind a picket fence to keep the sheep and goats from eating the precious greenery or to confine a few hens. The pickets (stellegans) are made from the thin trunks of small evergreens and for that reason are not straight. They are carefully trimmed and spaced. The effect is a charming one of a studied regular asymmetry. Here and there among the smaller houses is the larger but never pretentious establishment of the merchant or the minister or the man who has returned from the States. The two principal churches, the United and the Church of England, dominate the skyline of the south and north sides respectively. The Salvation Army Barracks and the Pentecostal Church lie rather more modestly near the Tickle Bridge.

Scattered along the roadside are many shops, running from little one-roomed cash businesses to the large general stores of the bigger merchants. The House of Ashbourne is the biggest business in the harbor. They maintain three premises for the fitting and supplying of their schooners and the outfitting of the small fishermen whom they carry on their books. They have been here for a long time. Their Upper Room, their buildings near the tickle, is said to be full-studded. The upright joists are in contact with one another so as to form a wall of solid wood. The lumber was all cut on the island. Now there are only a very few trees that would yield a single two-by-four. Once they even cut "any stick you were a mind to." That meant masts for schooners. You can still buy Wellingtons. They are knee-length leather sea boots with a flap projecting up in front to protect the knee. They haven't been manufactured since the invention of the rubber boot.

At the north end of the Tickle Bridge, housed in the front of the square, yellow, two-storied courthouse, is the telegraph office. There is a good system of communication with the world by cable, landline, and short-range radio. The government is our source of news and every weekday the filtered bulletins are carefully inscribed in longhand in a ledger. It makes a nice break, on a call, to drop in and read the news and exchange a word with the genial operator.

The telephone system is another matter. It has nothing to do with the outside world but is our own inbred family affair. I shouldn't use the word "our," for being there only five years does not admit you to the fraternity that can make sense of the phone. In ten years, one might begin to catch on to the technique which calls for a peculiar high-pitched toneless voice and a special auxiliary vibration of the false vocal chords. There are about 35 parties on the single line that circles both the islands. The phone in Little Harbor is the source of most of our trouble. The relatives of the sick in Herring Neck bring their boats to Little Harbor and then call us on the telephone. In bad weather they come to Purcell's Harbor and walk the mile and a half to Little Harbor to that same phone. Some supernatural force takes a hand at times and they can't reach us from Little Harbor. In that case they call the long-suffering Bert Pardy at the foot of the hospital lane and he or Mrs. Pardy relays the message that last two hundred yards to the hospital. I don't know what the trouble can be. It must be that in Twillingate electric impulses can't go uphill. My father had heard me speak of the telephone and had the bright idea of calling me up on Christmas Day. He enjoined the New York Telephone Company to contact me. The nearest they could get was Foynes, Ireland, on their way back from London. By this time, the bill would have been something like $123.00, so father compromised by sending a smoked turkey.

Although there is no moving-picture house in Twillingate, there is an interest in the cinema. The hospital owns two ancient and favorite films—*Captain January* and *When a Man's a Man*. Every time some hospital organization wants to raise money, these two museum pieces can be depended on.

On the South Island, midway along the harbor margin, set up on the side of a hill, 200 yards from the water, is the hospital, a big square-fronted, three-story structure of concrete block. The rafters in the dormered roof and the woodwork were all sawn from the timbers of a wrecked schooner. To the left of the picket-fenced lane leading up to the hospital is a long story-and-a-half concrete building that harmonizes with the hospital and houses the power house, machine shop, carpenter shop, storehouse, and morgue. A little further along are the turf-covered vegetable cellars that supply us with an only too inexhaustible supply of cabbage, parsnip, potatoes and turnips. To the left of the hospital and a little to the rear squats the "Cottage," a comfortable, much-added-to, two-story wooden building with a glassed-in porch on the front with a garage under it for the motorcycle. The director lives in its roomy lower floor. Upstairs live a few nurses. To the right of the hospital rises the nurses' home, a nondescript mid-western suburban sort of a house that used to be over on the North Island. One winter's day they sawed it in half and launched it on the ice to drag it to its present mooring.

The hospital too has taken on pleasing weathered tones and blends well with the town. The whole aspect is one of snugness and independence. The town and its three thousand people look to the sea. They and their schooners and their homes are good to the eye and the heart.

When one looks on our incredibly beautiful expanse of barren rock and marsh, shorn of trees to the last stick—tiny, laboriously tilled, fish-fertilized gardens, one wonders how life is supported. It hardly is. Here life is artificial in the extreme. Even firewood is hauled to the island in "turns"—sticks eight feet long and five inches through. They are brought with great difficulty, thirty or so at a time, over the ice by dog from New World Island. A small family will use five hundred a winter and any conservationist's heart bleeds to see that each turn means a tree. It is such a problem that many families move to the wood supply and live the winter in a one-room tilt, tar-paper lined, five-foot ceiling, and a door four feet high.

Well-directed industry could grow more produce than the few potatoes and cabbages that are reared here. The deliberate inertia of these Wessex and Scotch-Irish has prevented much change during the four centuries of the islands' inhabitation. Speech, agriculture, and mores tend to be Elizabethan. A woman often proves her fertility before she is an acceptable spouse. It is so difficult to accumulate enough money to provide for inactive old age brought on prematurely by rife tuberculosis, malnutrition, and beriberi, that many children are needed to help out. The homes are small and snug with the inevitable iron pot on the squat kitchen stove and a pleasant mosaic of hooked rugs. The homes and the people are reasonably clean in spite of the obvious difficulties in the way of bathing. Even the rare wealthy have no running water. I know of one merchant family reputed to have made a million dollars in the fish trade. They send their children to England to study music. They buy countless gadgets and trick bric-a-brac from the mail order houses, but nary a bit of plumbing.

It is an unusual fisherman who sees fifty dollars in cash a year. The fisherman ordinarily has no equipment. He fishes for a merchant. The merchant advances supplies and equipment, putting it "on the books." This is taken out of what he pays the fisherman at the end of the voyage. By the time more supplies are advanced for the winter, the fisherman is often in debt and devoid of bargaining power.

It is just as bad in the industries. A sawmill will pay twenty five dollars a week for a short season. This is paid in scrip while the money is drawing interest for the company elsewhere. The scrip can be redeemed only at the company store.

I went through one sawmill while on a typhoid survey. It was an old rickety shed impossibly full of lurking open hatches, unguarded flywheels and naked, rapacious power saws. I was not at all surprised when the shingle cutter turned up at the hospital with a nasty gash in his hand. "You are insured?" ask we. Proudly, "Oh yes, the government makes them insure us." "How much are you being paid now, until you can work again?" Without a sign of resentment, "O, nothing, you see, when I showed 'e to himself he says it's too bad insurance doesn't cover flesh wounds."

This calm acceptance of such tricks of man and fate is characteristic. There is no general unrest and complaint so long as dole is easily available. They have become so inured to the dole diet of bread and tea and salt pork that it represents a satisfactory form of living. A fatalistic philosophy has flourished in the poverty and hardships until everything is attributed, calmly and with finality, to the "will of God." It must be confessed that in the unhappy eventualities of medical practice, it is comforting to have this phlegmatic attitude to fall back on, though it may tend to make the patients uncooperative.

It is with this same calm that they accept the, to me, miraculous presence of the hospital. Shortly after the First World War, Dr. Charles Parsons, trained at Hopkins and Vienna, of an adventurous turn of mind, became associated with the Grenfell Mission. Sir Wilfred Grenfell had long felt the need for a hospital in this large Notre Dame Bay, supporting as it does on its thick archipelago and along its tortuous shores some thirty thousand people. The operative cases had to be sent to St. John's, perhaps a week's journey, or taken care of in a little shack by two local practitioners hampered by a life-long feud and no equipment. They still boast of the number of ruptured appendices who recovered. No one knows how many were never seen.

During those lush post WWI days when brisk Mediterranean and South American markets brought eighteen dollars a quintal (112 lbs.) for dried fish, Parsons and Sir Wilfred Grenfell raised the money to build this modern, well-equipped, hundred-bed hospital.

John Olds, also from Hopkins, took over the directorship in 1935. He was confronted by a $3.50 market for fish and the utter collapse of Newfoundland finances. Newfoundland had just given up her dominion status and become a Crown Colony. There simply was no money. Dr. Olds evolved a form of prepaid medicine which enables us to run just about even. It is one of the very first health management plans on record anywhere.

If a whole community takes out a "Blanket Contract" for forty cents a year per head, any member receives free hospitalization, free consultation at the hospital, and free medicine. If a patient has to be hospitalized for two years for tuberculosis, his bill may be as high as twenty dollars. Surgical patients are supposed to pay for operations: five dollars for an appendectomy; five dollars for a single hernia, and seven fifty for a double. Brain surgery may go as high as fifteen dollars.

If a settlement can not get well enough organized to take out a Blanket Contract to cover all its members, then each person is allowed to take out an "Individual Contract." This carries the same benefits as a Blanket Contract but costs sixty cents per head per year. House calls are, of course, limited to the families that are within a reasonable distance of the hospital. We seldom are called more than fifty miles. It may take half a day or it may take a week to make a single call. For our own islands and the ones near us we have established an organization known as the Medical Center. This costs five dollars a family on Twillingate. For this the doctor will visit the home whenever he is needed. Medical Center service on New World Island costs ten dollars a year.

New World Island lies between us and the mainland. It is semicircular in shape. Twillingate lies in the concavity. Main Tickle is between and a nasty bit of water it can be. Most of the calls to New World Island take a whole day and frequently several days. I have had to walk thirty miles through six-inch snow for one of these calls. Dr. Wood, a local Tufts man, works with us at the Center but does not ordinarily work in the hospital.

In addition to the Contract system and the Medical Center, the hospital maintains a traveling clinic. For this service, the hospital owns and operates the *M.V. Bonnie Nell.* She is a fifty-foot, twenty-five-ton, ketch-rigged motor vessel. She has a high billet bow that gives a large forecastle with plenty of headroom. Her draft forward is very slight and that fact, coupled with her high forward deck, makes her pound like fury in a head wind. The doctor and nurse have, respectively, two small staterooms off the Saloon. The Saloon is inclined to be a bit of a jumble. It is living quarters for all hands in the evening and a clinic during the day. It is cluttered

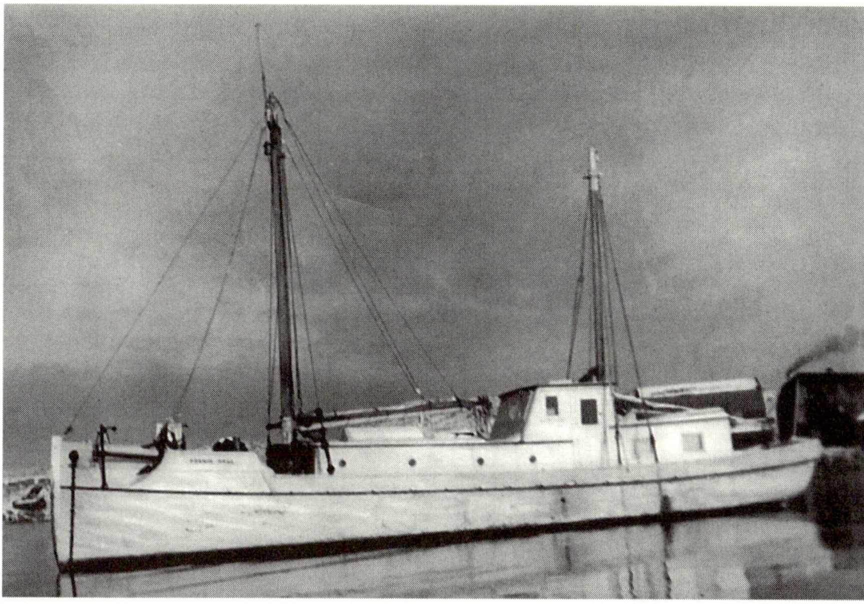

Peripatetic clinic *Bonnie Nell.* Author's photograph.

with the bottles and instruments and laboratory equipment, and all the other materials that go to make a fairly complete doctor's office. The patients are seen here and at the end of a rainy day when fifty of them have tracked in the mud and the wet, our evening cocoa does seem to take on odd flavors.

The Skipper, Elijah Dalley, and his helper fill out the ship's complement of four. We have seventy-five ports of call—all the points and harbors around the whole bay. This extra service is not covered by the contracts, but to the holders of contracts a complete physical examination and the ordinary laboratory procedures cost a dollar. Teeth are pulled for a quarter apiece. In order to strengthen the contract system, non-contract holders are charged double. This penalty charge is still less than comparable service by local private practitioners. This boat trip is very important to the people of the bay. The uncertain fall weather often makes it very exciting for the doctor. It brings medicine to many who would never come to the hospital unless they were very ill. Many whom we see are referred to the hospital for treatment and many are taken care of on the spot. This spares them the expensive trip to the hospital.

An effort has been made to promote infant health. This we do by sheer bribery. If, of a Wednesday afternoon, the mother will bring her baby, sick or well, we will provide it with clothes, food, medicine, and medical attention—all for free. This, unfortunately, is not enough of an enticement, and we rarely have more than seven or eight old standbys. I think we lost most of our customers when we told them turnip water had vitamins in it.

The baby clinic is run by contributions. The boat trip is run at a loss. However, by the Contract system, and the Medical Center, we raise half the yearly fifty thousand-dollar budget. The government gives us about twenty-four thousand dollars a year but takes ten thousand back in import duties on equipment and medical supplies. This, however typical, has always seemed a little incomprehensible to us. In some respects our expenses are not great. A ten-dollar-a-month job as a maid is one to be scrambled for. The laundry bill for the hundred beds and staff of twenty-five is under four hundred and fifty dollars a year.

A considerable portion of our work consists of outside visits for the Center. Usually the patients provide transportation. Men will come twenty miles by dog team or boat to tell you that Mrs. Bulgin has broken her "laig." It is useless to tell them they should have brought her with them. We have to go back with them perhaps just to tell her she will have to come to the hospital. Like as not she will refuse. Even if a six-year-old refuses to come it is final. The children tend to be rather undisciplined. Many a baby has lain home and died because it would "fret" or "grieve" in the hospital. Piercy Elliott, eight years old, was discovered lying on a board bench in a winter tilt trying to make up his mind whether to cover himself with one thin cotton blanket or to lie on it to make the couch softer. He also had a ruptured appendix. Examination (sounding) and conference with his mother, the luxurious Clemmy, produced the following mother-son exchange of sentiments. Clemmy: "Do 'ye wants to go to the hospital and get operated on or will 'ye bide home and die?" Piercy, brown-cheeked, and bright-eyed: "I'll go long with the doctor." Piercy became one of our favorites. His belly was too much of a mess to get the appendix out at that sitting and a year and a half later it ruptured again and was removed. If he escapes tuberculosis and beriberi, the normal life expectancy is his.

Most of the time the ones who come for us have no information as to the nature of the illness and we have to go prepared for anything. When it means lugging your forty pounds of equipment through four miles of bog, you like to know what to take. The routine answer to our question, "What is the matter with her?" is, offended like, "That's what we wants `ee to tell us."

Rather too often even the patient can tell us no more. "I can't tell 'ee exactly how I feels, doctor. I finds a sort of a dead pain, you know, a hachin' an a smurtin and a burnin. It starts here and runs around here and stops here by this little spot where me gun exploded six years ago. I only finds it when I works and if you don't mind would ye give me a 'tificate (dole) so I can git a bit of food for me 'n the old doman."

The population seems full of sick people who call you too late and won't come to the hospital, and people who aren't sick who call you out at all hours and besiege our doors with minds made up to bide the winter with us and perhaps have brought a baby along for us to take care of too. They are smart and come on the last fall boat; it is something of a problem to send them away.

Dr. Olds, or "Dr. Hose," as they call him, was sent for one night late in the winter when the ice was breaking up. He walked endless miles through a foot of slush, jumped from pan to pan of rotten ice dragging a punt to ferry the open swatches. Then more pans and swatches and slush. It was a hazardous and dreadful trip in the pitch dark. He arrived exhausted to confront old Aunt Mabel comfortably knitting before her fire. "I just wanted to know if I should come down in the spring to be examined when navigation opened." The twenty miles back to the hospital that night left little time for bitter reflection on the behavior of the upper class native.

Many, of course, are the bona fide cases where you are only too glad to drag your heavy feet through miles and miles of ten-inch-deep slob, the soft salt-water ice that gathers on the surface of the frozen bay. The dogs can barely budge the komatik, even empty, so tenacious is the murderous stuff. Then there is a swift run over the three-mile neck of Trump Island where you leave your exhausted driver and dogs and are handed on, frozen and hungry, to another waiting team for the second half of the journey. You arrive in such a state that you can do nothing but sit in front of the stove and tremble while the officious midwife plies you with hot tea and cheese. The groans from the next room, or for that matter the same room, tell you that the woman has not given birth but you are helpless even to look at her until you regain your senses. The joy then is great when you have been able to do a little to ease three days of agony. Your reward may be to have a little red Newfoundlander bear the dubious label of

"Hackie" tucked into his name somewhere. That is the closest most of them come to my name.

You don't mind hours crouched in the cuddy of a thirty-five foot skiff with every wave coming over the bow, you gaining little comfort from the skipper's firm avowal that no skiff has ever turned over. You can hardly believe that the vicious wind-lop isn't going to do the trick at last. You know perfectly well that if this quarter-century-old coffee grinder propelling the craft should give out, there is no friendly Coast Guard to come look for you as you drift towards Ireland or macerate at the foot of the cliffs.

I had the pleasure to bring the "New Doctor" and his wife down from Lewisporte, forty miles by dog team. We did it in a day but the mail team leaving only an hour behind us was a week getting here, so fast was the ice going rotten. The rents between the fields were three feet wide and as the dogs leaped them, you could see the blackness that two hundred fathoms gives the water. A hundred times our feet went right through to the knees as we walked or ran to hurry the dogs. The only light touch was the immersion, through a swatch, of the "New Doctor for Fogo" when his slide just sort of sank through the ice and he sat there clutching the slide with one hand and his new reflex camera (under water) with the other, while all eight drivers of our cavalcade yelled and ran and stumbled and fumbled at retrieving him. A cardboard box of Lord and Taylor hats floated unharmed in the swatch.

While he dried his clothes, the grateful wife passed a five-pound box of Bon Voyage chocolates around to the gentry who had assembled from nowhere. I daresay it was the first time the folks at the bottom of Virgin Arm had ever tasted Schrafft's and they seemed to like it to see them fill their fists. Zeke Burton allowed as how it was too bad we hadn't fallen through the swatch near his house 'cause then we could have come in and examined his wife ("sounded the ol' doman"). I expressed regret but didn't tell him that it would have afforded me little pleasure to see his wife with whose hopeless tuberculosis I was already well acquainted through countless previous visits made usually in the early hours of dawn or driving storms.

There are many pleasures in working here with these brave kindly people but the note struck by the whole setup is not one of hope. A few dreamers have visions of the fishing on a rational basis: factories and free ports that will make Newfoundland not wealthy but at least able to supply a living for its small population. When you see that a country the size of England, possessed of the finest fisheries in the world and on its mainland rich forests and mines and untold water power, has been unable to find work and decent homes for 70,000 employable, you realize that something must be wrong. It is a strategic country from a military point of view. It is the airway key to North America and neither Great Britain nor the United States can afford to have it weakly independent or possessed by any other country.

Though it had been no pleasure to me to work that brief period in New York, it was a valuable experience and I was grateful for the chance to see private medicine rampant. I didn't feel for a moment that what I saw in New York was a fair example of private medicine. I have seen too many honest doctors literally give their lives to their practice. But if every doctor were a saint and if every hospital were run only for the patient, I would still feel that our Twillingate system is better for the patient's welfare and the doctor's soul than anything that private medicine may have or has to offer. It is all very well for the honored physician to proclaim that he gives a third of his time to the free clinics—that only gives him the unfair advantage of feeling noble. I am unimpressed when the mayor boasts of the free city hospitals and I'll grant that the free city hospitals of America are in many cases as good as any in the world. My point is that there is no need either for reactionary nobility on the doctor's part nor for charity from the mayor and his supporting citizens. Even considering the Newfoundland standard of living, the cost of medical attention is so low that only the smallest handful of people find it outside their means. The patient pays only enough to make him feel that he is not receiving charity. The hospital is a community institution that the people can feel they have a real part in. The Twillingate hospital would still be able to swim without this prepayment socialized system, but it would have an entirely different flavor. The few who could pay well would have to be charged heavily and the rest would have to accept a free government service. That would change the whole aspect. The greatest joy a sincere doctor can have is the opportunity to look on a sick fellow human purely as a problem in healing. As soon as the patient becomes a financial prospect, both the doctor and the patient have to contend with that element in their relationship that can not help but cloud the situation. The patient who expects to pay a big bill has every right to bargain and question. He is probably eager to spend money lavishly on every conceivable means of hastening his cure or making his demise comfortable, but he is not always interested in buying a new sterilizer boiler or endowing a new wing under the guise of medical charges. On the other hand, the private patient with restricted means shouldn't have to balance an operation against taking the children to the country for the summer. He shouldn't lie in his sick bed wondering if he would get well more quickly if he had a special nurse or private room or a consultation that he knows he can't afford.

It is a great comfort not to have to consider money when you deal with a suffering patient. None of this reprehensible business, so common with the rising surgeon, of taking tonsils or hemorrhoids out in the office because a hospital bill would render the patient unable to pay the doctor. In our plan, if Mrs. Burge ought to stay in bed another week, she stays in bed. If she needs to be alone, she is put alone in a room. If she needs six x-rays, she gets them. If she needs special nursing, she gets it. The only limitations are those of our personnel and plant. The result is that the poorest fisherman has available a medical service and hospital privileges of much better quality than many of my friends or family could afford in America, namely, those unfortunate people of modest means who would hesitate to go to a city hospital and would be ruined at a private one.

There was nothing holy and noble or especially ideologic in the evolution of the Twillingate plan. It merely evolved as the best practical means to get enough money to run the hospital and bring to as many people as possible the best medical attention available. Not a single directive came from Moscow. The terrible evils posed by the reactionary opponents of socialized medicine have failed to materialize. The government supplies half the money necessary but its heavy hand has been entirely missing. All we get from the government is an occasional social visit and invitations to come to St. John's. There has been no complaining that the people can't get the doctor they want—when a patient enters the hospital, he gets all the doctors we have. I do not feel that the doctor's initiative fails because he is on salary and not scrambling for a patient's favor in wild, undignified competition.

It is true that many outside calls are made which, in the doctor's opinion, are not necessary calls. It can't be said that these calls would not have been made had there been a fee to be considered. It can be said, though, that I saw recently a very successful private physician in the United States. He fell exhausted into a chair about midnight and said he had made eighteen calls that day and in only two of them was a doctor actually needed. His disappointment at the other sixteen was assuaged somewhat of course, by cash emolument. Our average, I am certain was better than one in nine. The doctors won't get rich in Twillingate but they live better than the richest merchants in the area.

CHAPTER III

Journal from September 1937

(Editor's note: Dr. Ecke kept a journal of his activities at Twillingate from September 1937 until he left in late 1941. The journal was written in spare moments such as evenings after work or while traveling by boat from island to island. Sometimes days were missed and at other times a single entry covers several days. As mentioned earlier, his recollections in preparing this journal for publication were enhanced by reviewing letters, notes, and various papers he kept from those years. While the journal has been edited somewhat for clarity, it appears substantially as originally written over sixty years ago on the rugged coast of Newfoundland.)

Mid-September 1937 was a busy time for the Notre Dame Bay Memorial Hospital at Twillingate. The summer rush of patients was at its height. The two students who had come up from Hopkins to work as interns for the summer were frantically finishing up their records and preparing to go back to their fourth year at school. The permanent staff consisted of the Director, John Olds, and "Rube" Waddell. Waddell was just getting ready to take our clinic boat, the *Bonnie Nell*, on the last part of the trip around the bay to see the sick. Howard Ives had been here for the summer and would be staying a few months more before returning to Yale to take a graduate appointment in medicine.

September 13, '37. A good chance to catch up on a week of notes. The trip down was a good one. The auto ride through Cape Breton was fun with my sister, Kay, and her friend, Dorothy Houghton, even to crashing head-on into the lawyer from Halifax, breaking his patella, ruining both cars, and spraining Dot's wrist. The MacKenzies in North Sydney were wonderful to us and stowed me on the *Belle Isle* for St. John's because I had missed the *Caribou* for Port aux Basques. They introduced me to the captain at the rain-swept gangplank. The trip was a stormy one and the waves broke over the bow continually. The propeller raced a great deal. St. Pierre-Miquelon, after we finally got in through the fog, was interesting. I bought some stamps, a beret, and a quart of champagne, which I drank lukewarm before supper with no effect at all. Miss Hart, the only other passenger who appeared for every meal, was entertaining and we walked together to the Cabot Tower our first morning in St. John's. The doctors who examined me for my license were amusing and rather eighteenth century. I don't know if I passed their exams or not. I hung around, called Mrs. Kearney, got in the mud to my knees back of the hotel, and caught the train Sunday morning in the rain. The Pullman was too crowded for comfort, but the first class, like our day coach, was commodious. Meals were adequate but not cheap.

I fell in with Lady Walwyn on the train, to write a prescription for her son, the aide de camp to the governor. Dr. Cluny McPherson, the dean of St. John's medicine, had told her I was on board. Cluny is world famous. He invented the gas mask canister. A patent would have made him a billionaire. A couple of hours out of St. John's, the steward had mumbled something to me. I didn't understand what he said but I gathered that someone in the last car wanted to see me. I was in an old corduroy suit and a shave wouldn't have hurt. I combed my hair and made my way aft. I was a little bemused to note that my goal turned out to be the private car, *Terra Nova*. The last time I had seen it had been three years before when Dick Mirick and I had offered to share our forty-ounce bottle of Canadian Club with Sir John Hope Simpson, the empire strike breaker, and, in retaliation, he had invited us to dinner in this same car. The trip and the bottle had ended just as we reached Port aux Basques. The *Caribou* was waiting for Sir John, dressed in all its flags, and the last we saw of him he was on hands and knees, looking under the table for his shoes. Well, here I was in the *Terra Nova* again, and seated regally in the rear center was a slender woman obviously in control of the situation. I said who I was. She asked if I would write a prescription for "this creatchah heah" indicating with a long forefinger a lean lad in a navy uniform sitting next to her. It seems he had the "summer complaint" and she tied my hand by adding, "Don't give him any dope—he's dopey enough." What he needed was opium or the equivalent, and he had lost a prescription.

With some misgivings, I agreed. I wasn't afraid of poisoning him but it had been three years since I had written a prescription and my last two hundred and fifty patients had been monkeys. I asked for a piece of paper and after some scratching around she found a large blue sheet with a crest and Government House written on it and half covered with tea stains. At this point I began to wonder who this woman was. I asked for a pencil and a short stub was found on which I chewed a point, discreetly putting the splinters into my handkerchief. Then I started to write. I covered the page with long division and finally evolved a simple prescription for Bismuth, half in the metric system and half in the apothecary system. As the labored minutes wore on, I could see my patient's confidence waning. When I had to ask for another piece of paper on which to transcribe my voluminous script I knew I might just as well not bother. However, I finished bravely and was dismissed. I hurried to the porter to find out who she was and was a little confused to learn it was the lady of His Excellency, the Vice-admiral, Sir Humphry T. Walwyn, K.C.G., etc., etc., Governor of Newfoundland, late of the Indian Royal Navy.

The shuttle took us to Lewisporte where I visited the George the Fifth Hotel for a good tea and then to bed on the *S. S. Clyde*, glad to be near the porthole and rid of my roommate on the *Belle Isle*, who kept shutting it all night. Oddly enough, I had never seen my roommate. I only knew he had been there because every time I opened the porthole, he would get up and close it. It was exciting the next afternoon to round Long Point and see the hospital.

Everybody seemed glad to see me.

It had been three years since I had seen John Olds and he said he wouldn't have known me. I guess that is because that last year at medical school took fifteen pounds off of me. I would have known him though. He was unchanged and I suppose will never change. He is four years my senior and the few gray hairs don't show up in his full head of wavy light hair. He is slender and well formed with an aristocratic bearing of the head. His eyes are large, long lashed and clearly gray. His nose and mouth are straight and classically modeled. He is serious, gentle and determined. He can turn out a bearing on his lathe with the same facility that he removes an obstructing prostate. His manner has never taken on the ponderous quality it might have from the vast responsibilities which are his. He is the breath of this whole institution. It is his flavor that makes this hospital the social instrument it is. His bravery is legend. He climbs any cliff, he will ride a horse on ice so thin that a dog wouldn't venture on it. He will face any weather in any boat. He is good to drink or play cards with or to hunt caribou with. His chess is fun but monotonously successful. He drives dogs well and shoots well. He reads everything. He is quite human though and there are moments of moods, sharply unpleasant though understandable. Once in a while I choose to avoid him. Operations have gone on without a word being exchanged. There was a certain violence of temper which reminded me of my father. My mother tamed those in him and I often offered to put Mrs. Olds in touch with my mother for instruction on this course. I was never sure that John was amused by these dinner conversations.

I never saw him doing what one would call loafing. He would seem to sit quietly doing nothing in the bottom of a small boat while crossing the bay. Suddenly he would snap his fingers with a pleased lighting of his face—he had solved the problem of how to make surgical towel clamps in the machine shop rather than buy them at an outlandish price. His interests were wide. He had charts to prove that Twillingaters could grow a much larger portion of their food. He proved there could be more variety in the vegetables grown. He tried to promote the use of local peat instead of imported expensive coal. He tried to promote an aeroplane for hospital use. He is reported to be the only male intern that Dean Lewis, Professor of Surgery at Hopkins, President of the American Medical Association, ever personally asked to stay on in surgery. John came to Twillingate instead.

Betty Olds, of the quiet amused inward smile, was a good wife for John. She is beautiful, graceful, and a magnificent hostess. She was untouched by sudden uxorial storms. She understood the quiet reading moods of her spouse but she could ski with him as well. She ran her pleasant home and often did the housekeeping for the hospital with the same ease and warmth. She was also a Hopkins-trained nurse and frequently worked on the wards—often as the chief.

As I started talking to John a figure ran past us with his arms full of shotguns, coats, blankets, gloves, boots and binoculars that, John explained, was "Rube" Waddell, a young doctor working at the hospital who was just about to take out the traveling clinic aboard the *Bonnie Nell* for a month. Rube was busy getting his impedimenta aboard. Soon the cycle roared up the lane—a few shouts were heard outside—a door burst open and then slammed shut and I was introduced. This was Waddell—almost six feet, solidly built, red cheeks, bright gray eyes and lots of long straight black hair falling over the corner of his forehead. The smile was wide and warm. His resonant voice held a real Virginian accent. The clasp was warm and strong and the manner wide and breezy. Rube is to be reckoned with at every juncture. He knows his way about and I suspect he knows yours too. His persuasive manner sweeps all before him.

Considering the smallness of our hospital group our social life within it is extraordinarily complete. We have friends outside the group though and we enjoy them. At the foot of the hospital lane with its back to the harbor is the home and shop of Burt Pardy. He's a tall, lean, husky, experienced man of around forty. His earlier years were spent in strange northern places. He worked for the Hudson's Bay Company on the Labrador and around the north magnetic pole where his compass would describe a complete circle on a ten-mile uncharted trip. He worked in the far northwest Yukon around Aklavik, too, and has even been to King William Land. He likes to play poker even if he does seem to be burning up a box of matches to light his inevitable pipe just as it is his turn to deal. It's fun to drop down for tea (the evening meal) with him and his pleasant hospitable wife. We don't seem to play bridge at the hospital but Burt likes it and so do a couple of his neighbors—many's the pleasant late, fought-for rubber by his stove while the tide lapped audibly under the kitchen floor and the wind howled through in his chimney.

I grant that everyone might not enjoy weather. I don't mean enjoy good weather, I mean take pleasure in the very idea of it. If you like it, we have plenty of it for you. It is of vital concern. It is part of everything we do. It is part of our moods. My wide bedroom has three windows. From two of them I can see the harbor. The other one is on the level with the ramp leading down from the back door. I keep that one closed because dogs and rats come in if I don't. The other two though keep me in contact with the weather. A nostalgic sound was the slap, slap, of the flagpole halyard as the northeast wind whipped the ropes. I love to lie abed of a windy night and listen to it. The wind used to roll up the linoleum away from the windows and the same wind piles the snow six inches deep on the bedroom floor. When I am awakened for a night call off the island I lie still a moment in the dark orienting myself to the weather. I listen for the wind or rain or the snow. I listen for the fog horn on Twillingate Long Point. I sense the temperature. By the time I get up I have planned my equipment and my costume. We follow all the changes, we can't help it. We hear the reports of the temperature at Crow Head, over on the exposed front of the North Island, where they have the worst weather. We watch the harbor sish over with thin ice and then clear and then sish over and clear until it finally catches. Our mail, our travel, our patients, our leisure—a great deal hangs on the weather.

The permanent Waddell left on the *Bonnie Nell* to scour the bay. Today Waddell's cases started to be harvested: abdominal fluid, post partem, and a beautiful pair of rachitic shins to be fixed.

The weather has been beautiful and warm. Millions in the outpatient department, lots of calls, lots of operating, and some rain. The students left in a high wind and we don't know if they caught the *Fort Amherst* at St. John's. We never did hear they were lost. I am the port health officer and I visited one ship. I took out tonsils today and they bled and needed two sutures. Took out one rotten appendix with drains the other night.

The governor came on an official visit. We met his doctor and were invited to tea but were held up by a patient. Home calls are interesting, mostly for the summer complaint, but I got one appendix and a possible typhoid out of it. Saw a boy limping on the street today, told him to come to the hospital but his dull old man, Lambert, just leaned on the fence and watched his pigs with obviously more interest than he had in his child. Have pulled teeth and have ridden a motorcycle and have been out almost not at all. Plan to keep good records and get some exercise.

A quiet, very busy day, part rain and fog, fine and warm this afternoon. Lots of OPD (Out Patient Department) in the A.M. and P.M., Brett has a phlebitis or at least a thrombosis. I took out his continuous intravenous. Tea at the Cottage where John and Betty live now. Upstairs are quarters for four nurses. Made two calls down on Twillingate Arm with Ives. The crud is better, the second probably has typhoid, but I can't feel the spleen. My tonsil has a "wonderful" sore throat. Flos French was over last night for a second with Gilbert Osmond, who claims I said to him the last time I saw him, "I hope I never see your face again." I don't remember it. Replaced Walter Cole's gastrectomy tube today. Walter is only eleven, been here over three years, since I was here as a student. John is building him a new esophagus to replace the one Walter ruined by swallowing lye.

September 15, '37. Awakened rudely by Miss Kelly, the night nurse, who

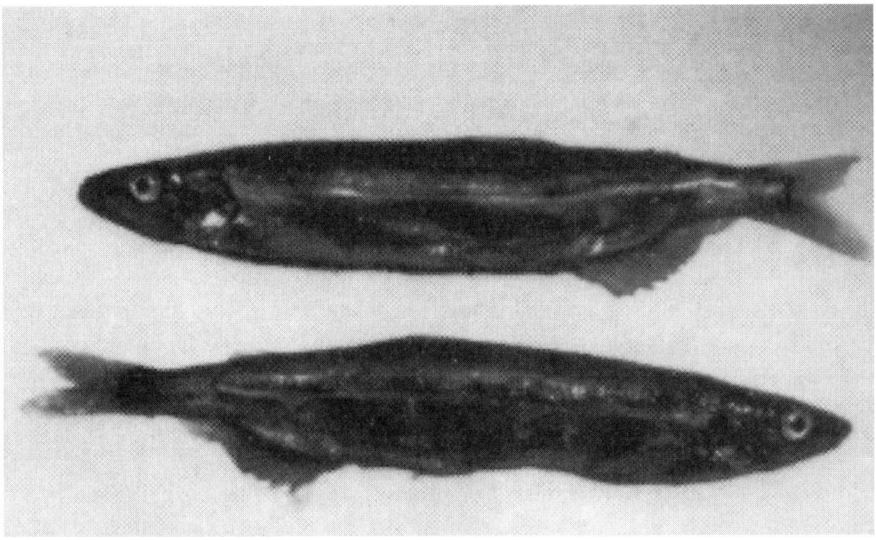

Capelin.

announced that there was an outside OB, refused by Doccy Wood and John. I went down after a hasty cup of tea on the ward. Mrs. Gillette, who had had a terrible time with her first two babies, twenty-five and fifteen hours respectively, had burst her waters at 4 A.M. I hung around and hung around while she dilated. Had tea with her mother-in-law and lunch the same. I gave up finally and came home to tea and when summoned hastily, returned taking Joyce, our anesthetist. She was dilated then and carrying on. We draped her and waited three hours. She wouldn't do a damn thing but scream. We gave her lots of chloroform and ether and I dreaded to use the forceps for the first time. But deep as she was in a feather bed, we put them on and pulled the baby through the perineum to the tune of a small second-degree tear. Such carrying on. I sewed her up while two held her and Joyce poured. She was going to die—talked about pigs and capelin (a grunion-like fish). Billy, her brother-in-law, came in. He had skippered the *Grace B.* to St. John's in the record time of nineteen hours. Meanwhile, I visited next door and in French Bay.

September 16, '37. Not much, fooled around the OPD. Couldn't put Skipper Young's hernia back and sent Ives down to try it. Another warm day. Seven outside calls. Mostly crud.

September 17, '37. Another hot day. In the A.M., I lost a toss with Ives and he had the pleasure to go and see Mrs. Herbert Gillette with a "quart of chill" in her stomach. I helped John do an Albee spinal fusion and it was much easier than I thought. I then did the twenty-second operation on Mary Earl and grafted her face. She had had an x-ray burn (not here) requiring repeated grafting. Lots of calls in the OPD and after dinner went down to the bottom of Virgin Arm to Carter's Cove on New World Island to see a little girl with the crud. Also saw two cases of impetigo, one of athlete's foot, and one of scabies. Had tea at Max Burt's, who has a kyphos (hunchback). It was a good tea and a nice house. Back late to tea at the nurses' home. Went down to see Skipper George Young, whose hernia, replaced with great effort by John yesterday, is causing him to vomit. Last night I was awakened at 3 A.M. to catheterize old Hines and went back to dream of Sommers (the fellow intern who had died in Baltimore). I held his head on my lap after he was dead. I was very much depressed. I thought of him all day today. Made rounds alone and was happy to feel greater interest coming with greater responsibility.

September 18, '37. Some rain. Fooled around the OPD in the morning. No operating. Made ten calls on the Arm, saw three cases of measles. Tommy, the head nurse, went with me. My perineal repair doesn't look very good. And James Gillette's little girl is no better. Tea at the Cottage and sat around and talked for a long time.

September 19, '37. Sunday and a lovely morning. Breakfast in the sun in the dining room. Saw several patients in the OPD and made three calls in the morning. Picked up a belly which I told to come in. She did and though the findings were minimal, had an infected appendix which John and I removed. The girls went to the Tilt for a picnic, but I couldn't make it. Made another call late at night and we had our teacups read in Joyce's room. She told me I was scared, near enough to the top of my profession but lacked the confidence five more years would give. Then to bed late. I'm trying to read some clinical stuff a bit. A cerebral accident came in and died. (The Tilt is a sort of recreational cabin we own on the other side of the island.)

September 20, '37. A pleasant day. Morning spent as usual in the OPD going at it. The afternoon was a windy rainy one, and I made nine calls

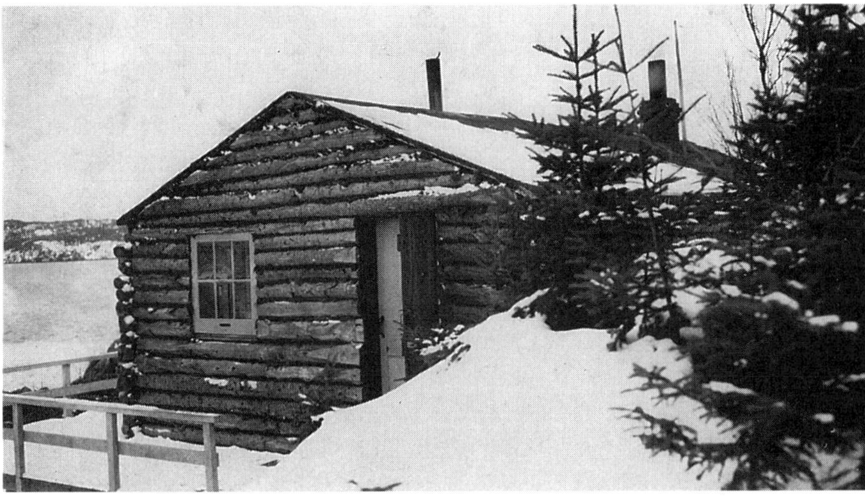

The Tilt. Author's photograph.

mostly on the Arm on a very cranky cycle. I saw two rectal prolapses. Old man Hawkins is much better. In the evening, I had just retired when a call came to go to Pike's Arm, which I did, with Joyce. It was a gorgeous, cool full moon of a night. Crossing our island to Little Harbor, you could have driven without a light. The boat was a nice new open skiff. The old man, Josiah Stuckey, had an occlusion, I think, though his temperature was rather high: 102.6. I digitalised him and supplied him with morphia. Then I had to see his daughter-in-law who rushed into her bedroom and grinning, took off her clothes, telling me she had hot flashes, feelings of things crawling, spots on her legs, and water running in her. I reassured her and came home through the canal and Gut Tickle, after a touch of tea. It was a lovely time, and I had more tea with Kelly on the ward before turning in.

September 21, '37. It's blowing a gale as I write this. Several doors have blown shut so hard the glass was broken. Worked in the OPD all morning and afternoon. My jodhpurs came and we had tea at the Cottage. I must remember to write this every night because I don't remember much if I don't. We left the Cottage because the Board of Directors came for a meeting and I lay down for a minute until Joyce offered me some tea. I've started my yoga and really would like to do a lot of it. One really keeps busy here. I'm so tired at night that sleep is a joy and difficult it is on these brisk mornings to rouse oneself.

September 22, '37. Up early to pump out Mrs. Perry, who we think might have pernicious anemia, and we have her on hydrochloric acid at least, having sent for liver. Helped Ives take out a tonsil, took out three teeth on the same fat lady and before that revived another caesarean baby. I wish I had the courage to merely let them lie just to see if they wouldn't breath anyhow. Now to do an incision and drainage on a buboe, which is probably a rare luetic one. More work in the OPD until a cup of tea at Edith's. After tea I made a call, then the *Bonnie Nell* came in and we had to do an appendix. After that, I opened the worst hand I ever saw—full of pus to the mid-arm. Then more tea at Joyce's.

September 23, '37. Started out as a very lazy day. I did little all morning, made six calls this afternoon. My perineal repair is fine; all the crud cases are clearing up. Mr. Clark is on the skids. I spent quite a while cleaning out his catheter. His old wife was a little mournful when I told her it wouldn't be very long. I think she was right when she said the next world would be better. Had my first moment of nostalgia this morning. I thought during breakfast of the Baltimore party at Sarah's, when Clark and his girl and Woody and Betty Washburn were there and I brought the gardenias. I should like to see them all again. Waddell is with us now and I helped him put on some casts this morning. Then I pulled one tooth. Just before tea I saw some chickenpox with Waddell and they were ready for a caesarean section when we returned. John and Ives did it. The baby breathed quickly, but it's still blue. Mrs. Roberts, yesterday's caesarean section, is crazy as a bag of hammers and is running a very low blood pressure. Some nice tea and stuff in Edith's room and I'm going to bed very soon because the lights have just gone out, but I think that I will start a letter first. The 120-volt generator is turned off to save fuel. A water wheel takes over at 60 volts. If you aren't careful, you blow the bulbs.

September 24, '37. Not much of a day. Watched Waddell try to open a TB peritonitis and he had a hell of a time until he found that the peritoneum was very thick and pebbled but perfectly free. They cystoscoped Green and proctoscoped him and he had too much paraldehyde for he looked like dead the whole day. Mrs. Roberts went bad and "like to died" several times during the day and that's too bad. Though she's a primitive, she has a lot of charm. Made several calls during the afternoon and had tea at the Cottage. John suggested a motorboat ride and I went with him. Damned if he didn't go all around the North Island right out in the ocean in a miserable 12-foot outboard and him not knowing where the rocks are. Off Long Point it was dreadfully wet and I got frozen even in my brown coat. John involves me in foolhardy things, I think just to scare me. I refuse to react. I'm the only other person willing and able to ride his bucking, kicking stallion, Jack. The moon came up just as we were off the lighthouse. It was more than lovely. Came home to find Mrs. Roberts bad again. I was sort of put out to see Waddell operating alone but it must be true that he's had a lot of experience someplace.

September 25, '37. Up, to no operating. Fooled around the OPD, fixed a broken clavicle, then got Jack out for a delightful ride. Warm as a summer's day. I went down the Arm and back over Carter's Cove and Carter's Head. Jack is a good lively stallion and the sea was bluer than I have ever seen it. I lost my jacket on the way back and went back in the cycle after dinner with Tommy to find it. Dot Burden had found it and I'm going after it when I have a reward. Then I saw another patient. Went for a swim and lay in the sun for a piece and it was swell. Back to work in the OPD. Made rounds and then to the Cottage for tea. Betty et al went to Purcell's Harbor in the *Bonnie Nell* to put it up for the winter. We had a nice tea and then to the Arm with Joyce to give caffeine to Peter Clark who is Cheynes-Stoking (irregular terminal breathing) and will not last the night. Back to practice piano duets with Bud, our technician, and then a long tea at Edith's where I talked with Ives who is a swell guy. He had to go to Bridgeport on a typhoid case and I to bed.

September 26 to 29, '37. I don't know how I've neglected these days so much; I have been pretty busy. Outdoors a great deal. Riding the horse. I went for one very long ride all the way to Purcell's Harbor to open an abscess in the neck of a boy from Friday Bay. I dropped my bag on the way over, broke the syringe and spilt the antiseptic. I took Kelly to Herring Neck on a dull, cool day and saw six patients. William Hawkins had a stroke. John Powell came and got me for his wife. She has a breech and ought to come into the hospital, but today is too rough for her to come. She lost her last baby because it was a breech. I went to Tizzard's Harbor too, to see a bad cold and stayed for a nice cup of tea. Came home to poker and won two dollars and fifty cents. Last night we all went to the courthouse to a dance. Ives and I got involved in a quadrille, which is indeed a very strenuous performance. Ives is a tall, lanky, redheaded, handsome, Portland Maine socialite who certainly held up his end. Came home, six of us on the motorcycle and did a bit of eating, drinking, and singing in our apartment and really had a very nice time. Mamie Roberts was very attractive at the dance. Went to bed at 3 A.M., which is quite wild for this part of the country. Yesterday I was stopped at Manuel's Cove on the way back and damned if there isn't a case of meningitis. Ives went back with me after tea to see her and suggested sulfa. It is the Hines family and a terrible, sorry one. The grandmother is one of those officious birds who know everything just before you say it. She makes me examine the baby when I don't want to.

Talking to Waddell about sex around here and he agrees that the possibilities are very remote. Ives reports that Waddell is not too appreciated by the natives. They do not understand his Virginian breeziness. Ives is a very thoughtful, generous, and kind guy.

September 30, '37. A fine southeaster all day backing around to northeast by evening. Cold and strong winds, the harbor full of whitecaps. Really a beautiful day. I helped John take a stone out of a ureter this morning and helped Waddell take out a prostate, which was rather fun. After lunch, we just sat around until I went to see my meningitis, which is a little better. It was gorgeous out on the cycle. Too much canned lobster for tea and I was kind of sour. I went with Waddell on some calls and he is indeed casual with the populace. The cycle broke down and we walked back stopping in at the Orange Hall where there was an amateur concert in progress. We listened to some very provincial singing and playing. No real folkstuff, just rather poor, everyday material. I was scared though, when the portly Mrs. Blackwell hit the high notes of *Oh, For the Life of a Kerry Dancer*. I know her blood pressure is 260 and I expected to see the top of her head come off. A grand walk home in the wind and the rain.

October 1, '37. While at breakfast, a call came from Herring Neck for me to see Mrs. Powell whom I had diagnosed as a breech two days ago and advised to come to the hospital. This is her third such and she lost the last. I couldn't get Joyce to go, so I started out in a taxi for Purcell's Harbor. There I was met in a little skiff in which we assayed the few miles to Merrit's Harbor. The sea off the tickle was tremendous and when we turned to take the harbor, I was really worried by the broadside swells that drenched and froze us. We crossed the island and went down the neck with Hussy to find the waters had broken but she had no pains. I waited in the house a bit and climbed perilously around the cliff with her son, Bob. Then gave her some quinine. I made some calls on a depressed, agitated idiot, a back-paining female with no periods, impetigo, and food poisoning. I saw old Rebecca Woodford, a great character. Returned to find my labor had begun. At 4:30, the cervix started to dilate and was fully dilated by 8:00, but not any descent. The rectum was full of feces, the bladder full of urine and a great rectocele. I waited on her until about 12:30. Meanwhile, I had eaten bread and tea and a bit of boiled dinner and starved in the interim. Mr. Hussy had carted me around the Neck looking for cigarettes, in the course of which Joe White waved us into his office, where I did not get a root of rum but did get some terrible Gold Flake cigarettes. Joe was a moving force in Herring Neck. He manages Carter's fish business and commutes each weekend from Twillingate. He returned to his native Newfoundland after being in the States long enough to build the chutes at Luna Park, where I as a kid slid down the slides. Fifty years old, burly and hearty, he makes a good team with his lean, dark friend, Malcolm Simms, the telegraph operator and unofficial mayor of Herring Neck. Between them, they run the place. Joe is a great friend of the hospital, is a member of the board of directors, as a matter of fact.

October 2, '37. By 1 A.M., I was ready to do a vaginal whereupon I found the child very high. I ironed and ironed but the rectocele was in the way. In well above my glove, I finally identified the genitalia and managed to get one foot. It was ten minutes more before I got the other and exerted traction. I dragged the patient to the edge of the bed, the old midwife poured the chloroform, I pulled pretty hard. The butt bided but finally descended. The shoulders gave a little trouble, the head none. It breathed at once and was the fattest damned baby I ever saw—12.25 pounds. The rest was easy but my hand was scrammed from fighting that tetanic uterus and I was wet as if I'd had a dip. The uterus remained high and I retired to sit up in one of those short, lumpy, not too clean beds with a great big bolster and a little pillow. Rose at 8:30 and after tea and bread was taken by skiff up Goshen's Arm, walked the two miles to Indian Cove, and over the Neck to Lobster Harbor. Had to row over to Purcell's and walk to Little Harbor to telephone for the cycle. It passed me and came back. It broke down and we blew the "snorf" out of the feed line and got home. Dinner, pumpkin pie at the Cottage, nothing in the afternoon except the meningitis which is much better on sulfa. Tea and a snooze and a fried chicken party that was exceptionally dull. Not a word was spoken.

October 3, '37. Up early after dreaming of Professor Warfield Longcope sitting on my bed while I complained to him about my typhoid injection. Breakfast, letters and the journal. Felt lousy all day—my shoulder hurt at every move. I spent most of the morning writing to Bob Barrows, with minor interruptions. Pulled the bag out of Hines' prostate. Wrote in the afternoon and somehow, oh, I read too, the afternoon passed. Snowed like hell and was cold. Funny, round, hard flakes like hail. I almost went to tea at the Cottage but remembered that the business manager, Wyn, had asked me down to his house for tea. I went over full of codeine. Dope that is. He had forgotten and already eaten. So I had tea in his wife's bedroom by the fire. She is sick. Sat around until 9:00. Then home and I read till 12:00.

October 4, '37. Grievous is the day in spite of a wire from Marianne saying she is throwing up her job to come here for four or five months. Marianne's expected arrival is a good light on the horizon. She's a type that I know will fit well into our economy. She can waltz like crazy, she rides horseback like mad, she has the enthusiasm of a hep-cat, only it's for symphony. She's an intelligent omnivorous reader and besides that there is a good probability that she is one of the best anesthetists in the world. When I was obliged to do anesthesia as an intern and my patient turned blue or behaved in any peculiar fashion I would quick call Hopkins and get Marianne on the phone. My plea of "what do I do now" always brought a resolving response. In the face of accomplishment she has not sacrificed any of her femininity. When she swoops in, tall, dark and slender in a black velvet off-the-shoulder outfit, the favorable reaction is quite apparent. She has arrived at a point in her job in the States where world famous surgeons vie with one another to have Marianne do their important cases, but that has made no difference when the charms of Twillingate were brought to her attention. Three days of pondering has elicited the laconic "Arriving Lewisporte 3 November."

After tea, I saw patients until a call came to go to Moreton's Harbor to see a slight fever and pain in the "born on arrival" who hasn't done well. The bight was extremely rough—every wave in the face. Landed at Tizzard's Harbor. Just as I was leaving the hospital, a cable came from Ed Barrows, older brother of my fellow camp counsellor Bob. A Dartmouth student, Bob met with a fatal auto accident Saturday night and died Sunday A.M., Services Wednesday 11. I wanted to be alone and think about it but had to go on this damn call. Had cocoa and cake at Locke's and walked a beautiful six miles

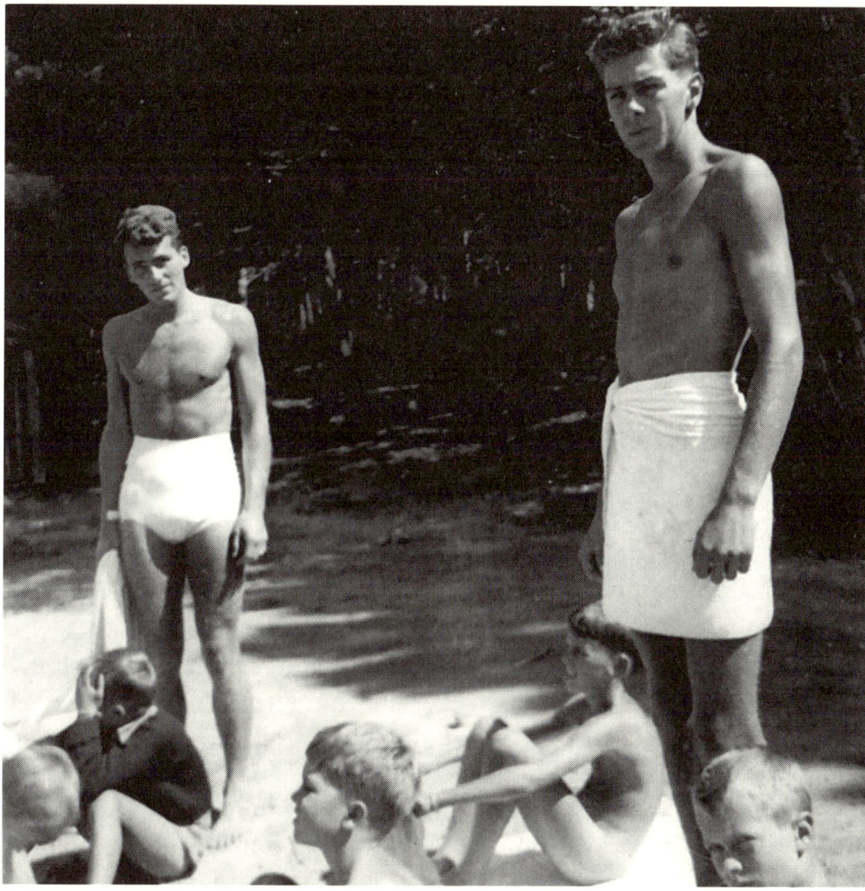

Dr. Ecke and Bob Barrows, as counsellors at Camp Winona, Summer 1937.

back in the dark. Had salt meat soup and tea with goat's milk. Back to drinking and poker. Lost a dollar and a quarter. Read some *Tristram* and my letters—a nice one from Sue Burnett. Cousin Jean is an Alpha Delt. I felt low. It's a little mysterious to see why Bob should be killed, though I felt his future was rather obscure. He had a frail, blithe spirit that was bound to be hurt. I'm glad I knew him and will miss him. I wired his mother a dozen red roses. (Bob's father is governor of Maine.) [Ed.note: Ed Barrows himself died on D-Day.]

October 5 and 6, '37. This was a rainy, cold day with nothing to do. I didn't stir out of the house all day. I was too awake from inaction last evening, so

I read till 2:30 in the morning when I was suddenly called upstairs to see a woman who had been in labor only an hour or so. I was surprised to find the head on the perineum and she was barely cleaned up before it started to look serious. Waddell came up and told me to put the forceps on, which I did, and eased the babe out, with no trouble except a small tear in her hemorrhoids. Why the hell I took his advice I don't know, since I know more about it than he does. The baby had a small mark from it. To bed at 4:30.

Wednesday was busy in the morning. I helped on an operation and the A.M. was beginning to look dull when John asked me to do a cystoscopy. I did so, but left early to go to Moreton's Harbor on that dreadful, big, official boat that the magistrate uses. It rolled like one possessed, putting her rail under at no sea at all. I went below to keep from being thrown overboard and had a nice sleep for myself. I woke in Moreton's and Gilbert Osmond took me to the Salvation Army Captain, who walked the two beautiful miles with me to Western Head, down the long steps, over the cliff above the cove. It was extremely beautiful. We spied a man ahead of us running like the dickens over the rocks with a chair in his arms. He got into the house just before we did and it turned out to be the chair for me to sit on. I saw a baby in a very poor shack. Waddell had looked in on it before, when he had been on an OB case. When I saw her, she had a full, solid right chest with her heart displaced to the left. Pulse and respiration fast and a moderate temperature. She was sick as hell with a tender mass in the right lower quadrant and the same in the right upper quadrant. I thought they were TB abscesses and advised admission. The captain walked back with me to a house where a whole family had scabies. I told the woman to get some flowers of sulphur and mix it with any old fat she had around the house and heat it. She seemed to be struck dumb by this, but after a moment of incredulous hesitation said, "Oh, Doctor, I couldn't do that. It would taste awful." I had forgotten the Cockney torturing of the letter "H." She thought I meant for her to eat it and I agreed with her that the taste might leave something to be desired. She finally consented to use the concoction as an ointment and not as a comestible. I was ferried over to Osmond's where I was royally entertained. Good tea, good homemade beer, and a game of Auction 45, that local combination of Old Maid and Rummy. The old man is a charmer, a boisterous W.C. Fields. The children are bright and charming. It was a nasty night, raining hard and I had gotten soaked. Gilbert cut my hair in the kitchen. It was one of the best haircuts I had ever had. A good bed. They had a funny indoor can with a chimney.

A fine breakfast and a good trip across the Bight, through Shoal Tickle in the big cabin skiff with a rough following sea. We saw a lot of bull birds (little auks). I massaged Gilbert's prostate and found a negative smear, but gave him prontolyn anyway. Opened an abscess and did a tonsil on Locke.

October 7, '37. The morning was hopeless. It rained and was very gray. I read the whole morning and started to do the same in the afternoon, but no end of patients came in and I worked like sixty until 5:00. One bad TB and I made a vain attempt to pass filiform sounds. I pulled a hard tooth. At 5:00, I took Jack, the horse, and Joe Bat, Waddell's nondescript little cur, and rode over to Manuel's Cove. It was a calm and beauteous eve, a yellow to red sunset and a glorious new moon. The nights are coming on much faster now. I saw an obscure fever, my meningitis perfectly well, a chicken pox, and an erythema multiforma on a little girl with a neck abscessed from louse bites. At night I conferred with John about tomorrow's trip around the bay. This is to be O.H.M.S. (On His Majesty's Service). They've had a typhoid scare in the lumber camps and the Health Department has requested us to tour the bay giving typhoid inoculations. Captain Stone will take us in His Majesty's cutter *Number 2.* He had no help so I take Elijah Dalley along. He skippers our *Bonnie Nell* in the summer time. Two captains will make a fine crew and the boat is a very neat, impressive, forty-five foot, two-engine craft. It looks like a miniature destroyer. There are several catches. The engines are almost impossible to start. There is no clutch and no reverse and that's no gear to go down the Straight Shore with. Besides, this is a fool's errand, because there is no advance publicity and no one will want to be immunized.

I was interested to see in Bob Barrows' letter written at Dartmouth two weeks before his death, that he says he feels like a guy who had his pants slit and his head shaved for the last trip, but he thought he would survive. What a grim joke.

October 8, '37. Dawned a magnificent day and I was in much of a stew getting off. I didn't know Skipper Dalley when he turned up, but judged it was he from the context. Finally packed, we went over in the cab, stopping to buy shotgun shells and bargain leather gloves with the lining gone. Skipper Stone came along and we were off in the very comfortable, but rolly cutter. It had been decided not to do any clinical work on this trip, but at the last minute being at heart an obstetrician, I had grabbed my stethoscope and the extra OB bag. I sat on the forward deck with the gun over to Herring Neck and took one shot at a cloud of bull birds but didn't get any. Reached Port Albert in good time and catheterized Mrs. Bennett and got two liters at least. We gave one shot of typhoid and on to Horwood where we went through the sawmill and gave one more shot. There the men work for two bucks a day in unguarded machinery and get only scrip and have to pay company store prices. Mr. Hoddinot was kind but indicated that he was averse to giving men time off if the shots hurt. I made flapjacks for tea but for the most part, we seemed to eat salt meat. The night was cool and people sat around the cutter until late. We made a couple of calls on a bad heart in a smelt fisherman's hut and a child with a feeding problem. I wished I had charged but didn't. It rained on us coming back. The northern lights were swell. I may be able to help this bad heart by tapping the dropsy. I'll wire for a trocar tomorrow.

A lovely morning and Skipper Stone got breakfast. I sent a few wires and went for a walk because he didn't want to sail on Sunday. He relented though, and got off to Victoria Cove just before dark after a hell of a struggle with the engine. Got here for tea. I made some biscuits and an apricot-orange marmalade turnover, which was very good. We were looking for the local authority, Mr. Oak. As the people came aboard, Dalley looks at them and says, "Everybody but Oak, eh?" The skipper rigged a riding light on a broom in the rigging. It seems that a broom in this position means either a great naval victory or that an auction sale is going on. We had some tea, toasted a few rolls, and I'm going to type and read before bed. We finally had to go ashore to see Mr. Oak. Mr. Hoddinot had given me his last drop of rum.

October 10, '37. A very quiet day. I rose early. The sun was so bright and I felt so grimy that I made the mistake of taking a swim. I trailed a line off the stern in the swift current of the Gander River and dove in. The frigid shock sent me scrambling madly for the line and any old way to get out of that arctic clutch. I clambered up over the stern getting liberally smeared with the black grease around the exhaust. There was nothing to do but clean my shivering form with gasoline and dive in again. A good breakfast restored my senses. I vaccinated about 18 and sounded three. I'm afraid I condemned one to go to work. We had a good dinner of embalmed willy (canned corn beef), canned tomatoes, bacon, and cracker crumbs all baked together. Mr. Farrell came aboard last night. He is the operator from Clarke's Head. He is an old polio case, tremendously developed in the shoulders but a bad lordosis (spinal curvature) and I never saw such shrunken lower limbs. He can build a house or dig a ditch all the same.

We made Clarke's Head and did a little work in the evening, but the notice of our arrival came the same time we did, so we spent the night here to give people time to know of our presence. I made a chocolate pudding—not so good—and pancakes—worse, for tea. The fire was not so good and we are running out of coal. I visited a kid or two tonight and came back on board to the tune of quite a blow. We dropped a second hook and all is snug for the night, though there is quite a precipitation of heavy snow. I'm enjoying the men I am with. The skipper is quite a humorous old guy and Dalley reports that he likes him very much. The men are notable for their weak profanity and lack of vulgarity. Mr. Peckford of the Gander store is bitter and seems to hate Mr. Saunders who went down to Twillingate to take the boy I cystoscoped to St. John's for what he considers may be better treatment. It's quite cold and I don't know what tomorrow holds.

October 11, '37. Some work in the morning and off to Mann Point, where Mr. French runs the sawmill. It was getting rough. Dalley and I went ashore and got some wet wood. We were going to walk to Mann Point but I forgot the vaccine. French stopped the mill and I made a speech on a pile of sawdust concerning the virtues of immunization. A few came for shots but it was blowing so hard that the skipper wouldn't wait. We steamed to the lee of the far shore to ride out the storm. I've learned to bake very good biscuits and did. Mr. French was most cooperative. The weather shore we left is as dreary a spot as I ever saw. Not a soul. Not a house. Not a sign of life. I expected to hear wolves howling there all night. It was cold and blew like hell.

October 12, '37. People from Victoria Cove came aboard before breakfast but we were off to an early start. Went back to Mann Point where it still blew. I did quite a few, including Ray Hodder, whom I recognized on deck by his voice. He came aboard singing *I Wish That I Could Diddle Like the Man Who Played the Fiddle*. I went ashore to see a woman who had been in the hospital with beriberi three years before. Then Hodder's old man with a bad stomach and another guy. I hurried and we set out for Carmanville where we arrived just as the *S.S. Segona* did. She's a beauty, 1,200 tons, does the whole coast out of St. John's. We had seen her at Frederickton the day before, where we had stopped for dinner. My friend, Ted Drover, came aboard and we boarded the *Segona* to have a beer with Captain Knee in his cabin. I climbed up the tall, sheer sides of the *Segona* on a rope ladder much to my dismay, and down again too. Ted left on his fast skiff for Alder Harbor. We had a quiet rainy night. We learned that the *Kyle*, the *Clyde*, the *Home*, and the *Segona* had all been storm-bound Monday and three schooners had gone ashore at Surprise only a few miles from where we rode out the storm. We got some of the survivors to get water for us.

October 13, '37. This day we planned to lay up to give the skipper's crud a chance to heal. No typhoid people came aboard, but a few came for examinations. Some people walked all the way from Frederickton. I seem to be doing more and more clinical work, although I planned not to do any. Dalley and I tried all over the place to get coal and failed, until someone mentioned the post office where we bummed a hod. Mrs. Hicks came down to get me and I went to her nice, clean, widow's house to examine her for a pension. She was well. I retracted the grandson's foreskin. They wanted to pay me but were too nice. I took instead a pie, a loaf of bread, and some preserve. They were all good, even if I did have to hold the baby while the pie, which is not a pie at all but a layer cake, was being baked. It rained like hell all day. We saw Mr. Woolfrey, whose mill burned down the year before. He said he was rebuilding because so many depended on the mill to make a living. He said fire insurance on the mill was so expensive that it was cheaper not to insure providing your mill didn't burn down more often than every five years. Towards evening, we were beginning to think of going over to Alder Harbor when Ted Drover hove into sight to pilot us. We did not start until late and approached the difficult entrance after dark. It was pelting rain and the guarding rocks made Alder Harbor look anything but hospitable. We found anchorage though, and it was a good place. Went ashore with Ted to his snug little bungalow and there was Jessie, his wife, a very charming lady indeed. I was royally entertained with a good chicken dinner. She set about making cookies and gave me a lesson in piecrust. They have their clocks an hour and three-quarters ahead to save on daylight. Ted is an artist and knows more sea-lore than anybody I ever knew or heard of. He speaks with an English accent and looks like Brian Aherne. He is most kind and considerate to equals but perhaps a little hoity-toity with menials. Alder Harbor is a temporary summer village holding only the sawmill, which Ted runs for his father. He could not do enough and I would say is a perfect host, as is Jessie. About 4 A.M., I heard some stewing at the door, but that will go for tomorrow. I slept in the storeroom in a comfortable enough bed, but there was a pan of smoked fish under the bed that smelled strongly. The head sawyer lives with the Drovers and snores and sings in his sleep.

October 14, '37. At 4 A.M., above the sound of wind and sleet, I heard the noise at the door and thanked God that no one knew where I was and I wouldn't have to be getting up. Ted came in his bathrobe and apologetically told me there were some men from Musgrave to see me. They had come the 20 miles down the Straight Shore in a small open motor boat and had been to Carmanville looking for me. A woman was in her third day of labor and needed a doctor. I thought I ought to go right along with them, but I was afraid of their small boat. I sent them on and said I would come in the cutter as soon as it was daylight. I had breakfast and to my great joy, Jessie offered to go along to help if I would bring her back. I accepted. The cutter was already alight, the men having looked there for me first. Ted started to pilot us out of the harbor with his skiff in tow. Alder Harbor was too small to turn around in. Sweating, Stone started an engine in reverse. Here's where we wished we had a clutch. We went stern foremost towards the rocks. We shouted to Stone to throw the switch and try to trip the engine into forward motion. She caught, of course, in reverse and we gathered speed towards sure destruction. Dalley had the presence of mind to throw out the anchor and we brought up short with a jolt close enough to the rocks for Jessie to touch them with an oar. We couldn't have had more than two inches to spare. We got off finally and it was rough indeed. Stone was not at all enthusiastic, said we shouldn't look at the water on a day like this. I got kind of sick, but made breakfast for the crew and lay down. Everything in the aft cabin was loose and on the floor. We passed Green's schooner. She was lovely heeling over to the gale. We made Musgrave Harbour, which has no harbor at all. This whole Straight Shore is nothing but a shelf of boulders. We tied up to a collar in the lee of one of these boulders and hurried ashore in the dory to the exhausted Mrs. Guy, who was indeed in her third day of labor. The midwife had ruptured the membranes two days before. The bladder was big. I had to push up the head so Jessie could catheterize her. I felt some cervix that seemed to be prolapsed cord. I couldn't hear fetal heart and thought the babe was dead. The forceps wouldn't lock properly, but I went ahead. Jessie poured the chloroform. The babe appeared with no great difficulty. It was covered with meconium (fetal feces). Certain it was dead, I was about to roll it under the bed but routinely put my finger in its mouth and it nipped me. Everything turned out well. Jessie and I borrowed bicycles to go several miles along the shore in the rain to see some patients. We returned to find Dalley frantically looking for us. The wind had changed and Skipper Stone was blowing the foghorn and making wild signals for us to get back on board. Much to Dalley's annoyance, I took the time to examine a possible appendicitis on a lad lying on the floor of the general store. On the rough trip back to the cutter, I will never forget Jessie sitting calmly in the stern of the dory, while I held on for dear life thinking each moment my last. Stone heaved us on board swearing he would have left without us if he could have managed the engines alone. We needed to get out into deep water fast. We were in difficulty without a clutch. We couldn't loosen our mooring until we were sure the engine was going and would stay going and every time an engine started we would slew around and head for the rocks and have to turn it off. We let her fall away until she was headed for the channel, then just as an engine caught, I slashed the mooring with a butcher knife and we precariously limped off, broadside to the sea and parallel to the rocks, making leeway until Stone, red-faced and swearing, got the other engine going. I lay down and worried until I fell asleep, like Jessie. I went on deck when it got dark and I was certainly happy when a tossing light loomed suddenly ahead. It was Ted out looking for us and we never could have gotten back into Alder Harbor without him. One of the great joys of this life is to feel the water suddenly quiet under you as you come into harbor. Got supper and talked and went to bed more convinced of the charm of my hosts.

October 15, '37. The skipper refused to sail today so I had the chance to do 25 injections. Then we just sat around and talked before turning in early.

October 16, '37. Dalley and I started off right after breakfast to walk to Apsey Cove, although there is no road to it, just seven miles of boulders. I shot a Tickleass and he got a plover, an 'ant sarey', and a dozen tiny snowbirds. A stranger took us in for tea. Then I did eight injections among the sparse population of that place. We started back on the run and covered it in a little over two hours or almost an hour better than any native. I got wet. I was very tired, had a good tea and we sat around till late. Jessie fried the birds. We stayed by the stove smoking and warm in borrowed slippers. The Straight Shore is a dreadful place; the ships do well to give it a wide berth. Ted cranked the gramophone and played his beloved *La Traviata.*

October 17, '37. An early farewell breakfast, delicious beans and then over to the cutter with some cookies and gift tobacco. Off and a pleasantly rough run to the Indian Isle where I saw, of all people, Mrs. Perry. After a shore call, as I was climbing down off the wharf, the patient's mother ran down to me with my stethoscope that I had left behind. She had put my "zounders" (stethoscope) in a paper bag, which I stuck in my pocket. When I went to climb from the dory into the cutter, the dory pushed away from the boat and as I stretched helplessly trying not to fall into the water, my stethoscope fell out of my pocket, whirled once or twice on the surface and leisurely settled on the bottom where I could see it for a moment—12 feet below. The whole village turned out to retrieve it. They put cod liver oil on the water to make it smooth. They peered through fish glasses. They grappled with boat hooks and grappling irons. They jigged with codfish hooks. They put down the lead with butter on it and finally a stranger lashed three oars and a gaff together and hooked them for me. It's a lovely but bleak place. There isn't a piece of land higher than six feet. Saw a tumor of the testes which must be a cancer, then on for a lovely run to Stag Harbor where we shot off the gun several times and blew the fog horn but no one came because there was no public notice of our mission. We pulled up and went by beautiful moonlight to Little Seldom Come By where we left word that we would be back the next day and then on in the dark through the tickle to Seldom Come By. There we tied up and I made some griddle cakes. We stole what looked like a scuttle of coal from a pile on the wharf. I asked the skipper if he knew what it was and he said it was Epsom salts. I'm going right to bed now because I think I'm getting a cold.

October 18, '37. A rather too quiet day to ever finish this job. Up early enough but no business. Dalley and I walked across the Neck to Little Seldom, but none there, although a few came over later. I visited a mewling brat and set off for Wild Cove late in the afternoon. It was so rough over there we couldn't land but lay hove to where it was too deep to drop the hook. It also appeared to be too late and dirty to try Cape Fogo so we came back. We did the worst tossing so far. I cooked some meat rolls, according to Jessie's recipe. They sure were good. A not too intelligent local character came aboard and we had to throw him out. (He couldn't understand we couldn't pull teeth without instruments.) I saw a man who may have typhoid, but his temperature is too low. We had to get out of our berth to let the *Young Hood* come in, a handsome 80-ton schooner. She's lying beside us now as we bump against the wharf.

October 19, '37. I saw my patient again. His liver is not large but his spleen is very large. I'm almost certain he does have typhoid. The people never said a word about pay and the wife is so hopeless that "she has her rugs hooked for her." I bought a lovely colored but poorly made one, for which I had to pay a dollar. I will never get rich if I give my patients money instead of collecting. I saw a couple of children, but nothing the matter with them. These people are a little spoiled about doctors. They don't realize with what effort medical attention is brought to them and how lucky they are. We did get off to the Cape and I fell asleep, missing the lovely trip around. Dalley even shot at some turrs and at some bull birds flying in clouds like swallows over the water, but I didn't hear him. I awoke as we came into Tilting, a land-locked harbor. It is a Catholic settlement and seems very snug and neat and prosperous. An old duffer came out in a punt and told us that 130 men had gone into the woods to make money and 34 women were also gone. Where to, God knows.

As I was finishing my letter Tuesday, I heard the *Segona* whistle. Dalley got out the dory and we rowed like fury over to her. It was fun in the swell. I scrambled up the ladder. Found Captain Knee having a snack in the pantry. He recognized me and was pleased to mail my letters. At Tilting, the *Hood* caught up with us again. We hurried on to Joe Batts' Arm where we arrived early in the evening. The skipper went off to see a friend in the cold storage plant and got some smelts for breakfast. We walked over the hill to Barr'd Island, a lovely settlement with two huge, unfinished, concrete churches which must have cost thousands. Money more ill-spent could not be in the midst of this penury. We had a quiet evening on board, reading and writing. I enjoy every minute of Dalley's company. He has been around a lot, has lived in the States, and is a strong, fine-looking guy. He is very nice to me, gets me water and builds the fire in the morning. I approve of him highly.

October 20, '37. An old codger came in this morning from Little Fogo. Said the priest had seen his son and said it would cost a hundred dollars to get a doctor from Twillingate. He obviously is against the hospital. The man said he had a very sick little boy. He described the symptoms of ureteral stone and said the pain went down into his little privates. This was the only baby they had left. A boy of twelve had gone out on the ice after a bird and when they looked his way, he was gone and they never got so much as a little mitten. I was surprised that a child so young should have a stone but got into the motorboat and went across the arm to a wretched little hovel with rags stuck through the broken windows. The baby was 19 years old. Absolutely treating him like a four-year-old, never letting him speak a word for himself. They had him plastered with religious medals, crucifixes and beads. He was highly neurotic and it was very difficult to get a decent story. The pain went down the main vein, whatever that is, to his legs and up to his head. I think it's a stone all the same, and advise coming to the hospital. I spoke to the public nurse about this case. She told me that this particular man was always sending for her but had never contributed to the Nurse's Fund. On being asked for money, he said he was sorry he couldn't give her any but all his spare coppers had to go to the church. Father Jones had told him the church was in particular need of every cent now because the Italians were having such a hard time of it in Ethiopia. It seems kind of rough to me to take money from this windowless pauper for the glorification of a greater Mussolini.

We hurried on and came to Fogo by lunchtime. No one there to see us. We tried to get the constable to round up some prospects, but he was too engrossed with his own troubles. He had lost a two-and-a-half-month-old baby the week before, and a thirteen-month-old baby was showing the same trouble. I went to the courthouse, where he lives with a wan, young, pretty woman with a faraway voice, hair coming down, stockings coming down, cotton bathrobe, and slippers. She was wandering vaguely around among the wreckage produced by eight children. "I have too many, Doctor," she says, "I don't know where they all come from." I then went to see the Postmaster's Ruby. She had a bruised leg and when I got her to straighten it out, they thought I was a miracle worker. I collected a dollar and hurried back to the boat and we were off to the impoverished Hare Bay, a perfect little harbor with three narrow exits. I saw old Skipper Tom Nipper with erysipelas of the face and got a loaf of bread from him. There was a funeral in town. An old skipper had died in his eighty-sixth year. A white rag of a flag was at half-mast and the six pall-bearers wore white bands on the weather arm and all wore rubber boots. The girls came back singing. One girl came to the boat, a pretty one, never out of this spot in her life. Beautiful teeth and her clothes full of gewgaws, beads, pins, coronation medals and what not.

We left the harbor through a fine, narrow, swift-flowing tickle. The skipper was very apprehensive. He was afraid that the man who told us to use that tickle wanted us to get wrecked so that he could get salvage. We made a course straight for Change Island, westward, through a lovely mellow sunset. I couldn't but think of Bob Barrows all the way over. I'm still unwilling to accept his sudden death. It's too vicious and abrupt. It seems like a gigantic hoax.

Big, stout, affable Billy Earl came down to meet us with a message from Mr. Hoddinot that our dropsy case at Horwood was dead and also brought the trocar to fix her up. He wanted me to go see a patient and I went down through the main tickle to Mr. Abraham Coles, sick a fortnight with an obstruction. All I could do was to give him some morphia out of the OB bag and tell him I would take him to the hospital the next day. I went back to Billy Earl's house to tea with the minister, a very engaging Scotchman. Mrs. Earl, or Trixie Elliott as I knew her three years ago, is very much the mistress of the mansion. I stayed and talked fish until 1:00 and promised Billy some smelts. He has a grand house up on a hill with a view of the ocean three ways. Not without reason it is called the Four Winds.

October 21, '37. Up to a late breakfast and Billy brought down an 86-year-old protégé with a hernia. I went down the tickle to order a bad corneal ulcer to the hospital and on to Abraham Cole's, who had had his first night's sleep in two weeks, from my OB morphia. We got him hoisted onto the top of Earl's boat and at the worst part of the tickle, the rudder broke, giving us a bad moment. I saw Mrs. Torraville, a cultured Scottish nurse. Her child's heart was touched a little by scarlet fever. Trixie invited me to dinner, but the fog had lifted so we made for Twillingate with three cans of duck. A fine trip back and we sat in the sun on the government wharf, the three of us, to smoke a final pipe. Captain Stone promised me a berth in his new schooner. He thinks I would be an able-bodied seaman after a time. John was glad to see me. Tea, after a long bath and reading ten letters. Tonight there's a party and I will go soon. People are glad to see me back and said so. They say I'm thinner but I feel better. My family was shocked by Bob's death. I don't blame them.

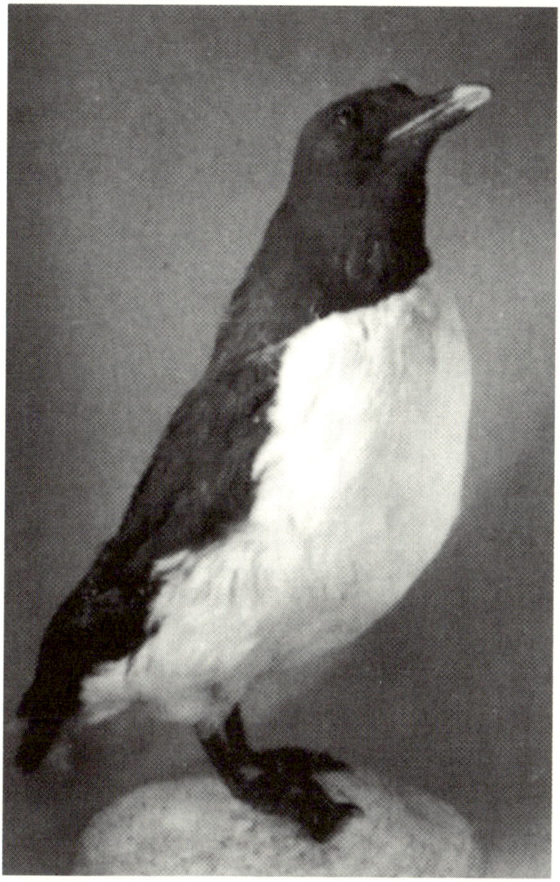

The Turr.

October 22, '37. The morning was a little dull. I sorted and reread mail. In the afternoon, I made three calls with the motorcycle with Joyce over to Crow Head and Back Harbor. I will never get used to the variety of gates. Went to the Cottage to tea and ate two turrs. They're a delicious and gamey bird, but not so good as plover. We ducked out because of the directors' meeting and I'm given to believe that something important to all of us was discussed and passed, but they won't tell. I was reading in my room, when Ives called me to go to see a woman who hit her finger with an axe. I thought it was nearby and started to walk, but found it was way down by Jenkins Cove. Over the cliff, I got a splendid view of the best northern lights this fall. A fantastic arc of sheer gossamer flame, of pale translucent green, festooning across the zenith. I found the bleeding had been stopped by a man who said he could stop any bleeding and could also charm teeth. I found my patient sitting frightened in her little kitchen with at least 15 people sitting around in stony, commiserative silence. When I brought her back, the OPD was full of Ives treating a four-year-old for lockjaw. We gave him intravenous, intrathecal, intramuscular antitoxin, but he died in convulsions. The parents took the news as if I had told them he had a bad cold. They seemed annoyed when I stopped them to tell them. They were impatient to get down to the Harbor View Hotel to go to bed. This is characteristic of the people's attitude in the face of serious illness or death. This apathy is ruining the place. There is so little singing, no folk stuff at all.

I found the finger almost off, but sewed it back on to give it a chance. Used base anesthesia for the first time.

October 23, '37. A gray, dull day and I was depressed all day. Did a bad job on a tooth I should have left alone. Went to tea at Wynn's with Edith. Talked to Ives and Waddell when I came back and came to the conclusion that the latter is going to screw me out of doing any surgery this year and my time will be wasted. On top of that, I listened to a broadcast of *Men in White*; tripe that it is, it started me thinking about careers and how mine is going to pot and I can't help but be discouraged. I wrote a couple of letters in this mood and am sure that the recipients will consider it bad form to go to them with my complaining. But people like those better for whom they can feel sorry. The strong ones are strong alone. Read *Pinocchio* today and liked it.

October 27, '37. I got a letter from my sister and a note from Mrs. Barrows saying that Bob's friends will be theirs. It does look as though Waddell will do me out of what ought to be mine. He is clever, covers guile with southern glamour. I did get to do a hernia today and felt a little better. I've been in a depression the past few days, but feel my manic stage coming on. That cancer of the testes that I diagnosed in Seldom turned out to be a perfectly benign hydrocele and I fixed it this morning. The boys did a posterior gastro-enterostomy on a diagnosis of ulcer. I had not thought he had cancer and was pleased to find out I was right. I haven't been out of the house in a long time and if it kills me, I'll get a long trip soon. I've been working hard in the OPD. Great crowds of patients came from the Straight Shore these last few days. Ives left Monday for his Yale appointment and I miss him—I feel we have much in common. I once in a while doubt if I will ever amount to much in surgery. If left alone, I can muddle through, but the presence of betters disturbs me. Tea at the Cottage with one of Susie's famous pumpkin pies. I don't think I should operate if there is a better surgeon available.

October 28, '37. A good day except that I did not set foot outside of the hospital. Waddell was already gone to Lobster Harbor on a suspected diphtheria when I arose rather late. I did an appendix with John and the silk was possessed. I sewed in a nerve and it took all morning to get it out. John was a little caustic, like the old days but exercised pretty good self-control. Then helped with an appendix and a very successful cataract. Gilbert Osmond was waiting for me to massage his prostate and then it was time for dinner. The OPD went like sixty until 5:00. I pulled about 15 teeth, some out of old Mrs. Gillingham. I saw her the day we almost wrecked the cutter at Musgrave. She has a mouth full of scrags and a peculiar, small grape-like tumor that seems to be attached by a short pedicle to the lower right gum. We are cleaning her mouth up before attacking the tumor. After rounds Waddell offered us a drink, his new favorite, blueberry wine spiked with rum. Dinner was soon over and I lay down for a minute when he came in to get me to go to the masked ball. He said it would be sad if I couldn't get into the spirit of it, for the poor girls have been in a tizzy over the ball these two weeks. We had a few drinks and never did get to the dance, just tossed the turd. The odd-job man, Stanley, the child of nature, wandered in. I am treating him for syphilis. He always claimed that his primary lesion resulted when the head of a match blew off while he was lighting his pipe while lying in bed. He must have been raped, for he's as simple as the day. Annie, his cohabitor, is a sloven wench. He had just come from a Salvation Army meeting at the barracks and was loud in his praise of the preaching. He admitted it was as good a pastime as any.

I saw Skipper George Young, whose hernia gives us so much trouble at times. He was carrying lumber around with his one arm. His bride of a year was sitting on the platform knitting in the sun. He married her to save paying her as a housekeeper. They are both 70. She had a no-good son who came to spend the night. The skipper threw him out and he went down to sleep at Clemmy's, that elegant fishwife, who wanted us to keep her children so they could eat. Her husband came home and broke every dish in the house and burned the family Bible. "He's not a Christian," said Clemmy, "Goddamned if he is." Clemmy is curvy and full of style and manners. She developed St. Anthony's Fire once on the ward from running doses of ergot. No permanent damage.

October 29, '37. A pretty good day. No operating. Waddell dictated and I seemed to have the OPD to myself. Mrs. Elliott slipped into uremic convulsions and I passed the morning on the ward giving arsenic and pneumothorax treatments. Pulled the second installment on Mrs. Gillingham's teeth and had dinner at the Cottage. More ward and OPD work and I'm sure tired of men who are nervous and run down and have self-avowed heart trouble. Waddell relieved me and I took the horse for a lovely slow walk way down around Bluff Head Cove where I've never been. It was just dusk and very blue and gray. The horse cantered all the way back and there was a fine, warm, horse smell. Gave some glucose at 3:30 A.M. to Mrs. Elliott. She seems a little better.

October 30, '37. Up at 7 A.M. to give more glucose and then a leisurely breakfast in the bright sun. A full morning of OPD and operative notes. More glucose at 1:30 P.M. and a quiet afternoon with a little reading and another tooth installment; some OPD. Tea at Edith's and a call to the Cooper child, who had a temperature of 105 degrees with nothing to show. Back just in time for a drink with Waddell when Cooper came for me again to see his child's spasm. I hurried down and the spasm was over but he had had a fine loose stool and seemed to be breathing—the crud. I left some paregoric.

October 31, '37. A grand day. Blew like hell with sleet and rain the whole day just a little above freezing. I rose at 5:30 to find Mrs. Strong with the baby's head on the perineum. I summoned the staff, scrubbed and applied the low forceps, and brought forth the child with great ease. It breathed poorly though, and I had to work on it for hours before it would keep going on its own. It stopped about 4:00 and couldn't be roused. The mother, a former aide here, took it well. "Make the brute breathe, if you can," said she. Her husband, Roy, is here bleeding from the lungs with TB. Ives christened the baby after me, Jeanette Roberta.

Just at dawn while we were in the operating room, the sun broke out from in back of us, making the far shore of the harbor stand out in gold relief against the gray. A glorious rainbow stood out from Long Point. It was beautiful and gone in a minute. To the Cottage for a grand dinner. The rest of the day was quiet and restful.

November 1, '37. No operating. The storm continued with sleet and rain and a full gale. We did little but try to keep warm. The morning had a few hours of clear sky before it closed in. I cycled over with Waddell to Long Point to the lighthouse. A great wind lop was throwing spray clear up onto the cliff. We couldn't stand against it so didn't go near the edge. Stopped for a call at Manuel's Cove and back to the hospital for a fine tea at the Cottage. We had lobster, great platters of it. I had the crud today. To bed early so as to rise early for turr shooting with John.

November 2, '37. Woke to a gale of wind that rolled up the linoleum on my bedroom floor. I rose with justified misgivings at 5:00 and had breakfast on the ward. I put on long winter underwear, turtleneck sweater, my "B" sweater, leather vest, leather windbreaker, a scarf, mitts, my hat, two pairs of socks, rubber boots, and a complete suit of oilskins. The half-witted Stanley and John and I squeezed into the little punt with the outboard, putting it way down by the stern. I was terrified before we left the harbor and asked John to please let me out as we went through the tickle. He just laughed and we plunged into the bight. The lop was stupendous, 10 and 12 feet high, cold as the devil and I was in dread. We got seven turrs, but each moment I was convinced was the end for more than one reason. The weather was bad enough without having Stanley wave his shotgun in my face. I found that you could steer if you waited until the boat was perched on the top of a lop. Afraid to turn around, we drifted down stern foremost, with me at the oars, tired and cold. We turned to go into the tickle for refuge, but were going too fast. We sped along the top of the lops but would suddenly plunge with a wild twist that threw the stern under. We shipped lots of water and it was a glad person who scrambled stiffly up onto Blandford's wharf. I had to go right to the operating room, smothering in my long winter underwear. I started to cut out Mrs. Gillingham's tumor to find it was not on the jaw, but deep in the floor of the mouth. By much dissecting, after a mandibular block, it yielded. Then to the OPD and little else until tea. Played poker with the Ranger Sergeant, who is not especially bright. I lost $2.50, my first loss in a year. I would give my shirt to beat John. He wins all the time. Found a nice tray of chicken salad by my bed.

November 3, '37. Up early to a full morning of operating. First a double hernia. I was allowed to do the side with the small sac. Waddell is not an easy person to work with—inclined to be arbitrary and didactic. Next was a bad cancer of the breast, a foul, stinking thing and the woman had nursed a baby on it only a few days before. Then I opened a bad breast abscess. After dinner I saddled Jack for a quick ride to the North Island. I was much surprised to find the patient was 90 years old, a hefty woman who had had a "turn." She wasn't sure whether she was sick or not. Next, to an old couple, 75 years old. The man had a coronary. He came to the door with a streaming, wet face. "Have you been washing?" say I. "No," says he, "I was just having a drop of tea." "You must have poured it on your face," I said. He allowed as how he always perspired like that. He should have been in bed. He couldn't stay there because his woman is blind or nearly so. She had had a cataract done eight years before by an itinerant M.D. from St. John's, and it looks like a horse's blind eyeball, sort of blue. I then went to the telegraph office to wire Marianne that we would come and get her. She is marooned in Lewisporte and fed up with the whole business. I will go if the weather is fine, but I can't afford to get stuck for two or three days. For tea we had the turrs we shot the other day. They were good. The horse was in wonderful spirits. He pawed and neighed and kicked out with both hind feet and tried to bite me. He knocked the fence down and tore up all the ground in front of the office.

I am moving in with Waddell and I shifted some of my stuff before going to bed. I've had the crud for two days and there seems to be some pain in my calcified hydatid of Morgagni (never mind what that is). Tonight the weather looks bad for our trip to Lewisporte.

November 4, '37. Up early to call Skipper Frank Roberts, but he wanted to wait and see what the wind was going to do. It was doing too much so we didn't go to Lewisporte. In fact, it blew like fury and the bight was white with breaking waves. A prominent minister and a divinity student were drowned in Bonne Bay when their engine gave out and their boat drifted on to a sunker—a submerged rock. She swamped and broke up.

I did a cystoscopy and had a lot of trouble finding the ureteral orifices. They were hidden in folds of a shaggy bladder. The right kidney turned out to be pretty badly shot. I moved more of my stuff before tea and called on my nonagenarian. I fell asleep about 7:00 and woke to give an intravenous and do a catheterization, and fell asleep again and woke at 1:30 to go to bed.

November 5, '37. Up at 4:30 to see Bobby Cooper again, blood pressure 235/140. He's had something like a stroke, probably vascular spasms. I comforted him and he said he felt better whenever I came into the room. Back from my second breakfast and word from Skipper Frank that he would not leave before 9:00. I've had three breakfasts and am just about to start for Lewisporte for Marianne. I am full of tincture of opium for my crud.

November 8, '37. I become lazy, but this entry has been complicated by my moving in with Waddell. I feel like a stranger. His possessions are all over the place, and he is a domineering if not a dominating character. He leaves his junk anywhere and I feel as if I were intruding. This, of course, may be due to my own twisted personality. I've had a pretty good time this week otherwise. On Friday, a couple of traveling salesmen and I went to Lewisporte. It was the roughest trip Skipper Frank had ever made. We took every wave aboard. The roof and side of the *Little Grace* leaked like a sieve. There wasn't a dry spot on the craft. We hauled into a delightful little harbor to boil a kettle, but were soon at it again and reached Lewisporte after six hours, two hours longer than usual. Western Head was magnificent. At Tickle Ass Rock the waves threw themselves 20 feet into the air. It was punch all the way.

At Lewisporte, Marianne was depressed beyond words and ready to go home. I tried to cheer her up. At the King George for the night, we played two-handed poker and read. We were aboard the boat at 5:00 A.M. and made a quick passage back, watching the sunrise. The mental alarm clock is interesting. I sighted Western Head, went below to nap and woke just as we reached it. I sighted Twillingate and repeated the performance. Marianne was very quiet and frightened by the strangeness of everything. I took her on several outside calls. I examined old Mrs. Richardson, who caught the beriberi from her strict diet. She's boarding at Bobby Cooper's. I had to charge her $5.00 because he isn't on the Medical Center. That liar of a quack, Knapp, was her doctor. When her blood pressure was 180, he said it had gone down half. He brought a man here five years ago for X-ray. While in the hospital, the patient developed a temperature of 103, but Knapp took him home. "What has he?" we asked. "Oh!" says Knapp, "He fell into the harbor two days ago, he probably has a touch of the typhoid."

November 10, '37. Three long operations in the morning. Marianne gives perfect anesthesia. After all, she was the best anesthetist at Hopkins. I was in on all three. Afternoon was quickly consumed by a little work on the wards, in the OPD, and a couple of calls in the clear cold afternoon with the sun dropping into the bight behind Western Head about 4:30. The ponds are frozen on top and winter seems about on us. Rounds and tea of fresh herring, of which I ate innumerable. They're so sweet and innocent when you first eat them. Then a little work in the OPD and a call. Sat and talked to Marianne and John and was just going to bed but didn't make it until I fixed a catheter and had some jam and clotted cream and tea. Then to bed and had to get up twice to make discharge slips. Finally I am back in bed. Kelly came in to get a slip and I must say she is a friendly soul. She sat down and talked for a long time. I don't know. I don't know.

November 12, '37. Shouldn't commit myself to paper when feeling badly towards the world, and that is how I feel. It's disagreeable because one can be certain that the cause for such a feeling is always in oneself. The world is benign enough. I lost at poker and am tired of adapting myself to living with the sloppy Waddell. He has moments of great charm and generosity, but is so cocksure and superior in his medical manner that I have enough of that. John, on the other hand, is almost always pleasant and thoughtful. If he is crusty, it's for the good of the crustee or the crustee deserved it.

I wish I could write more regularly, but living with someone makes it impossible. Yesterday was Armistice Day. I helped on an operation or two, then while my colleagues smirked at the windows, I had to stand on the front steps to receive for the hospital a memorial wreath that a variegated squad of veterans brought up the lane to lay at the tablet. They were in formation with the unctuous Tom Ashbourne blowing his whistle at the head. They sang *God Save the King* too high. Then we worked around and played poker until 11:00 when we went over to the square dance. I was full of fun and enjoyed the strenuous quadrille very much. Today I did a tonsil and opened a dreadful breast. I'm worried about her. We settled ourselves in the room for a quiet afternoon, thinking the snow would keep patients away, but I tended the OPD, pulled a tooth on the ward, and had to go deliver the Bulgin baby. It was a little slow in coming so I returned to the hospital for tea and to get Marianne. We sat too long and I just caught the baby, getting the amniotic fluid up my sleeve and a small tear. Got back, getting stuck in a snowdrift with no light on the cycle, to tea at the Cottage. Poker to the tune of an $8.00 loss. In my blood mood, I will write a while and then see if I can get to sleep.

November 14, '37. Saturday was punctuated by an outside delivery. I was called to Jenkins Cove and hurried as best I could, but the snow was too deep and had to leave the cycle at the foot of the hill by the Arm and go around the cliff on foot. The midwife met us and says, "You are just in time, Doctor." The baby had already been born but like most midwives, she was afraid of the placenta. The bag was a mess: no OB package in it and no stuff for the eyes. Tommy had to boil a piece of string to tie the cord. It was the same patient who had erysipelas on the tip of her nose. We feared some complications from that, but she's well now. I've heard since that the baby has some water trouble and I'm going down tomorrow. Sunday was a nice, quiet day. We had a good turr dinner and sat around. I played chess with John. The first time in many years. I lost.

Monday and Tuesday I don't remember very much of. I did two tonsils, a hernia, an appendix, and pulled about 20 teeth. There are moments when I'm tired of almost everybody, and every day I wish I were back in my own apartment, where the dirt, at least, is of my own making. In here, there is too much mess to move around. Waddell is unbearable when he lets me operate. He talks to me as if I had never scrubbed before. Today has been all right, though. I went over to Herring Neck with Marianne right after I had finished a little ward work. It was a cold day, gray with a little sea on. Square across the bight, through the gut and across the Neck, with a bit of a walk over to a nice house. I frightened the baby on my way in. The old man of the house had slipped and hit his flank. He may have cracked a rib, but I doubt it. I strapped him and we were then bidden to a bit of tea and birthday cake from the spry old lady's sixty-seventh birthday. It was good and the people most kindly. I held the baby awhile. It had decided to be friends.

After dinner, I got out the horse, which is now wild, and really bucks and tries to unseat the rider. I don't have too much trouble and the natives are impressed by this bronco stuff. I trotted down the cliff road to Hart's Cove, and saw a crone with a headache. She was insufferable, indicating she was doing me a favor by letting me treat her for her hemicrania. Her husband had insisted on Dr. Olds and looked rather disappointed when I came along. Perhaps he doesn't think so much of me since I took him for that night ride in the cycle with no lights. We did go off the road over a bump too swiftly taken and down on the grass by the sea. It certainly is slippery stuff. He had to push me back on the road. Went on for a nice gallop and the horse was wet when we got back, though far from worn out.

All the snow is gone now and it is almost like a snappy spring. A lone bachelor's tea at the Cottage. Betty is in labor and the ineffable Suzy, the cook, had made a guessing cake for the church supper. She had gone over to see the guessing. I ate too much and wanted the boys to play poker. They are very slow to get started. I was strongly moved by the astronomy pictures in today's *Life*. I want to be an astronomer. I wonder if there are medical astronomers. I don't know any math though. It would take me forever to learn math.

November 17, '37. From the depths of indigestion, I write this. Too much lobster for tea, if that is possible. Suzy fixed it and she can fix even canned rabbit so that you eat too much of it. I bet she could fix canned seal. Last evening, Betty was in pain. Olds stayed with her so I had to go down to Bluff Head Cove on the cycle. It's a very wild spot and the road winds tremendously over rocks and through narrow places. The cycle hasn't much clearance and the engine gets hung on the projecting rocks in the road. Some day it is going to be knocked right out. The young husband came for me. I found a young, attractive, loonish girl of nineteen, doing a very good job of her first baby. I waited until midnight and finally had the old midwife pour some chloroform and all alone, I draped, held both legs on two mattresses, put on the hooks and got a nice male. The chloroform in the airtight little room almost got me. I fixed a tiny tear and in no time, I was home to find Betty just getting to work. It is disturbing to hear the involuntary gasps and groans of someone you know well, especially if you have known her as a stable, sound, composed, lovely person. It took a team of five to deliver her with low forceps and I had just done the same thing all alone. I had to laugh—the self-important Waddell saving himself for the difficult task of backing John up. I went to bed late while John drank in our living room to his new son.

November 18, '37. Started off by helping Waddell on a hernia. Then I did an orchidectomy and a tonsil by myself. Waddell did a normal appendix that he should have let me do. He's really selfish and hard, but covered with gloss and plantation ease. I tried to fight with him about his leaving orders on *my* patients. He agreed with me perfectly although I am certain he is guilty.

After dinner I had to make a few outside calls. I took Marianne and we went to Manuel's Cove, Crow Head, and Jenkins Cove. They are very far apart so I hurried. I spun around corners and skidded. All went well until, coming back in the dark with that poor light that shines just nine feet ahead of the motorcycle, I dashed through that narrow spot where the road just squeezes between the building of Ashbourne's lower trading room when, square in front of me, was Joe Bulgin sitting on his big two-wheeled cart. I jammed on the brakes and tried to duck to the left but only succeeded in putting the sidecar, with Marianne in it, under the big wheel. Joe was tossed off against the building when the horse and cart flipped neatly upside down.

The cycle leapt forward sideways and end for end. I preceded it by about 15 feet. There I was lying comfortably in the ditch against the fence when I noticed Marianne coming right at me through the air. I had time to hold out both my arms. She landed on them lightly and took off again, putting her face through the picket fence. It seemed to take hours for the accident to finish. Finally, I stood up. The cart was ruined. The wheels were off, a broken shaft was between the horse's legs, the harness was in pieces. The horse seemed to take it well. Bulgin was limping around giving me hell. The wheels on the cycle were still spinning. An ominous black puddle, that I at first feared was some innocent bystander's blood, turned out to be only ergot from my call bag. I apologized and offered to pay. Marianne had a split lip while I, a bruised knee. No great damage.

Thanksgiving, '37. We will soon have to abandon the motorcycle and take to the horse or dogs. That gives me great advantage over our Resident, from the old south and full of it but paralyzed on a horse. The horse is nice enough although he does playfully bite you and kick out with both hind feet when you go near his stern. I talk him up as a bad animal and that saves him for the director and me.

I propped myself up against the stove and got ready for a long discussion of sealing and fishing when there was a whoop upstairs and I got there just in time to catch a female child. The mother waved the chloroform away scornfully and went right to it. Even in the short time I was in the room my feet became numb from the cold. You couldn't expose the patient at all. All you could do is practically get into bed and pull up the covers over both of us. I'm sure I looked more like an old fashioned photographer than an obstetrician.

The northern slob came in this morning on the tail of a northern gale. That is not what or whom you suppose. It is made up of the ice pans formed along the Labrador and brought down by the arctic current. There is no travel until it gets here because our own bay is too rough to freeze. Though this northern ice is solid enough to travel on, it has the disconcerting habit of suddenly making up its mind to go someplace else. If you happen to be on it at the time you may find yourself down off the Grand Banks waving your undershirt at passing steamers. Some men have lived as long as forty days in this predicament. Grenfel himself made a famous voyage on an ice pan. He killed his dogs and wrapped himself in their warm skins and made a staff for a signal flag from their thighbones. He later erected a bronze monument to the memory of the unwilling but effective help of the canines. Tyson and seventeen others spent from October 15 to April 1 (1871) floating on an ice pan and covered almost 1,300 miles before being picked up—without a fatality. Their party even increased by the birth of an Eskimo baby.

I am afraid I am getting old. For the past two days I have had lumbago—a fine ailment for one in his prime. It is a visitation of the Lord. I was coming back from a little trip across the tickle. It had been wet and cold and as I drove the motorcycle along I was right chilly and I says to myself, "It is silly for people to blame so much on chills and drafts." Here I am in the worst possible conditions of meteorologic environment but a quick warm tub will fix everything. Not an hour later I was bending over the bed of a patient doing a dressing when I almost scared him into acidosis by clapping my hand to my back and giving an involuntary but substantial yell. It is quite well now and I have taken to woollies.

For a call to Moreton's Harbor I dressed warmly and I counted four pairs of socks showing above my boots—brown, black, pink, gray and white in that order. Some socks have two colors, so the count is correct. It was dark coming back and they were unable to land me where they had found me, so I had to walk a couple of miles to the cycle. If it hadn't turned to a wet cold rain in the meanwhile, the cycle would have spent the winter at that spot. As it was, I skidded home just in time to join the Thanksgiving festivities. You would never have suspected hinterlandedness if you could have seen our board—caviar, martinis, anchovies with capers, mushroom soup, roast goose, and fine imported cheddar. Of course, it's no trick to have imported things here. If you depended on home products, life would consist of rope, pulpwood, turnips, and potatoes with codfish.

Last night at 4:30 a woman came in to have a baby. We had just (at midnight) finished an emergency appendix. There wasn't a bed in the whole place for the obstetrical patient so we had to put her out in the main hall. Just as she started to kick up a fuss my tetanus patient started to have convulsions. A young woman who came in a few days ago with a headache which proved to be tuberculous meningitis was excited by the confusion and started her act of crawling down the hall on hands and knees. Our insane patient, hitherto reasonably quiet, also appeared on the scene and required a bit of catching. The babe came at 5:30: push, push,

push, snip, squawk, a nice little boy. Everybody got a portion of morphine and quiet reigned once more.

November 28, '37. Had to go to Change Island on one of those O.H.M.S. mercy calls and we had a little ten-ton cruiser. Every wave came aboard. We huddled in the cabin where the roof and walls leaked so much that the fire was put out. There was not a spot where water didn't spurt at you every time a wave hit us. The skipper said it was the worst he had seen in 35 years and "I was on the *Hetty* when she went ashore in Bonne Bay in the worst storm ever. She was sister ship to our *Clyde*, 600 tons. She was water logged and making only 4 knots. 'Go below' says the Captain 'and tell the passengers to put on life belts'. 'Hell' says I. 'They'll never be able to swim in this—I'd rather tell them to put anchors around their necks!'—She was driving dead for a reef and in anticipation I could feel the grinding crash as her spars go over and her back breaks on the rocks. But, no, a huge seas lifts us clear of the reef and over it, depositing us on the soft sand with hardly a stir that would knock a glass off the saloon table. There wasn't even a sprained ankle on board and to this day she sits intact 20 yards above the water's edge. A wave hasn't touched her till this day and that was 25 years ago."

December 3, '37. It is impossible to remember back three days, not that things are so routine, but there is a tone and consistency to this place that wavers very little. Saturday I do remember. Waddell and I were sitting around with nothing to do. I set about putting up my thermometer. I was out only a minute in the lovely, crisp, spring-like sunshine when he appropriated, without conference, a call to Pike's Arm. I brooded around a while until dinner with Marianne at the Cottage, did a couple of pneumothoraces, and worked in the OPD until Waddell's return. I was much relieved to find he had gone to see Ives' patient with the "ice-water" kidneys. I noted that the carts now give us a very wide berth when they see us coming on the cycle. My reputation as a cyclist is permanently ruined. I offered to drive Waddell over to Little Harbor, but he refused.

December 4, '37. Supposed to go birding with Saul White, but it blew a gale and we didn't make it. A quiet day. I looked forward to playing poker in the evening but lost $4.00. Joe Bulgin was up for a long, fruitless dissertation on our accident. He hasn't counted the damage yet.

December 5, '37. Dull rainy day. Got out the cycle to visit Bobby Cooper. His blood pressure is suddenly down to 185 which is not good either. I make free visits to the woman boarding with him just to keep her pacified. She is a financial help to the Coopers and I like them. Went for a brief walk in the rain. It was lovely up on the hill. You could lean 20 degrees against the wind. I ran around on the heath and got wet and sweaty. I could see Old Harry Rock breaking in the sea off Burnt Island. I even sat down in the rain. It made me feel clear. I tried to walk along the dam but the wind was too strong. Dinner was too good at the Cottage and John started to play chess with me, but quit suddenly. It is extremely unsatisfactory to quit a chess game. I felt punk about it because it may be that I'm too slow for him. I sat around and read about the New York elections until Suzy gave us tea in our room. I just read *Famine.* It's a wonderful book. Twillingate is in some ways like Ireland. No landlords here though, because there's no money to pay them. The people are in about the same fix. A famine would be hard on this place.

December 9, '37. I don't know where all the time has gone. Meanwhile things have shaped up pretty well. It is apparent that I will never become a great surgeon. I can tackle any tooth, I can take out any tonsil, and open almost any abscess. I feel pretty confident opening a belly. If I were left alone, I could blunder through almost anything. I've been reading quite a lot, but nothing of note, mostly detective stories.

I've made two lovely trips—one to Gander Bay with Skipper Frank Roberts. I was marooned two days at the Herring Neck Hotel where we tied up beside the *Bessie Marie.* Joe White runs the hotel just so he'll have a place to live. Here I got a bed that was too short, with two cotton mattresses on it, and six layers of thin, heavy cotton blankets. Unfortunately, the only other marooned client was an insurance salesman. He worked on me for two days and when my guard was down, I bought $2,000.00 worth of unwanted insurance.

We punched on to Horwood because it was too stormy to get into Gander Bay around Dog Bay Point. We took on so much water that though I was sitting on a table in the cabin with a raincoat and hat on, my feet got wet. It really did toss and it's a mystery to me what keeps the damn thing afloat. Finally on to Gander Bay, though at Horwood I diagnosed a placenta praevia by her history. It was a normal pregnancy, except for two spells of daylong bleeding, a fortnight separated. My patient in Gander needed intravenous glucose. It was quite a job to give it in a home with my equipment.

Went for a long walk to Brown's Cove where the aged, pink, bright Mrs. Roland lives, aunt of our office manager, Wyn. She has a very elegant house for these parts. It has graceful arched ceilings and is set among lovely trees. I collected two bucks and at the behest of the schoolteacher went on to see an ex-hospital patient, reputed to be covered with sores. He complained that while he was in the hospital, someone had stolen his stove, bedding, and everything else. He wasn't so bad, only absolutely filthy and grousing about nobody being able to take care of him. I asked where a bed could be found for the night and was directed to what I supposed was a boarding house. I stalked in and sat down and demanded food. The widow Harris, still wearing black after seven years, bustled around to feed me. I asked for a light in the living room and unsuccessfully tried to play the organ. After the night in a good bed I was embarrassed to find that I was a guest and there was no charge. The charge at Herring Neck had been thirty-five cents.

Skipper Frank always gets you up at five in the morning. It was a beautiful sail home on a clear blue day. I missed two easy turr shots and Skipper Frank, a fine mariner with a strong, clean face said of me, "No good with gun."

Yesterday I went to Bridgeport, leaving in the late afternoon thinking that if I saw only one patient, I could get back for tenderloin tea. We hit New World Island just as the sky cleared for the sunset. The road wound in and around the sharp rocks, passing by the reflecting ponds with their sheer, abrupt, pine-clad banks. The sky was full of deep pink wisps and there was a roseate unreal glow with the color intensity of an overdone Kodachrome.

The woman had a burning in her head and was angry when I called it a headache. The husband sat around belching to get my attention. It seems that he had had typhoid four months ago and was still on the diet and the rest of the regimen, because no one had told him he was well. I told both of them to get up, though the woman had a great big kidney. They both wanted me to see their mother though they hid the fact as long as possible that she was related. She was 75 and in bed believing in tumors and taken care of by a woman just a little younger with only one leg. I got her up too and refused tea in my hurry to get back. The *S.S. Marine Trader* was at Osmond's wharf loading fish. The big freighter completely filled Moreton's Harbor. My heart yearned to drop everything and make a trip, which makes me think that I'll never amount to much. I slept on the hard board seat on the way back, arriving just in time for Suzy to salvage me the last bit of tenderloin. I am trying not to eat at the Cottage because I'm up to 182 pounds and want to stay lean. Wrote letters till late. Someone is taking the mail into Lewisporte today because the *Clyde* can't make it for more than a week.

Today was a fair day. I worked in the OPD and almost made a call to New Bay but Doccy Wood grabbed it. Since he is a local doctor, his arrangement with the hospital allows him to keep the money he collects on these long trips. The patient is crazy and has a bad heart. Nobody can help her and certainly he can't bring her back to the hospital. Wood is a good doctor. I like to listen to his long tales about his feud with Doctor LeDrew. It reached its height about the time the hospital was started. Wood wanted the hospital and LeDrew thought they didn't need one. Libel, lawsuits, assault, and general perfidy are all mixed up in it.

Waddell and I went shopping, he on the cycle, I on the horse. I must ride it more often. It's a good horse and we both need exercise. I got some long winter underwear and some old English Christmas cards that have been lying around in the dust for 40 years. I'll have to make envelopes out of wrapping paper. It was warm out and we are all wishing like hell for snow. They've had it everywhere else in the world but here. I got 500 Benson and Hedges cigarettes that dad had sent from Canada, but we can't fool the customs that way. I still had to pay $5.00 duty.

I must be a nut. Waddell is turning out to be a very fine guy. I am very fond of him and take back any criticism I have made. He is generous and magnanimous. I am glad to live with him if I have to live with somebody.

December 10, '37. Up at 3:00 A.M. to see Mrs. Stuckles who had burst her waters. She is a large placid woman who has had many children. Syd Boyd, Skipper Frank's cabin boy, came for me and I took him over in the cycle, with his bicycle around his neck like a tuba. She was not dilated at all so I returned to have a cup of tea with Kelly on the ward. A call came in at 6:30 for me to see Bobby Cooper. I went as soon as I could but not until they had called again. He was in terrible shape, smelt uremic. I gave him strophanthin and morphia. I returned to have a hard time in the OPD. Dole neurotic after dole neurotic. Every Gillard in the world was there. One had a vague assortment of unrelated pains. I gave him aspirin and yeast to get rid of him and he counters with, "How about a dole certificate?" I demurred. He says, "There must be something wrong or you wouldn't

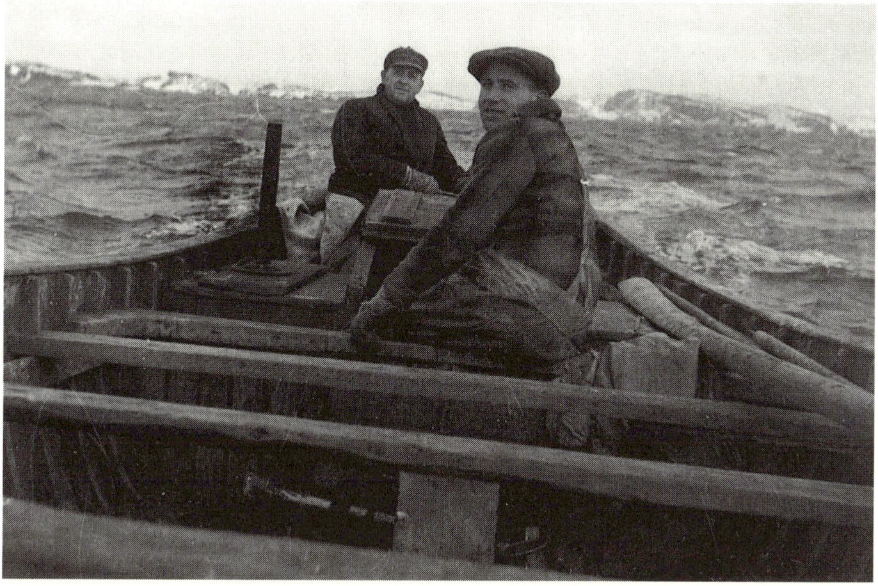

The Doctor's escort for a house call. Author's photograph.

have given me the medicine." I admitted defeat and came across with a certificate. Just before dinner, Burt came in a great stew for a doctor to see his father at once. He hadn't been "satisfied to come to the hospital." He'd been clipped under the chin by one end of a board when the other end engaged a power saw. I gulped some dinner and got dressed to ride in an open boat. We sat on the floor in the rain all the way to Fairbank. There I found an old man with blood in his ear. I sewed up the chin, while the son was all for knocking me down because I hurt his father. He'll be all right in five days if he doesn't get meningitis. I charged $10.00 and they made it seem like the last money in the world. There were many able-bodied men around and they own a busy sawmill. Then the bombshell was delivered. They wouldn't bring us any nearer home than Gillard's Cove. This time I slept on a bag of wet sawdust. I walked with heavy suitcase and blanket through deepening mud for three miles. I was flagged down once to see a woman with a pulmonary hemorrhage. Then home and dinner after a grand drink, tub, shave, and reading of the mail. I was waked at three to go see Mrs. Stuckles. I fell asleep, was roused again and the baby was born when I got there. I was covered with chagrin. The woman said, "Be you married?" I shook my head no. "If you were, I'd say you hated to leave she."

December 11, '37. Early to Bobby Cooper's and he is better, wanting to know if he will get well. Back to send the 40 year-old Christmas cards, the ones with the legend "Keep your pecker up."

December 12, '37. This was a nice quiet Sunday. It rained and was wicked outside. A late breakfast and a big dinner at the Cottage. I lost two games of chess to John. I get worse and worse. I always let him into my backfield. The afternoon sped by like nothing. After rounds I went down to check on Bobby Cooper and came back for two drinks in the apartment with Waddell. We dropped over to Edith's room for a cup of tea with the others. The rum flowed freely and what with one thing and another we polished off two and a half bottles. We all of us amused ourselves by zipping and unzipping the back of Edith's dress. Then things got a little rough. Betty broke the lacing on the back of my dungarees and I tried to jump out of the window. John grabbed me by the belt and Edith, to get me free, snatched a knife and cut the belt along with the top of my pants. Thereupon, I fell out of the window. She also cut John's hand. I came back in and put some orange marmalade in Joyce's shoe because she pulled my hair harder than it was ever pulled before.

I suddenly felt that I had to go to bed and retreated about 8 P.M. I put my finger down my throat and fortunately had imbibed enough that I fell right to sleep and was spared the tossing of my bed. I was awakened when my friends climbed in through the window to see if I was still alive. Waddell shooed them out and gave me moral support for another application of the finger. Then suddenly it was morning, though still dark.

December 13, '37. Right after breakfast, a girl came in demanding to be given ether so 12 teeth could be taken out. I looked and she had only three bad ones but "Pa and they" had said she might as well have them all out because they all ached. She wouldn't even have the three out unless she had ether. I refused to use a general anesthetic for such a minor performance. She then said she'd wait for Dr. Wood but he upheld me. After endless harangue and much weeping, the three offending molars were extracted with benefit of deadening medicine. More teeth in the afternoon out of a young man with badly advanced arthritis. I'm afraid he's going to be a hopeless cripple. Mrs. Torraville says he is a hard-working worthy person with three small boys. Tea was served at the hospital because the water pipes have burst at the Cottage. Afterwards I pressed my pants for

I'm off to Fogo the first thing in the morning.

Japan has bombed one of our ships. I wonder if we are going to war. This may or may not be a peaceful spot—with a big airport nearby. English airships coming to America would have to come by here.

I took a big bottle from the closet, put creosote cough medicine in, and then saw it was labeled poison. I'm afraid there might be some left in it, though it was supposed to be clean. I'll take it anyway and see what happens. I can't waste all that creosote.

December 16, '37. Up long before dawn to a breakfast on the ward prepared by the admirable Kelly, who is a good nurse. Syd took me down to the *Bonnie Nell* on a very cold morning with the sun nowhere in sight. There was a good fire going in the cabin and we were off at once to Burnt Island Tickle. I succumbed at once to that tendency I have to fall asleep the minute I get on a boat. Enough of the water we were taking aboard froze so that Skipper Frank's craft didn't leak from the top as it usually does. I lay on the starboard bunk and when I sleep in this bunk I suffer from a disease known (to me) as Bilge Souffle or Rough Water Halitosis. (Souffle is not that delicious egg dish, soufflé, but the medical term, soo-ful, for the sound of moving liquids). I don't have the disease (at least no one has said so)—the boat has it. Bilge water seems to collect in all boats of any size. I have heard it is good for a boat—I don't know. It is more or less contained between the watertight outer skin and the inner sheathing or covering of the ribs. This inner sheathing is not tight. In some boats the bilge is "sweet." In some, it is not. Our bilge has taken on an abandoned sort of bouquet. When the boat rocks, the bilge surges up in its space and forces air out through a crack in the wall near my pillow. The said air whistles softly with the haunting nostalgic sound of the call of water fowl winging sadly south on a darkening autumn twilight. It stinks though and I don't know what to do about it. If I sleep with my head at the other end of the bunk, my face is in a dark hole separated from the engine by only a few inches and a match-board partition.

It was rough off Port Albert and the skipper kept turning her head into the lop to stop the roll. We went right through the main tickle at Change Island to Seal Cove and through the tickle there, under the bridge, into Fogo Harbor. At Mrs. Furze's wharf, the bank manager met me and took me at once to the widow Furze's house, where I met my breezy hostess, who sputters and laughs heartily at simple statements until she gets quite out of breath. She was heartbroken that the house was so cold and it certainly was.

It's a well-built house with bare beams and ceiling and the longitudinal sheathing is paneled lengthwise in a very attractive way. She got me out a very nice cup of tea while I made some toast by the Franklin stove.

The lackadaisical Mrs. Waterman, who threw hysterics for Dr. Waddell, served me sullenly but cheered up enough during the day to tell me all about her aches and pains. I sat for a minute until a man came to take me a mile or so to the Catholic settlement where his wife had post-measles pneumonia. Next door was more of the same in a child, except that it was complicated by tuberculosis. This house was full of children. They just sat in the messy kitchen eating bread and tea every few hours. I prescribed and climbed the lovely hill behind the house where a cascade comes roaring off the plateau. There was a nice col on top, a lake, and a few sharp peaks farther off. I climbed the highest for a magnificent view of the sea. Then I walked back, speaking to all I saw.

Mr. Fitzgerald called me in for his son and invited me to spend the winter. They all thought I could collect at least $5,000.00 a year. Old Dr. Mackenzie used to go a week with his shoes untied. I sat until 11:00, after a cold supper, when I decided to see Payne. He is a widow's son, struggling to support the family. He is reported unable to lift an arm and I was afraid it might be polio. I walked clear around the harbor to their cottage. I met a boy at the tickle bridge and sent him in ahead to tell them I wouldn't charge. I found a very nervous frightened young boy just getting over the acute stage of rheumatic fever. I persuaded him to come to the hospital. It snowed all the way back and the *S.S. Segona*, anchored in Seal Harbor for the night, was very lovely with its blaze of distant lights. Mrs. Furze had provided a very comfortable featherbed and was up, to speed us in the morning. It was an uneventful trip on a clear cool crisp day, except just as we rounded the Rock at French Head the motor started to give out because of water in the gas. There was a heavy sea on and we would have been lost with all hands if they hadn't been able to nurse it along. That night we tried to ski a bit but succeeded only in getting hot. I tried to let the dogs pull me. Got left in the OPD Friday, and the *Clyde* came in with a full cargo of patients. I never saw more in less time.

December 18, '37. A walk to the stores with Marianne this morning. It's easier to get into heaven than to get waited on in one of those general stores. Went to the customs house to get the Smithfield ham that father had sent from Virginia. To see me chat with my old pal, Arch Peyton, the customs collector, you'd never guess how much we hate each other. The walk back in the snow was strenuous. While working in the OPD a call came for Waddell to go to Back Harbor but I took it because I can ride Jack. It was further than I thought and the skittish Jack shied at everything. Every dog team with bells scared him. As we came up over the cliff someone fired a gun at a turr right under us. Jack got into deep snow and floundered around like a jackrabbit.

After seeing two light cases of white mouth I came out to find Jack had slipped his halter and was disappearing up over the hill on his way home. I was afraid they would worry at the hospital when the horse came back without me. I cut down behind the customs house to Lynfield's store and my heart failed me when I saw how public the phone was. There were at least 50 Christmas shoppers mulling around the store. I couldn't raise the hospital anyway. But I did find that Lynfield's son had captured the horse and tied him up with fish line—a brave, bold act. [Ed: That son was to die on D-Day] I replaced the bridle on Jack and was home without more ado. Waddell had left at 5:00 for a mild case of chickenpox and got back at 11:00. We had started to play poker. I'm happy to say that John lost three bucks. Mr. Chaulker would have lost $15.00 if we didn't have a $3.00 limit to losses.

December 19, '37. Nice lazy day. Planned to go out but didn't make it. I did have a tub, put on my jodhpurs which I wear all the time. Dinner of fried chicken was a failure. Tea was late. I knew the boys wanted to get drunk but I felt kind of *triste* and didn't join them.

About 11:00 at night John talked me into buying a pair of sealskin boots that don't fit me. Then he suggested skiing and we all bundled up and went out into a strange night. It was bright but there was no moon. We sped over the frozen ponds and across the crusted snow, over the tops of the low trees, for an hour or more. It was like an arctic night, enough light to see all the hills but eerie and unreal. You could see your companions ahead of you and then they would suddenly disappear. Back after 12:00 for some canned oysters and then to bed.

December 20, '37. Up to help John do a laparotomy, help Waddell do a hernia, and do a hydrocele myself. I hate Waddell when he helps me operate. I thought I was going skiing but a call came in and someone had to stay so Waddell went. I was surprised today by five pieces of mail. The

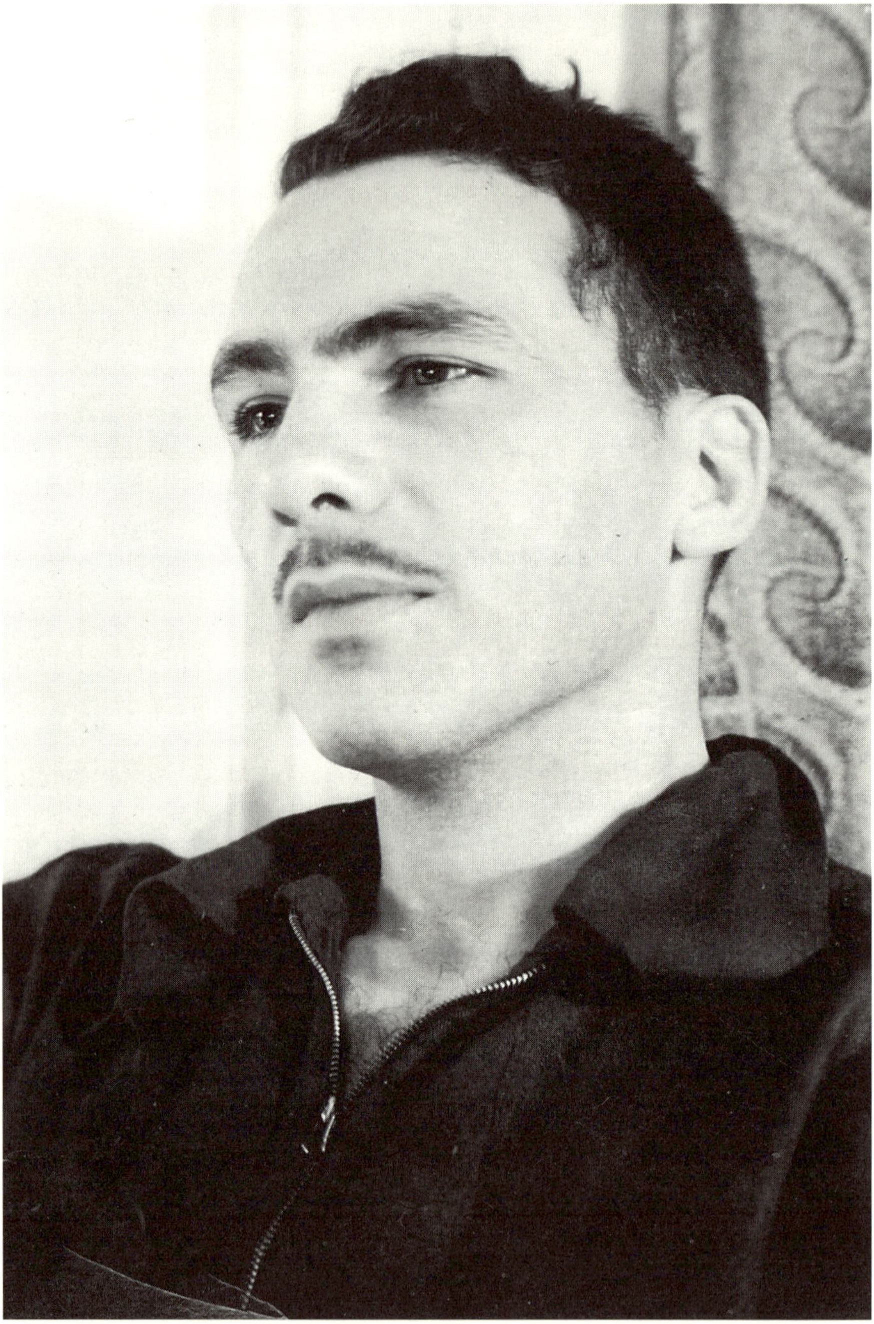

"C'est Moi." R.S.E. with 17 ounces to go.

church letter said in part, "Albert Dekker (Albert Ecke) first member of the cradle roll, can be seen at the local movies, etc. His brother Robert is the Head Surgeon (sic) at the Notre Dame Bay Memorial Hospital in Twillingate, Newfoundland, a hospital founded by Johns Hopkins." I'm going over to Edith's now for a cup of coffee, but I'm determined to eat nothing having lost two pounds and want to lose five more. I've decided that my stock in trade is looking romantic and you can't do that and be fat. Besides I like the lighter feeling on your feet. I'd give anything to get to Alaska or above the Arctic Circle. I hereby make my declaration of that intention. I had a nice long talk with Joyce this morning. She and I see eye to eye on lots of subjects. She is a fine girl even if she does have depressions, when she stays in the bathtub a couple of days at a time.

December 21, '37. A good day, though the shortest in the year. The sun set around 3:30 P.M. I swore last night that I would do all the surgery today and it worked. I said to Waddell, "Isn't it about time I was due for an appendix?" I did the appendix and Waddell was very quiet. There was only one slip. Just after putting in the purse string, there appeared a string of some dark stuff on the needle. I inspected all the stitches and none seemed too deep. At any rate, we closed it and took out her tonsils, which were a lot of trouble, being small, deep, and rotten. I sutured both sides. Her sister's tonsils, the next case, were just as bad. Then I did a cystoscopy and catheterized the left ureter. The kidney, by three pictures, is bifid in the upper pole.

After dinner we went to the north side of the harbor, I behind the horse slide (a kind of sled) on a pair of skis. It was cold and darkish. Stanley drove and went down the hill so fast that he overturned the slide and threw Waddell out on the beach. Back for rounds and a tub. This is funny water we have here. It's brown and whole leaves open out on the bottom of the tub—it smells like a Florida swamp. John had suddenly to go to Moreton's Harbor. The wind is blowing hard, the bight is rough, and it's cold. And yet he has to go over to see an old crock who can't be helped.

December 22, '37. Wednesday, a swell day. It blew a living gale the whole time. Snowed a little and was cold even by local standards. The afternoon, John and I got out the skis and went for a grand run over to the Little Harbor Road. I took the two dogs half the way. It was good sport behind them; they don't really pull the whole time but if you keep your feet moving, they increase your speed a good 30 percent. They're remarkably docile and it is hard to believe that Sport, the 90-pound oaf, was condemned for being a "man-eater." He's as playful as a cub and as ungainly as an elephant.

Tea was an uproar. John and Waddell, after an aperitif, decided to put up the French doors between the living room and the sunporch. Tea was all ready but they insisted. The doors were stowed in the cellar. They had to take out the icebox to get them up the kitchen stairs. Suzy bet them $5.00 they couldn't do it. It took them a long time and a lot of hammering and maneuvering. Joyce, Betty, and I sat around the fire and griped and fumed. We got out some rum to console ourselves while tea was spoiling. Joyce decided that I was depressed and poured about six stiff ones into me. I got scared and quit.

When the doors were finally up, Betty had had enough rum to be her most amusing. Tea was a grand success despite the delay and I played chess with John afterwards. I should have won but rum is not good for chess.

December 23, '37. Waddell and I got Christmas presents together for the girls. A rolling pin for Betty, a girdle for Mildred, a rocking chair for Agnes, a damper for Marianne, and a dried-up ovarian cyst for Joyce. Waddell went off to Bridgeport for a girl on whom "the measles failed to come out." The afternoon was dull and now at 5:00 I am writing this while John skis.

December 24, '37. Christmas Eve. A bad day from beginning to end—not really bad but the kind of significant badness easily overlooked if you're not sensitive to it. I had sat up and read so late the night before that it was nine this morning when John invited "You bastards" to get up. After a hasty breakfast I started to help him on the abdominal obstruction that Doccy Wood had admitted the day before. He was a kind of screwball with 52 congenital anomalies, among them a prolapsed umbilicus. It developed that he had a patent Meckel's diverticulum with diverticulitis and a volvulus around the adhesions. It was obviously hopeless and he died during the afternoon. I was all thumbs and felt extremely stupid. Waddell scrubbed then and kind of took over my place when I dropped out to give an intravenous. It left me exceedingly depressed and I failed to recover all day. We sat around and wrapped presents and drank and drank.

Martin our mechanic was funny. He came in with his cousin who is the engineer on the *Bessie Marie* and is going to bring Waddell some rum from St. John's. On the last trip of the *Bessie Marie* he was locked in the engine room for three days. The only way to get out of the engine room is up to the deck and it was so rough they were afraid to open the hatch. They had a drink or two and the cousins started to tell us about some of his trips. He was in Skipper Frank's crew when Skipper Frank owned the *Grace.* The pilot ran it aground in the Strait of Belle Isle. They managed to get off in a boat and were picked up by the steamship *Hetty,* sister ship to the *Clyde.* Soon they were in trouble with ice. The flag halyards were three inches thick with it. A bull in a pen on deck was above his belly in solid ice. They were so sure to founder during the night with her engines almost gone that the captain chose to beach the ship as the best hope for survival. She skidded on the bottom a quarter of a mile off shore and drove on in to within 150 feet of the beach. A miracle had guided her between the reefs on the only course that would save her. If she had hung up on the bar, she would have slipped off into deep water and all would have been lost. They tied a small line to a life preserver and the story has it that a Newfoundland dog swam out from shore to retrieve it. A breeches buoy was rigged and all seventy-five souls got ashore, including a six-month baby done up in a mailbag which went under water three times as the ship slacked on the line. All of them got into two shacks on shore. A trader on board with some fur had run down into the steerage begging for a preserver. They were rotten and the straps came off. The mate said to him, "You might just as well tie that piece of iron around you." The women were begging and screaming for help, but the cry had gone up "every man for himself"—this excuses you from helping anyone. The *Hetty* had been lifted over the bar and she is still there [Ed: she is *still* still there in Bonne Bay, the rusted, rotted feature of a provincial park].

Martin's cousin was later wrecked off Halifax by an eager beaver of a captain who, in order to get the title of captain, was working for less money than his engineer.

Martin came back and got very confidential and passed out. A Benzedrine by this time was making me feel better so we went up to the Christmas Eve party in good spirits. They were sitting in a dull circle. I sliced father's ham and it was good. At this point it was announced that Mrs. Ledrue was in labor. I didn't drink anymore and came down to watch her. Waddell gave her some paraldehyde and by 1:30 she was ready to deliver. I slipped on the forceps and it was nothing to lift the head over the perineum. The patient became inert suddenly though she had been given only very little sedative. The baby was very slow to deliver. The placenta came quickly and she literally poured. I yelled for Waddell and a uterine pack. The bleeding tapered off, but I thought I was going to lose her. It disturbed me so much I couldn't sleep. Suzy played the accordion at great length.

December 25, '37. Christmas. Not much of a day. Didn't feel very cheery at my late breakfast. Sat around and had a small drink, but nothing to speak of until noontime. Then I had a tub and we went up to dinner. We had a few martinis and were cheerful enough by the time dinner was over. Wine, goose, grapefruit, and pie with all the trimmings. Edith was very amusing and even threw a glass of water at me.

Immediately after dinner John and Betty went to the Tilt. I had a bit of a nap in the afternoon and a drop of tea at Edith's. We finally rounded up Pat Cody, who was feeling his ulcer and then arranged a game of poker. I lost the limit—$3.00. To bed late and I couldn't sleep.

December 26, '37. It blew like fury and snowed all day. I went down on the Arm to see Bobby Cooper again, although there was nothing new wrong. He was up. The walk was grand. Many times we could hardly stand up and the drifts were already four feet in many places, but in spite of great amounts of snow, there are still bare spots on the road. I wore my new skin boots with four pairs of socks. They are only fair. I will have to put something in them to make them keep the heel. Back to take rounds and another nap and tea at Edith's. A long listen to BBC concert. I write this and go to bed. Goodnight. I may add that on the way home, I saw the *Bessie Marie* tied up at her wharf and wondered if she were safe, but in all things the local people are more cautious than I am and God knows I am afraid of this water.

December 27, '37. At 5 A.M. Kelly woke me saying that Mrs. Walter Cooper was in labor and wanted me. We hadn't counted on her at all but had been dreading three others. I rose with some difficulty and remembering my lateness in getting to Mrs. Stuckles, hurried out into the snow and across the garden fences a hundred yards to find her only starting. I struggled back and had some more breakfast and they came for me again at 7:00. Meanwhile, word came that Mrs. Burton was in labor, way down on the Arm. I had been following her for a urinary tract infection. John was at the Tilt and Dr. Wood couldn't get down until 9:00, so I was faced with two widely separated patients. I got the orderly to bring a stretcher and a pile of blankets and we went across the gardens again to see Mrs. Cooper. I begged her to let us wrap her up and carry her to the hospital so that I would be free to go to the other case. I said she could have her baby in the operating room and stay in the hospital for 10 days and if she would do this favor it wouldn't cost her a cent. Some close relative, a bewhiskered old derelict, rocking by the fire, refused for her rather emphatically. He said he wouldn't ask a dog to go out in weather like this.

She wasn't making any progress anyway so I went to have a look at the *Bessie Marie.* She had torn her mooring and swung out into deep water just off Ashbourne's pier. It was too rough to get to her. Then she parted her small anchor and crashed on to the Point, breaking her shaft and rudder. They put out another anchor and swung her off to the channel between the Point and the breakwater. She was riding pretty free there but hitting her bottom in the deep troughs. Then they slipped her anchor and she beached right behind Burt Pardy's store.

I hated to make Mrs. Burton wait for me, but I had to get rid of the Cooper case first. I was glad to see Doccy Wood come plowing through the snow at 9:00 to relieve me. I put the OB "fitout" into small bags, donned my snowshoes and beat my way for the Arm. It was pretty strong weather. You could hardly stand against the wind and the snow was eight feet deep in places. The anxious father met me half way and guided me through the winter path. By the Academy the road was really not passable, but down over Dalley's hill the wind had swept it clean. I mushed on and got to the house where the sickly woman was in labor already. I did a rectal and felt a hard thing that seemed to be a foot but I didn't believe she had a breech.

I waited an hour and it was still the same. There had been no descent at all, so I boiled a glove and broke the membranes with a Kelly clamp. I was rewarded by a gush of water and a foot sticking into the breeze. I forwent the impulse to grab a hold and pull, and descended to the kitchen, leaving the able Mrs. Pilley in charge. I toasted some delicious dole raisin bread and had some tea. The stove was working in reverse. This particular wind always came straight down the chimney, they explained.

Upstairs again, the rupture had put her into more active labor. Both feet were wiggling at me. I put her to sleep and tugged on them and pulled all but the crown out with no trouble. I had the babe in Moreceau's position, but it was struggling to breathe. I got a little startled and really put some traction on and out he came with only a tiny tear. The was mother in good shape. I fixed up the baby and told them my first name so they'd know what to call it, but its feet were still purple when I left.

On my way home the weather was no better. I got lost even, and wandered way down by the shore. It really was dramatic weather. I finally got to the bottom of the hospital lane and in the lee of a shop stood watching the *Bessie Marie.* Laboring bravely in the deeper water, she rose proudly enough with each swell, but her sides were scarred. A tatter fluttered from her mizzen and withal she looked so brave and staunch that I cried a few real tears for her. She had six men aboard pumping. Home to a tub, shave, and rounds, and a superior steak tea. Poker was bad—I lost and hated every minute of it. Late to bed and slept poorly.

December 28, '37. Still blowing but much calmer. They got the *Bessie Marie* further off to a collar and she seems safer. I did nothing all day but read and eat. I went to bed right after tea but was disturbed by a party upstairs. I did get to sleep.

December 29, '37. The *Bessie Marie* has been hauled to the north side and is safe. I was glad to hear that the Terra Nova Insurance Company pays for part of the damage. Most maritime insurance companies insist on a total wreck. I helped Waddell close up Mrs. Pride, pulled two sets of teeth, and put some air in a chest—i.e. pneumothorax.

January 2, '38. Little to record. Thursday I took the Santa Claus outfit back to the Minty's. Up over the top of the hill the northwest wind really had power behind it. It blew steadily, as strong as the gusts that wrecked the *Bessie Marie.* At each step I was thrown off enough to expect to be hurled to the ground. The snow was so deep that I wound up by crawling on my hands and knees, even rolling to get over some of the drifts. They invited me back for New Year's dinner, which was pleasant enough. The meal was tremendous, but kind of staple. I sat around a bit and did all the talking. It's a very respectable house, with plumbing, and two very demure unmarried daughters who donated little to the gathering. The son is heavy of feature and speech. It got to be a drag. I played Ping-Pong for a while and made an adieu after a polite lapse of time.

In the morning I went to see Mrs. Hull, in bed this year with a bad heart. She was so symptomless except for induced belching that I ordered her up. It was such a glorious sunlit day that I went out in my intern suit without a coat. The mail Friday was gratifying—I got 42 Christmas cards, three telegrams, and three letters. The spirit at tea was like a fraternity just before a house party, as if everyone had been drinking or was on the verge of some happy event—hilarious, noisy, joyous. That's the way the rare mails affect you in this set-up. I went to tea at Wyn's with Marianne. It was fun as always, but there too you mustn't be disturbed by gaps in the conversation.

January 3, '38. A warm muggy day with a thick fog. The horn went all day—two blasts in five seconds then a fifty-five second wait.

Soon came a summons to the Arm to see a broken leg. They came for me with a large team of nine dogs. I rode strenuously behind on skis. We went fast enough. There was a curious lack of seriousness on the part of the driver who slammed the dogs around and even cut a bad one off, throwing him to one side. My patient had let a beached boat roll over on his foot. I put a good splint on his broken tibia and fibula. Twelve men hauled him home on a sled. I stopped at Mrs. Burton's to see my post-partem. Both she and little Robert are doing very nicely. A lot of children tagged along to watch the skiing. I returned across the inside of the island and the trail wasn't open. I can see why people get lost back here. I couldn't see a thing and if it were not for the foghorn going all the time would never have gotten back. As it was I was a little worn when I hit the United Church, quite a ways off the trail.

There was a dance at the Parish Hall and I had to go. The dance turned out to be fun but it was a hell of a walk around to the north side. The minister made some public crack about latecomers.

In the past week I've had two more deliveries. One was a "born on arrival" that would not have happened if Waddell had not butted in. He gave her paraldehyde and in half an hour she popped with a tear. I don't know if he is officious or trying to be helpful. He is kind enough and I'm very fond of him except when it comes to working with him. The other case was pretty good, except she was snug and I wanted to see how it would go without an episiotomy. I had to do some repairing.

January 5, '38. A good day so far. I read most of the *Times*, sorted my mail, and kind of got things into order. It's almost dinnertime and I am stiff from yesterday. In the afternoon I went out on skis with Marianne and had a lovely time. We slid up and down the hills and it was perfectly beautiful out. The clear spots on the pond were a delicate aquamarine in the white twilight setting. In the evening we got at our poker early and I won over $2.00.

January 6, '38. Another good day so far. I opened two hands, pulled five teeth, filled some prescriptions and made a list of my OB cases. Eight forceps, two breeches, two B.O.A.s, and one precipitous. This afternoon I'm going to ski down to the Arm to finish up some calls.

The skiing proved to be something. It was a dull day, starting to rain and freeze as soon as I got out. I followed the Arm trail with no difficulties. The Burton woman is okay. I came down the road and cut off along the shore to Bobby Cooper's. I found him about to die, hardly able to recognize me. "I'm afraid it's all up now, doctor," he said bitterly but with restraint. Fortunately he was too uremic to be entirely aware. From there I cut around the bottom to Bulgin's. He is in good spirits but still bleeding a little from his left lung. From there I crossed the fields through very deep drifts to Hawkins' house and then down to the bottom of Jenkins Cove through more deep snow, rain and darkness, to find the girl full of pain, though not much wrong. I came home in one spurt. It was dark as the devil and you couldn't tell whether you were going up hill or down until you felt the rise as you slid. It was quite exciting as I came down the cliff hill lickety split. I was dripping wet and worn to a frazzle. I must have covered ten or twelve miles.

I found some mail here, a card from Governor Barrows and my two polio papers that have appeared in the *Proceedings of the Society of Experimental Biology.* Then a tub, shave, and a drink, and down to Burt Pardy's where they tried to kill us by tea. I never saw such heaping plates of food. I hate to say I was damned uncomfortable afterward. Carrots, cabbage, turnips, potatoes, beets, parsnips, boiled meat, Yorkshire pudding, boiled pudding, Devonshire cream. We played cards for a while, interrupted by many a mummer. Until 12th night, the young people dress up and wear masks and go about visiting. They dance and sing at every house. Some were very good. The step dancing, a sort of gigue and tap dance was done by all and by many very well. These fishermen are light as a feather, even in rubber boots. Back late and to bed quite exhausted.

January 7, '38. A dull but beautiful morning. The sun was out, just below freezing. I oiled my boots with cod-liver oil, and am just about to go out for a few minutes before dinner. I've got to lose five pounds before I take the U.S. public health examination. I hear they will be given in Washington in the spring. They shouldn't be hard. After all, I passed them once before—eighth in a field of three hundred. Sometimes I think I shouldn't have refused their two offers of a commission. If it hadn't been so hot in Washington in June I would have joined up right away.

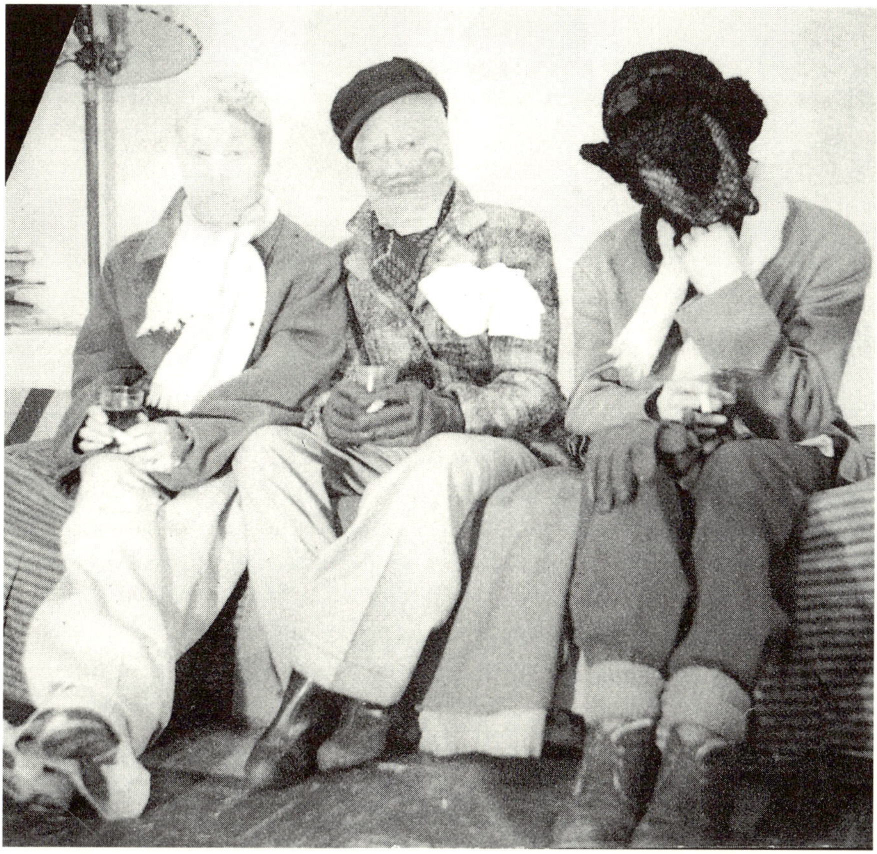

Unidentifiable mummers in stocking masks. Author's photograph.

January 8-12, '38. Not much of note. Lovely weather but cold in spots. I skied all the way to Little Harbor on a trip to Herring Neck. You can't dress light enough to be comfortable skiing and at the same time be warm enough not to be frozen stiff in an open boat. "I tried to get Dr. Olds and Dr. Wood, but I had to take this," said my host while he plied me with rum and his best. I skied back and was tired. I also had to go back to the Saunder's again for their "stun" daughter who has not changed a bit.

January 13, '38. Woke to a casual morn but a call came in for Tilt Cove. I tossed and lost and had to go but enjoyed it. Steve took me on his slide. He has a fine horse. They went like the wind the whole way. A boat waited at Purcell's Harbor and I was cold indeed. There were lots of seal about. At the house I found an old man vomiting and a nervous lad with pleurisy. The uncle talked a blue streak and was excellent though garrulous company. Back in the boat I borrowed a mat to sit on and a coat and blanket and was warm. On the sled we came along just at sunset. It was lovely to spin along behind a spanking horse. We took the winter trail. The horse went up to his belly once to let another pass. They're smart and won't leave the trail. By Minty's the slide turned over. I went out on my shoulder and was dragged along.

January 14, '38. I took out a tonsil and a tooth. It was a good job. Wheaton has syphilis, chancroid, and gonorrhea—just what the other contact with the same gal has. We will have to give him a job in the hospital to make sure he gets his treatments. In the afternoon I went out alone for a bit of skiing. I found myself on the top of the hill over the harbor just at sunset. It was superb: the pale pastel blue of the water, the hard sharp edge of north side cliffs, the incipient twilight in the east, the cold brilliant moon and New Bay Head and Cape St. John as clear as Western Head. It was an experience. With some vague sadness and unrest I came down slowly to tea. I'm starting a semi-starvation program today: Not a bite between meals—no seconds—no bread and butter—no milk.

January 18, '38. How have I allowed a week to go by? Is there anything of note? I must confess the days have taken on a certain oneness. They are gorgeous days meteorologically speaking—full cold ones with lusty winds. Ice forms across the harbor to be broken by the sea, to form again. It gains a little each time and today it looks as if it might at last make a bridge to the North Side and really seal us up for the winter. The sun sets a great orange or cerise ball, huge and glorious into the bight.

Saturday I skied with Marianne over to the Tilt. The Olds had gone on Friday. I did not know the way, but by good fortune came on John's trail made last night in the dark. Though circuitous, it made for the Tilt. We saw mute tracings of falls and slides. It was a grand day and we were tired. Poor Marianne's skis came off continually and she was provoked. I was disappointed in the Tilt itself. It's cut up into three rooms when you might get one good one out of it. The fireplace smokes. The Olds had made no effort to supervise its building and resented my criticism. I do not often offer criticism but I sometimes feel that I let too much slip by without comment. However when I try to take the bull by the horns and be an individual, I always offend someone in the doing.

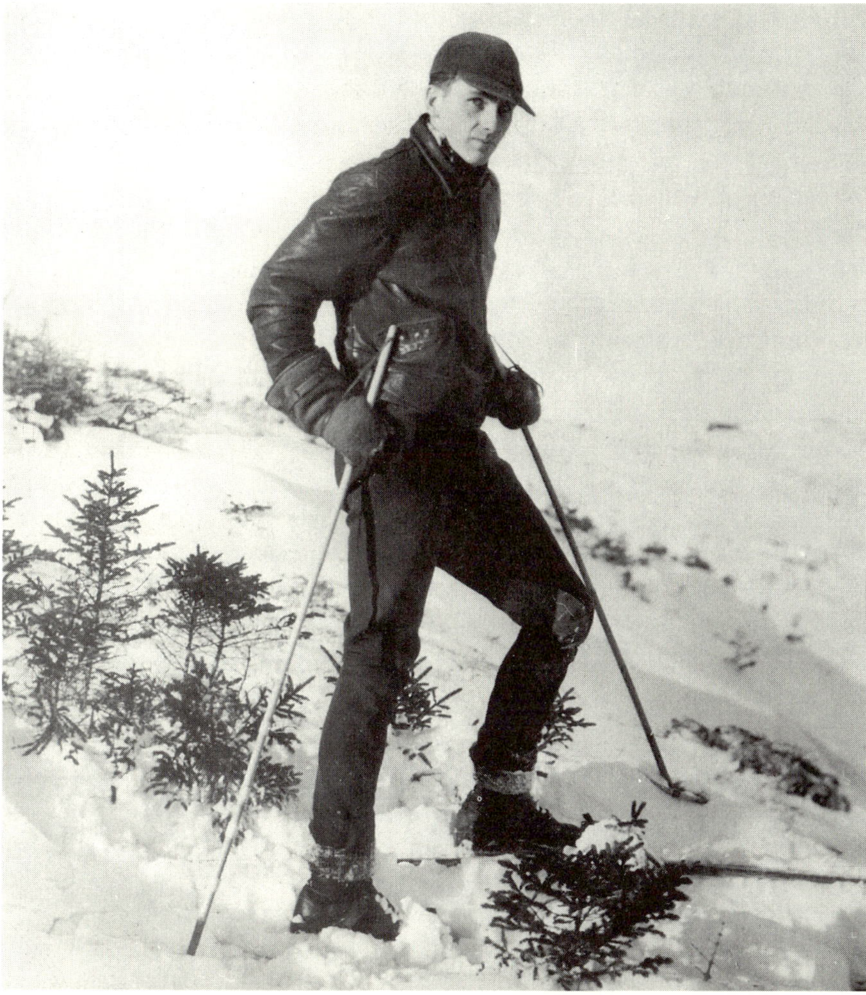

The Doctor pauses so Marianne can catch up.

We stayed all day. I read to them in the afternoon and we had lobster for tea. We expected Steve to come at 5:30 so towards 9:00 I went out to look for him. I found him in Purcell's Harbor, where he had been expecting us since 5:30. No one here seems capable of taking a direct order.

I skijored back behind the horse and having me trailing on behind frightened him so that he ran like a rabbit. I fell only once and that was while he was walking. My mind had wandered. I was thinking of something else and found myself suddenly on my rear. Speeding over the frozen ponds was a delight—you flew. The wind, under a full moon, searched out every seam. I certainly will have to get a zipper. Back to play poker until Waddell left to give glucose to a patient of Dr. Wood's. We had hoodwinked Wood into taking the case this morning because I wanted to go to the Tilt. He got into trouble with a first baby and the mother went into a bit of shock. It turned out all right though. We are going to Wood's for dinner on Thursday, though Olds won't go of course, but hides behind the time-honored excuse that someone must stay and watch the hospital. He is not especially fond of Dr. Wood and I'm not sure that I blame him.

I took out a tonsil this morning. I am fortunate that my post-operative tonsil patients don't seem to have very sore throats. The rest of the day was spent in doing nothing. I have this down to a fine art: I do a little Beethoven on the piano, read a little, find a task or two on the ward, drink some tea, smoke too much, go out for a spell, and there is no trouble—no boredom. This morning I made the anesthetist almost cry because I kept worrying if the patient was breathing. I reserve the right to question her at all times. In the final analysis the welfare of the patient is in the surgeon's hands. She got away with murder at Hopkins.

A half-hour after midnight a man came for a doctor to go to Manuel's Cove. I was reading in bed. It was cold as hell, snowing a blizzard and blowing a gale. He said she had just had her first pain and this was her first baby. I told him that the baby wouldn't come for ten or twelve hours. "You don't need a doctor now. I'll be down in the morning," says I. Says he, "I came for a doctor, I paid for a doctor, and I wants a doctor. If you won't go, I'll get Dr. Wood." "Don't get nasty," says I. "I'm not," says he. So I bundles up and go. He had a sled and an infinitesimal horse. I walked most of the way to save the horse. I found his wife dilating and settled down behind the kitchen stove to wonder how in hell I would pass the rest of the night when suddenly there was a yell from upstairs; I was only just in time to catch a female babe. She refused chloroform. There was a very small tear. My feet got numb in the bedroom and you couldn't uncover the patient a bit. The babe appeared in a cloud of steam. I burnt my boots trying to get warm by the downstairs stove. They loaned me a coat to put over my feet. I stayed on the sled all the way home, so cold I was sick to my stomach. Mercifully it was a short ride. I sank into a sort of stupor. It was a beautiful night but a stiff breeze blew off the water. At Crow Head they said it was 20 degrees below zero. At some of the coves the sea was breaking up the slob.

January 19, '38. Up early but I felt shot all day. Saunders came down for a doc. John and I walked down to shut him up once and for all. That daughter of his showed no change and refused a pelvic examination, so we left in a convenient huff, but not until we saw a case of Old's disease, or familial neurogenic pedal osteodystrophy. This case was in the third generation. The little bones of the feet slough out through sinuses leaving indolent painless ulcers. We walked out over the harbor a little. It was frozen to the other side.

January 20, '38. I didn't get out of the house until evening, when Waddell and I went to Wood's house for tea. They fair paralyzed us with duck, soup, cocktail, cabbage, potato, carrot, and trifle of sponge cake, strawberry preserve, and brandy with whipped cream. I was in intense pain at the end of the meal. Mrs. Wood is the only person in the world who can get me to sing really. In no other house have I been able to carry a tune.

After we'd sung a while, Doccy Wood recited his polemic encounters with Dr. LeDrew. LeDrew hated the hospital and fought against its founding. He inveigled Dr. Parsons into giving an anesthesia for him and signing a receipt for $5.00. Then he hauled him into court for taking money without a license. Parsons was fined $10.00 and Wood swore he would fix LeDrew's wagon. He urged Roberts to print libel in the *Twillingate Sun* and LeDrew sued. A big lawyer came down from St. John's; Wood gave him the lowdown on LeDrew—how he had refused to go to the drowned man because he couldn't pay and had left a delivery because they couldn't pay. The lawyer laid it on thick and reduced LeDrew to a scrump. Wood and he fought it on for years. They locked carriage wheels on the edges of cliffs and exchanged blows at the bedside. It was much in the spirit of R.C. Lincoln. We crawled home after midnight. I am still a little unwieldy in the abdomen.

January 21, '38. A fine day. The slob is spreading. Mrs. Chaffee is in labor. We had a circus taking an appendix out under spinal in a man who had had paraldehyde. He struggled and raved. He cursed and swore and we got Etty to smack his face. We finally gave him chloroform and Marianne had him in her lap when we were finished. The afternoon was spent in reading. Tea was dull enough except that I dumped a cup of coffee in my lap and Suzy insinuatingly said something about rum. John is in bed with a bad sore throat.

January 22, '38. Summoned from the breakfast table to see John who had really a bad throat. We did a smear and saw no diphtheria. It is all brown and nasty. I have been retained for the delivery of one Mrs. James Gillette. I'm afraid that I have to begin studying for the U.S. Public Health exams. I got some books together and am about to embark for the umpteenth time on a course of study. I wonder when doctors ever reach the stage when they don't have to do that. I am looking forward to our usual poker game tonight, but first we have tea and rounds. I lost $1.50 and had only a fair time. I was watching Mrs. Chaffee. Waddell suddenly went upstairs and ordered paraldehyde, three drams, for her. I don't know why exactly but it annoyed me beyond words. I sat dumb for an hour and fumed to myself.

January 23, '38. Waddell left early on a beautiful day to go to Indian Cove. He had to copy most of the Main Tickle. Copy is an expression peculiar to Newfoundland—the whole phrase is "skip and copy." It means leaping from ice pan to ice pan a la Eliza. Sometimes you have to keep moving to get off a small pan before it sinks under you.

I sat around and wrote until Mrs. Chaffee delivered herself of her breech. Had a bath, shave, and Benzedrine before dinner. I made some gin. At tea we were annoyed by the housekeeper's cat, the one that howls all night and everyone wants to dispose of. We captured it and Marianne put it under ether in the OPD so we could cut the vocal cords. I was all ready with mirror and knife. Kelly and Waddell held it. To our consternation, it died before I could operate. We put it under Mr. Cody's bed thinking no one had seen it. I pointed it out to the maid in the morning trying to act as if I knew nothing about it. In some mysterious fashion, suddenly everyone seemed to know what had happened. The housekeeper threatened to leave. The business manager wouldn't talk to us.

January 24, '38. More cat repercussions. We are definitely *persona non grata.* I fooled away the morning getting off my mail and application to the Public Health Service. I had to send a picture of myself, but the only one around was of me in the uniform of the Northwest Mounted Police. In the afternoon I went to Gillard's Cove with Stanley and the horse. I gave the family hell for picking the baby up every time it yelled. I ran all the way home behind the slide and got out of breath. I must be getting soft, although I don't gain any weight. Tea at the Cottage and some of my homemade gin. I beat John in two swell games of chess—one in six moves and one after I was lost but got a pawn to the king line.

January 25, '38. I tried to rupture Mrs. Penney's membranes but couldn't. I put a bougie in up to the fundus and gave her castor oil and quinine. Then I gave some air to Ruby Penney. She has such violent excursions that she inhaled the ink out of the manometer. After dinner I walked to Clark's on the Arm and found there an overdue pregnant woman. I came back to Hart Cove and over the new ice to the hospital. It was nice out. The sun seemed very hot. I saw a boy about ten driving a dog team by Ashbourne's. He was going hell bent for election, sideways and everyways, the way you do downhill, right among the dogs who were breaking their necks to get out of the way of what they are supposed to be pulling. His little brother, about three, was in a soapbox lashed to the slide. After tea we went to visit Joyce's aunt to play Auction 120. It was dull enough. On the way down though, the sky was as bright in the east as a well-advanced sunrise. The northern lights were brilliant, pale green and a real deep orange. There was a cluster of light right overhead, like amethyst crystal. The local seers say that red or orange northern lights mean there will be a war soon.

Waddell had given my patient Mrs. Penney paregoric to stop her stools, although she had had castor oil, quinine, enemas, pituitrin and a bougie. Her pains had stopped and during the night, I removed the bougie. There was also a call at 3 A.M. for Dr. Olds. The night nurse said I would go, but the caller said never mind, he would try Dr. Wood.

January 26, '38. A dull gray day and hot—temperature 36 degrees. Mrs. Penney was quiet at first but ruptured her membranes at 10:00. Waddell went across the ice but not before he told me how lucky I was to have the OB service where residents and so forth did not butt in. I didn't say a word. They did a spinal fusion this morning and I carefully stayed away until they sent for me to give an intravenous. This I did with dispatch and left, lest they go and leave me with the patient to take care of when I had nothing to do with it. A call came to see a child at Jenkins Cove. I plowed through soft roads to one Jenkins Cove only to find it was the other. I went all the way down there only to see an undemonstrable "strain of the side." The broken leg is much better. Coming back I saw that neurotic Saunders girl sliding down a hill. She looked pretty well to me. Mrs. Penney failed to produce.

January 27, '38. A colder day but the roads are still soft. Just before dinner

I went to see Fred Earl's daughter, with a pain in her side. I brought her in—urine negative, white count 17,000. I operated on her at once, with much direction and superfluous talk from the maestro, and took out her appendix. In the late afternoon Mrs. Penney really got down to work, cursing and denouncing me. Before she was in labor, she stated she had lived only for me. I gave her some paraldehyde during the night and she went completely nuts, proclaiming loudly that I had poisoned her and tried to kill her baby. We took her to the OR a little after midnight and she took the anesthetic easily enough. With a deep episiotomy, she was delivered by me of a male child. Waddell scrubbed with me and was most insulting quite unintentionally. He stood square in the way, but did let me put on the forceps like a kind master allowing his pupil to try something difficult. I couldn't help but recall the time when he had been unable to apply forceps to an aftercoming head and I had had no trouble.

January 28, '38. Today we started to examine all the school children on the island. The first installment was thirty. I found a bad heart and a myopic youngster who could read only 20/200. John picked up a tuberculosis. I have been in a blood mood ever since the delivery yesterday. I talked to my two superiors only with difficulty. John beat me hopelessly in two games of chess—that didn't help.

January 29, '38. The morning was cold and passed quickly in reading and letter writing. Right after dinner I took Marianne to Manuel's Cove to see an extremely dehydrated baby. The grandmother thought water was giving it the diarrhea and had withheld all fluid. It wasn't nursing either. We just edged out the Salvation Army adjutant who was coming to christen it before it went hence. This eventuality seemed unlikely to us, though the old lady was very pessimistic and saw no reason in trying to save it. It was a lovely trip even if I was feeling noncommunicative. I ran most of the way back and got here in time to hear most of *Tristan und Isolde* on the BBC before dinner. I lost $3.00 at poker. Waddell had gone on a nice trip to Herring Neck without consulting me. I suppose it's all right. I didn't sleep well.

January 30, '38. A cool brisk Sunday. I fooled away the morning and took a Benzedrine that did nothing to help; still depressed. I feel the fault is not all mine. I lost two games of chess after dinner. Read *Rich Man, Poor Man* all afternoon then got inveigled into going to the Cottage for tea although I had already eaten. Had a better time than I expected.

January 31, '38. A quiet day. The weather is extremely mild. Almost all the ice in the harbor has gone out and the ground is cleared of snow. There is a strong southerly wind with no sign of rough weather. This morning Marianne slipped on the wing porch and knocked off a vertebral transverse process. We put her in a body cast. I'm afraid that may restrict her activities but she can get around pretty well. Yesterday I had a long talk with the high school principal. His son has tuberculosis and we advise bed rest. He came up in the morning to tell me that his son wouldn't stay in bed at home—would we take him in? I said yes. The boy was admitted and in the afternoon up came papa to take him out again. He was not "satisfied" to have his son in a room with another tuberculosis. He claimed that if you put a hot stone next to a cold one, the heat would spread. He had figures to prove how soon the air in a room is vitiated by one person. He was afraid that Buster wouldn't get enough milk. He had all kinds of bum theories and wound up saying he didn't believe his son had tuberculosis anyway. He insisted that the right lung is different from the left (it is, of course) and would sound different to us and we couldn't possibly interpret that difference. He was willing to set himself up against us four doctors. Then he really lost face, as far as I'm concerned, when he quoted Mosdel, His Majesty's Commissioner of Health.

February 1, '38. This day has been good enough. In the morning thirty more school children were examined in the OPD. They're easy to deal with when their parents aren't around and are, on the whole, attractive children. Dinner as usual at the cottage. In the afternoon I did a couple of pneumothoraces and some syphilis treatments. Walked down the lane to Burt Pardy's afterwards, whither I was invited to return for bridge in the evening.

A fine wind is blowing tonight and a bit of snow is in it. The mild seems to be at an end. The harbor is beginning to slob up again. Perhaps we may get a glimpse of winter yet. I was shocked to hear that Mrs. Clark had delivered and had called Dr. Wood. The hell with them. Let them send for him the next time their brat is sick. Oh, yes, I was attended by a committee of young Church of England girls today who want me to lecture to them on health or something, a week from Friday next. I accepted and I'm sure I'll be sorry. At least it was I they asked.

February 2, '38. A fine day, dawning cool and getting colder all day. Now at 10 P.M. it is well below zero and blowing a gale. The ice was almost gone this morning and slob has been making all day.

I took out a quick tonsil before the school children came and we saw thirty more before noon—all girls this time. Where they get all the pink rayon I don't know. Dinner was over quickly and I returned to quite a lot of blood chemistry. A tooth pulled and the mail read. The latter consisted of two letters from mother, one from Mrs. Strong complaining of what might be a possible prolapse in little Robert, and the world's homeliest calendar from my old storm-bound friend, the insurance agent. Had a cup of tea with Marianne, who is able to get about some now in spite of her cast. I played a game of chess with John after tea; when he saw he wasn't going to win, he lost all interest and gave me the game.

February 3, '38. Up reasonably early. Waddell was scheduled for a repair and a hernia. I suspected that I would have nothing to do with it, but a call came from the North Side for him to deliver a baby so I was left. I helped John on the difficult repair of an old third-degree perineal laceration. He pulled over slips of the *levator ani.* He offered me the hernia and I did it in 20 minutes but I was scared at the start to begin. He seemed to be in a blood mood. When he started to fix the cystocele and found the patient hadn't been catheterized he staged a scene with Etty. "Do you mean to say you didn't catheterize her? Why not?" Such rhetorical questions and long staring. It was a little like old times. The radiators were all frozen at the Cottage, so we had a good dinner in the library by the stove. The afternoon was consumed in fighting everybody about admitting Mrs. Grenham. She took out her individual contract when she was already sick. She finally won but not until I had sided with Wyn and all hands had gotten personal. I suspect that the fact that she was championed by Doccy Wood had a lot to do with the resistance from Waddell.

I walked up on the hill before rounds for a look and things were lovely. The temperature itself was not too bad but the wind was just too much to stand on the face. The sun was bright and the ice was everywhere, except for lovely green open spaces just off Long Point and French Head. The ice goes clear to New Bay, 40 miles away. Rounds and tea and then I lost a game of chess. Then nothing much. I write this, will read a bit and go to bed. I have one OB case coming off soon and I wonder what midnight it will be.

February 4, '38. A good day. It started to snow in the morning and all day we had occasional glimpses of the North Side of the harbor. We had school children—twenty-two of them. They were very young—five to eight. It was amazing how well behaved and cooperative they are without their parents. Ordinarily not one of them would have submitted to examination without shrieks. Waddell grabbed a trip to Black Island and we were left kind of stranded. I haven't been outside to speak of for a week. The afternoon went quickly with study. Tea at the Cottage was pleasant, though the Olds have gone to the Tilt. We played four games of Auction 120 after tea, until Ralph Smith showed up and we organized a poker game. I lost only $1.20. Had it been more than two bucks, I'd made up my mind to quit, so I'm saved for further loss. I here declare that if I lose more than a dollar next time and the next, I will decide that a malignant fate is gunning for me and I will stop the game.

February 5, '38. A rather nice day, the landscape is too white to look upon. There was a low drift, thick enough at times to obscure the other shore. It is hard to tell whether it's snowing or not; I hope it is. I am going out this afternoon if it kills me. The boys turned up unexpectedly this afternoon to play poker again and I managed to recoup $1.50; that's more like it.

It was a dull, cold and cloudy day and in the afternoon Dr. Wood received a wire asking him to tend a delivery in Newstead. He thought about it until the telegraph office was almost closed, then told them he couldn't go. They returned a request for any doctor and I agreed to go. We couldn't get any dog teams. By that time, it was too late so we were to wait for a wire on Sunday. I read until one.

February 6, '38. The wire came at 9:30 and by 10:00 I had Alf and his six dogs and I was on skis. Off we went on a cold dull day. It was easy going over to Borden's Cove where we took the bay because the ice was too rough at Manuel's. The salt water ice proved to be smooth enough, but covered by an inch of very sticky slob. The dogs couldn't pull us at all. Alf would run ahead to urge them on but the minute you put a foot on the sled, it was too much for them. Soon it started to snow and for 15 or 20 minutes at a time, you couldn't see a thing. It was very slow and tiring. Once the dogs seemed to explode and, tired as they were, sprang ahead and knocked Alf down. That was because they had seen a raven. Alf kept up a hoarse running fire of "Caw caw, there he goes . . . Get out of that . . . Hiss . . . hiss . . . hoss . . . hoss . . . crow . . . crow . . . go get'n . . . giddap . . . yug . . . yug . . . grump . . . grump . . . sheep in the garden . . . sheep in the garden . . . go on . . . go on . . . hold in . . . hold in . . . keep off . . . keep off."

There were also all kinds of grunts and inarticulate noises. He would pound with a club on the sides of the sled and brandish it threateningly at the dogs where they could see it. "Keep off, keep off, hold in, hold in."

I thought we must have covered the six miles to the bottom of Virgin Arm when we reached Deep Cove Neck on Trump Island but it was only half way. Then a mile to Virgin Arm Point, then two more to the bottom, then it was three miles mostly uphill to Summerford. I stepped through the shore ice and got wet up to my nipples but it didn't seem to bother much. Going down hill was fun. You catch up with the dogs and there is a hell of a mess and confusion. Finally we rolled into Summerford and there was Mr. Brown. He said that Mr. Small was expecting me and had put out an extra cup. How was I to know it was the wrong Small's and knocked and opened and found a covey of fat women sitting around the table. I asked, "Is this the Small's?" They said nothing but motioned saturninely to a hunchbacked man reloading second-hand shotgun shells by the stove. "I'm with Mr. Brown," I said. "Down by the shore," says he. So I think, "To hell with you, I won't favor you with my presence." I retired. Brown took me, tealess, in a hurry across to Newstead where it was cold as hell and I was hungry like I hadn't been for years. Snow confused us and we got off the trail.

The horse stepped through a rent between the ice fields but we pulled in safely and I stumbled into the house, stiff and trembling. We were at once put by the fire and given bread and cheese with hot tea. It felt so good the tears came to my eyes.

The old grandmother, who had reared the girl since the death of her mother at age three months, was charming. Lots of relatives and a good midwife. The husband wasn't worth bothering with. I went in to the woman who had been in labor since Friday evening. The cervix was open but the head was high. She was standing it well but had been in the hospital for tuberculosis. I examined her, catheterized her, and shaved her. I smoked my pipe for an hour and then seeing she had done nothing, I got lots of help and had the midwife put her hesitantly to sleep. I dilated the cervix and put on the hooks. They wouldn't lock properly but I had to haul anyway. There were all kinds of ominous crunches and with a deep episiotomy a strangled babe was pulled out. I put in on the floor after it had gasped once. The woman holding the left leg fainted and I had to push her back on the bed with my foot. The placenta wouldn't yield. I broke the cord pulling and took time out to insufflate the babe; it worked. The infant was markedly molded and I had had the forceps over the forehead. There was only a little scratch.

The mother finally gave up the placenta but the uterus never did get very hard. I repaired her with gut and in a short time everything was jake, except the fainted woman was being qualmish and the grandmother had hysterics. The patient had a chloroform burn. I decided to hang around a while because the 23-year-old horse was tired. I stayed until 6:00 and saw the poor relatives—a young fellow with nephritis, and a girl with some neuropathy, probably advanced multiple sclerosis. Another daughter had a bad heart and consequent infantilism. Then over to Brown's house.

In the low kitchen, I was confronted by a big burly woman washing a few dishes in a little wash basin on the corner of a table with the plush cover rolled back a little. There never seems to be any proper arrangement for wholehearted household mechanics. She went into some peculiar gyration. Brown explained, "She wants to shake hands with 'ee.'" I boldly did so, to her and my pleasure. Then I saw some children next door. "Rickets," says the father. "Only too true," says I. "I gives 'em cod-liver oil," says the mother, "six spoons a day." I wondered if this would be the only case in the world of cod-liver oil resistant rickets. "How long?" ask I. "Since Thursday," says the mother.

Another child had a lot of small red papules like small pimples in thick skin which never come to a head. They're strange—never suppurate or show any special reaction. Must be mollusca contagiosa. Then back for more tea and bread and early to bed with sheets clean but too short and eight thick heavy blankets. I fairly sat up, my feet were cold and I didn't sleep well. By 5:00 in the morning I was stiff as a poker. More baloney and tea for breakfast, which meant nothing but baloney or tea for six meals hand running, beginning with breakfast at the hospital. Then over to my patient who was fine. When I made toast for breakfast, Mr. Brown marveled. "Do you like it?" asked I. "Yes," says he," but no one will make it for me."

The trail back over to Summerford was so sticky that we walked most of the way and it took over two hours instead of forty-five minutes as it had the night before. I had pulled something in my right groin and every step hurt and there were lots of steps. At Summerford I tried my old friends the Small's again. As I was knocking them up Alf appeared and told me I was at the wrong Small's. We left to go to Small number two, where we were treated well—bread and tea again, but I could have eaten more.

Then to the dogs. They were eager and barking in that expectant way they have, making wild starts in all directions but the right one. They hadn't been fed since two nights before. On the neck I met Dolph Berge who stopped me to complain that the yeast I had given him for his beriberi was curing that but had given him boils. I didn't tell him about the well-advertised Vienna specialists who all recommend yeast especially for boils. Then that terrible six miles on ice broken by Trump Island Neck. It was drudgery and cold. There was no running. It was worse than the day before. I dragged along my paining thighs those 6,000 paces. The headlands retreated as we approached and everything seemed to stand still. It was like a treadmill. Finally I got to Manuel's Cove and back on my skis, frozen stiff, hungry and sore. A bath, a shave, a Benzedrine, and at dinner I was sick to my stomach but recovered enough to get off some mail.

February 7, '38. Up early to see children until noon. Nothing in the afternoon. Betty is in bed with a sore throat and a face swollen from sulfa. I read until 3:30 last night so it's no wonder that I overslept and was late getting to the school clinic. I would like to adopt Piercy Elliott. After dinner I pulled teeth and took the baby clinic until 4 P.M. I met Bud as he was going skiing and went along with him. We had a great time falling in the snow. It was a glorious afternoon and we covered miles over towards the Arm. I have confused the days somehow so as to leave out Monday and Wednesday but they're all in here somewhere.

February 10, '38. I got left home all day. All I did was go out a minute early, to get some wool so Mrs. Penney could make me a pair of socks before she is discharged. John went to Moreton's Harbor with Bud, and Waddell went to Herring Neck on a very ill-conceived trip. He took his skis but the dogs were so poor he had to walk the whole way. Coming back he got lost and came home dead tired. Tea at the Cottage was fun. I read some Hilaire Belloc to Marianne and Betty, the latter still sick in bed. At bedtime it was snowing like hell; the bottom has dropped out of the barometer. I read *Introductory Lecture* by A.E. Housman that Goya had sent me.

February 11, '38. Blowing a gale and snowing like hell this morning. Everything was covered and you could hardly see the Cottage. I dug a tumor off a man's zygoma and got into the maxillary sinus doing it. Then very little until dinner. I prepared my speech to give to the Junior Red Cross but they didn't meet so I went across the harbor on skis. It was eighteen inches deep in slop just past the frozen-in schooners; I was scared. I waited until some dogs caught up with me so they could go ahead. It was grand out though. I bought some tobacco and wool for my sweater and saw a pair of three-quarter Wellington boots that I am going to buy at Hodges.

After tea I won a game of chess and talked a long time with John. Waddell has decided to stay here another winter so that he can go to the seal fishery in the spring. Stan Hardy is coming back to work here. If I don't pass the exams, I don't know what I will do—probably come back. I have finally stretched my sealskin boots. I wet them and put a pair of Waddell's shoes in them until they dried. I have been oiling them and they may prove fit to use. Right now the wind has veered to the northwest and you can't tell if it is snowing or not. It is blowing a gale and is much colder. I am due for a trip but I suppose I'll have to fight for it. Mrs. Gillette is due too, and I await hourly the summons to her bed. She is prone to having her babies in a hurry.

February 17, '38. A whole week almost and very little has transpired. A very unsatisfactory mail. A copy of *Citadel* came but I had already read it and so has everyone else around here. Notice came from the Department of Public Health that the exams are on March 28th. I don't know just when I will leave. Perhaps it would be wise to plan so that there would not be time to stay anywhere. The school children came yesterday and the day before, forty of them. They are amusing and have the Newfoundland habit of answering "yes" to all questions they do not hear or do not understand or do not know the answer to. One said when I asked him how old he was, "I be ten, zur, February gone." It sounded just like Thomas Hardy. One told me he had two sisters and two brothers, gave me their names and state of health. It developed he was an only child.

I fixed an inguinal hernia with a minimum of interference. My colleague is difficult to catch at a loss. There is no type of case he hasn't seen at least one of, most of the time it is scores—lactating women giving birth to children and all sorts of things. Tomorrow I go to give my talk on public health to the girls of the Church of England. I am going to include martyrs of thought, how to bring up children and how to treat a doctor—the things we are forced to do. It won't be easy to talk to eleven-year-olds.

Bill McConnell, my friend the guide in Portage, Maine, invited me to come in anytime for coffee, biscuits, and pancakes. I wish I could. I have just the right pair of boots to wear—high brogans with rubber bottoms. Last night I played bridge at Burt Pardy's. It was below zero and he let the fire go out. I almost froze to death. Waddell told a patient with erysipelas to put hot Epsom Salts on his nose. When he returned it was on his nose all right, but they had it in a hot water bottle.

February 18, '38. This was a good day. I spent the morning examining more than my share of forty-five children from Jenkins Cove. I hurried from dinner to outline my talk. Then I walked across the harbor. It was firm. There was a bitter northeast wind and it was cold though much warmer than it has been. Arriving a little early at the parish hall I went next door to dress Pierce Powell's foot. Then back to the Red Cross meeting conducted very parliamentarily by Mr. Harnett, the teacher. The thirty-odd children stood politely as I entered and were extremely nice. I sat while they read minutes and reports and a little girl read an illiterate naive paper on clean bodies, bowels, thoughts, and so forth. Another recited a poem about keeping the windows open. Then I spoke, introduced most flowerily by Mr. Harnett. I spoke for forty minutes or so starting with a declaration of Plato's ideology: forms are important and ideas exist only in relation to them; vice is ignorance and I then led them into a discussion of the difficulty of getting any new idea across. I spoke of Pasteur, Semmelweis, and Galileo. I went on to tell them how badly are doctors treated. It went well enough and I stopped before I fired all my shots. They were terribly polite afterwards and the Reverend Goodland made a long speech. I watched a little first aid demonstration and went home.

I had a nice midforceps delivery after tea. It was Waddell's patient but he has become very generous of late. I confess I am much better with forceps than he is. It made a full day. I finished *Tristram* while Waddell slept in the chair. He had been up all the night before.

February 19, '38. A miserable day full of odd jobs. It rained and got as slick as ever it can. I examined I don't know how many patients. It has gone quickly and I was very impatient to get started at our usual Saturday poker. Won $2.75—very pleasant after my late reverses, inasmuch as I paid Burt Pardy $2.60 only this morning.

February 20, '38. A dull cold day. A lot of ward chores in the morning but got done by 11:00 and went out for an hour of skiing after taking a Benzedrine. A tub, a shave, and a bit of gin put me into fine fettle for dinner from which Betty and John were absent. Joyce, Marianne, Waddell, and I had rather a profane, hilarious time of it. We wound up putting some of the furniture into the fireplace. We never did like that wicker chair. A kind of reaction set in after dinner and I had to take a nap though I did struggle through one game of chess with Waddell.

February 21, '38. A decent day. The boys did that gall bladder and it wasn't much fun. It was so bound down that all they could do was get into the sac. At any rate, a probe went into the stomach and the indication is that she had a spontaneous gastric fistula. I started to do a skin graft but the knives weren't ready, so it was deferred. The afternoon went I don't remember how and after tea we played a bit of poker. I read a bit of *Prayer for My Son.* It is good. I finished *Magic Mountain* and I suppose that there is no doubt but what it is great stuff. At the same time the Jesuitic dialectic is a little thick for me.

I forgot to say that Sunday night, or rather, Monday morning, I rose at 5:30 A.M. to deliver Mrs. Elliot. She was a terrible patient, carrying on dreadfully. We were obliged to put on the forceps just because she wouldn't push. She had been told by Dr. Wood that she couldn't have her baby without help and she was determined not to have it without help. The head hadn't rotated and I knew the hooks weren't in an ideal position but had to pull with them that way until the head was low enough for proper application. The baby did look a little like an old fedora but it was perfectly all right.

February 22, '38. Waddell was off first thing in the morning all the way to Herring Neck to see Carrie. We all know she is neurotic and without demonstrable physical disease. It is a crime, the attention she demands and gets.

The directors met in my study. As soon as Waddell came back, I skied down to see Andrew Grenham. He has a kidney stone and is vomiting—a bad sign. Mrs. Osmond looks bad. She has a pericardial friction rub, I think. I have used up all the veins in her arms so I got Waddell to give her glucose. I am going to start studying if it kills me. *Gott hilfe mir.*

February 23, '38. A lovely day and all I can remember of it is that Bud and I went to Jenkins Cove on skis to see a little girl with a gastrointestinal upset. It was fine out and we went down the back of the island. The hills were wonderful; the going was fast. The mail had come by dog team and ten letters were waiting for me. The one from Howie said that he thought we two had accomplished prodigious amounts of work during our one year at poliomyelitis research—more than three of them would do this year. Sister wrote asking for a present but I'm damned if I know what to get her here.

The Hospital Association met; Waddell and I paid our $1.00 dues and attended. There was much elation at the favorable financial report. The deficit was only $1,350 as against $6,000 for last year. Mr. Manuel supplied the usual diversion by asking a thousand picayunish questions. He wondered what we charged the outside help for meals and was horrified to find it was 15 cents at a cost of 11 cents. He allowed as how he would come over here and eat himself. He felt we should charge 25 cents. "Let them go home and eat—the way I do," he said. It was good insight into the character of the merchants. It was typical that old Skipper Watts, after being captain of a schooner for 20 years for Ashbourne's, had to go on dole when one voyage failed to make a profit.

Ned Facey, Pat Cody, Olds, Waddell, and Ecke played poker after the meeting. Oh, I forgot—just before we started, a fellow came in who had cut his foot with an axe up in the bay at 9 A.M. and had been traveling on the ice all day. He had it all swaddled up and when I undid the ten layers of rag, was greeted by such a flow of blood—a river—that I yelled for help and put on the blood-pressure cuff for a tourniquet. Waddell and I fished for tendons by the hour. There were three cut as was the tibial artery.

February 24, '38. This day was marked by a party at the Loveridges. They brought out at once the vastest collection of snapshots I have ever seen. They have a family of girls, who seem to be the same age, look the same, and sound exactly alike. We played Auction 120 after a while and were fed six different kinds of cake and sandwiches. We really had a good time. It was 13 below zero when we walked back across the harbor. Our host works for an insurance company and will show you a letter of recommendation from the firm if you talk to him for more than a minute. Waddell found that out on his trip from St. John's in the *Segona*.

February 25, '38. It was a cold morning. I was just planning to have an afternoon nap when they sent for me to go to Mrs. James Gillette. I got Stanley and the horse and Marianne and set out with dispatch. She has been missed before. We were in good time however, as the cervix was about six cm. I sent Stanley home with the horse and we were just settling down to a cup of tea when her waters burst, hitting the wall six feet from the floor. We returned to our tea and I read *Carl Grier* sitting on the floor by the stove. The sounds changed upstairs suddenly so we rushed up. Before Marianne could finish the cleaning up the head was on the perineum. It was a great satisfaction to watch a good obstetrical patient. It was wonderful to see her scrunch right to it and move that thing along with each pain. The babe was buried in the feather bed before you could say "dysdiadokokinesis." There was an insignificant tear. During this, the Rev. Mr. Vinum dropped by to ask us to come see his daughter the first time we were down his way. We agreed to come the next day.

February 26, '38. I worked the morning in the OPD. Right after dinner I got Bud and we went on skis down to Vinum's. It was a glorious day and coming back we skirted the other side of the mountain range flanking the Arm trail. We climbed all the peaks, I came down one steep slope like the wind. My left ski caught in a protruded branch that had looked frail but turned out to be solid. I fell like a plummet. My elbow hit the ground and my head hit my own propped shoulder. I thought I was killed. There were lots of good runs. The lowering sun was very bright. Each large snow crystal gleamed like a diamond flashing bits of red and orange and green. I have seen this only a few times. The sun and the crystals have to be just right. It is spectacular.

We had a late tea and then poker. I don't understand it. I won $11.00. Maybe Benzedrine helped. Ralph couldn't pay so he is discouraged. We ought to fund his debt and tell him not to come anymore. Bert Pardy called me up when he got home after the game. That scared me—thinking it was an outside OB call and I was tired. It was to ask me down to the tail end of his wife's birthday party. I wasn't too tired for that. I stayed down there until after two; couldn't get to sleep until after four when Waddell had to get up to go see some woman with fainting spells.

February 27, '38. Bright, clear, sun, with little wind. Temperature five below zero. Right after breakfast Marianne and I went down the lane to Alf Young's and he took us by dog team to the Tilt. We amused ourselves there by melting snow to get water. The spring was frozen. We couldn't get the fire to do much. I laboriously cooked some ham in coffee and fabricated some biscuits, but the butter was so hard I couldn't budge it and the fire smoked like hell. The meal was not very good. Just at the end of it I discovered a damper on the stove that had been closed all the time. After dinner we went out into the snow for some target practice with John Olds' twenty-two. It was bad because the bullets kept ricocheting from the rocks and whining all about us. We followed some of the bullet tracks through the snow and found them very little damaged by contact with the ice. Then back to the Tilt to clean up and have some tea. I fixed my skis and coaxed the fire to burn.

At 5:00 exactly Mr. Keefe turned up. He came right in and sat down by the stove and was not unwilling to recount for us his forty trips down on the Labrador. He's a charming, solicitous old guy. He hauled us home through a magnificent velvet night. He drove fast. As we passed a telephone pole at the top of the hill near Little Harbor, he told us about Sam Pardy's brother who used to own the land there. People were after him for years to move that pole. It was too near the road or in some way in just the wrong place. Pardy was too mean to do anything about it. One day they were moving a house down past there. He wouldn't help but stood around to protect his property. The house slipped and hit the pole, which snapped off and hit him on the head and killed him cold. On the way back, we slipped off the road twice into the harbor. Keefe didn't want to take any money but we finally forced fifty cents on him.

February 28, '38. A very busy morning, which reminds me that I forgot to say that on Saturday morning I spent a lot of time taking a small tumor out of a breast for biopsy. I thought it was carcinoma and when I carried it proudly in to John he says, "My God, I was going to take the whole breast off Monday." Waddell took it off this morning with the Greenough incision. Then John did an appendix which turned out to be retroperitoneal tuberculosis. Then I took out a red-hot appendix in the boy whom I had seen a month before with a bellyache. That brought us to dinnertime. After dinner I studied a bit and was getting ready to take a nap. I had a headache and a stiff neck, either from riding on skis behind teams or from my fall. Joe Bulgin, who has forgiven me for running into him on the cycle, came in with an infected thumb. While he was soaking it I bustled around in front of him, oiling the dental forceps. He followed me around with his eyes and after a couple of minutes said, "Gee, doctor, I wish I was as clever as you—so big, so strong, so fat." This gave me some hint as to the meaning of clever. To my disappointment it has nothing to do with brains. They use the word even to describe blustery weather. Anything is clever that is large and lusty and to be reckoned with, but there must be no evil intent.

February 29, '38. Started out expecting the Church of England children at the school clinic but the weather was too bad. We've been admitting patients right and left—carcinoma of the nose, lip, and penis and what not. We have seventy-seven in the house now. I worked almost all the day. I'm going to read some chemistry and go to bed nice and early.

March 5, '38. Not much happened this week. I've been disturbed a little by the floods of Los Angeles but I dare say my brother, Albert, can swim well enough to look out for rainwater. Bud and I went skiing over to Minty's where the slopes are the best around here.

March 8, '38. Did little all day and got raked into going to Burty Hodges to play chess. Burty is a tall thin fellow—courteous, hesitant, restrained, slow to offer opinion: withal a gentle almost tender host. He runs a bankrupt business for his older brother. They live in a great big gloomy house with high ceilings, coal fires, and heavy dark drapes. His brother came in at first, after I had been obliged to take off my boots and outer socks and put on a pair of slippers. He showed me all the pictures on the mantelpiece and gave me the life story of the family of Dr. Sterling, the first doctor ever to come to Twillingate—has been dead over fifty years.

The games were short and I gave Burty a little trouble in the middle of only one. I was fed too much as usual and I made a very cold trip back across the harbor at 1 A.M.

March 9, '38. Up at 7 A.M. to go to Herring Neck. I thought travel would be good because John had just come back from Change Island and the ice had been so slick that the wind blew them right up on their dogs. However, a little dry snow had fallen and it was below zero. The sled runners scroped, that's the way they describe the noise that snow makes in very cold weather. I tried skijoring for a while but it was too much for the dogs, so that each of us ran six miles at least. It was a perfect day with a bright sun. I had to wear sunglasses. I saw old Skipper Tom Blandford, 86 years old. He's had the arthritis for five years. His heart medicine ran out last spring and he seems none the worse without it.

We hurried back and passed Waddell on his way to Moreton's Harbor. John waited until 4:00 and then went to the Tilt. Just after he had gone a boy came from Indian Island with a broken arm. His sister has tuberculosis, his mother is dead, his father has some terrible disease that makes him swell, and they are certified paupers. The arm had been broken four days before. I started the x-ray machine and was setting both bones of the forearm when Waddell came in. He couldn't improve the position though it was nothing to write home about.

March 10, '38. Little in the morning. Out in the afternoon to Minty's farm for an exciting ski session. I enjoyed it so much I hated to come in. We had rounds and a drink or two and before I knew it, tea and it was time to play poker. I had started Mrs. Walbrunne in labor. She had tremendous swelling of the vulva. The labia were all out of shape—the size of a basketball. Her blood pressure was up too. She hopped right along and in the middle of the poker game protruded her membranes. I expected a hell of a lot of trouble. Waddell put her to sleep and I put the hooks on perfectly and with an episiotomy below the swelling withdrew a five and a half-pound boy with no effort at all and started the repair. "Is the uterus hard?" I asked. Waddell answered, "It's full of blood." He exerted a little pressure from above and to my immense surprise saw a funny white business that turned out to be the membranes for a twin, a breech. I punctured those as I had done the others and caught a three and a half-pound boy. They were both lusty and breathed easily and I have hopes of raising the critters. Back to the game and I lost only 50 cents. Ralph lost $2.00 and says he's going to quit. I hope he pays me my $2.75 if he does.

March 11, '38. Sunday and snowing like the dickens. I rose and did a few chores and fooled around trying to get Waddell and Joyce off to the Tilt to bring back Betty and John. They were slow because Waddell was not very anxious to go in the storm. We finally got Steve to hitch up our big truck horse, Mack. Just as they were leaving, Dr. Wood came in and announced he had seen Betty and John on their way back from the Tilt and the trip was forestalled. A bit of rum was in order and we had dinner at the Cottage after all.

March 12, '38. I don't remember much about Monday except a hernia and a hydrocele and John did a hernia and amputated a penis—the groin was full of cancerous nodes. I went skiing in the afternoon but didn't have a very good time because Waddell had broken one of my skis and John's skis do not suit me so well as my own. Bud and I built a ski jump. I went down it twice with success but couldn't stand up after that.

March 13, '38. Thirty schoolchildren in the morning, before which I hurried to the Arm to see a child that had spells. It turned out to be grand mal, I think. The paternal grandfather was always being picked up in a fit and the child had been having mild spells ever since it swallowed a duck feather this summer. This was the worst so far.

Tommy came back in the afternoon from up along. "Up along" means the States or Canada. This trip was to the States; she brought a lot of rum back with her and we had a party in the evening. I did not have a very good time. It was supposed to be for Waddell's fictitious birthday, our going away, and Tommy's arrival. It was discovered that Miss Kelly had a birthday so it was made to appear for her too. Waddell wanted to appease her because he had offended her when I had delivered the Catholic twins. She was determined to christen them before they died and Waddell didn't know why she was following him around with a glass of water. In the struggle, she got her feelings hurt. (P.S. They didn't die.) I drank very little. The party was quiet for a long time and then suddenly got noisy. That was late. I left at midnight and had just gone to bed when, lo and behold, everybody climbed through my bedroom window. It's the only way to get into the hospital after the doors are locked. Some were a little tight for navigation and wanted to stay in the apartment. I think Waddell would have let them if I hadn't gotten dressed and told them all to go home. I'm not sure what motives were involved but I suppose it was all on the up and up.

March 14, '38. Thirty more schoolchildren and the operating room is being painted. Dinnertime came soon and after I had seen ten babies or so, I lured Bud away from the laboratory for a long ski, having finally had my skis fixed. It was lovely out and we consumed two hours going way out to Codjack Cove by a roundabout route. It is difficult to conceive of anything more lush and full than these sunny afternoons with their rich rose coloring and great expanses of white snow, distant blue sea and hills. I seem to get worse at chess. I can't beat John for anything. I guess I am stun—that's local for stupid.

March 15, '38. Nothing much in the morning. I helped Waddell do an appendix and in the afternoon Bud and I went down the Arm to see Mrs. James Gillette. She was out, but her daughter volunteered to take me to her. She first had to get her sled, and take a few belly whoppers on the shore. I grew impatient waiting for this eight-year-old to get serious, and stalked off to find the mother by myself. She was having a spot of tea in a house built out of ships' timbers. The kitchen had a 12 x 12 beam running through the middle of it about five feet from the floor. This called for careful navigation.

The ranger sergeant and his wife came to tea—we had a bang-up meal. The ranger has two prisoners, a half-breed Eskimo and some local character. The Eskimo's only trouble was that he thought he was dead. His cellmate fell in with the idea and wrapped him up like a corpse in a sheet. He then sprinkled him with breadcrumbs and recited the Church of England burial service.

March 16, '38. I tried to get out all day. We had twenty-four children this morning. Finally, I sat in the sun and read though it was zero. The report is that this is the coldest winter in thirty years. A bit of a quick ski to the Arm to see Gladys Inge who has been enjoying ill health these six months. She resented very much the idea of getting an x-ray, but I believe she will haul her fat hulk down here. I can't hear much in her chest, though it may be she has TB. I fell down very forcibly on the way home and broke my harness all to pieces. I had to borrow a knife to cut the heel and half my sole off and limped back. A wire had come asking for help at Joe Batt's Arm for a woman in her twelfth hour of labor and her seventh fit. John wired that he didn't think travel was possible. Joe Batt's is on Fogo Island, well out to sea.

March 17, '38. Waddell rushed in after breakfast to say he was going to Joe Batt's Arm, that a man had walked up last night. I was miffed as hell and told him I thought I was being screwed. Until he went he was very quiet. I guess I am wrong in expecting people to give me my own and not take advantage. The trouble is I think I am peaceful and actually I haven't the nerve to grab for things. I want to do what is necessary. I don't want what is mere pleasure. Cooperation is fun when there is complete communion and equality of interests. When one is played against the other, as seems to be happening to me, one is only tolerated and gets leavings. He said I could go, but I merely became silent and sulked.

Went for a nice ski down to Jenkins Cove, then walked over to Tickle Point to the jail where I aspirated a knee of a prisoner. It had swelled up while he was doing hard labor, that is, scrubbing the courthouse floor. The prison is the most comfortable room in Twillingate, large, airy, warm, and clean. They eat with the sergeant so the food is good. The accused does not have housemaid's knee as advertised, but it is inside the joint and may well be tuberculosis. Back to a tub and a nice tea with bacon and eggs and pumpkin pie. I'm going to listen to the radio and go to bed as early as possible. I suppose I will have to get up again because Olds went off to the Tilt, leaving me in charge.

March 18, '38. Rose early to another pet day and my first feeling was one of envy for Waddell, out in such beautiful weather. Waddell's broken leg from Black Island came in and x-ray shows a bad break, healing well and with pretty good alignment. I put a cast on it and John came back. I wrote a note or two and a bad TB elbow came in. Then a call came to go down to Max Burt's. I know all about him. There was little sense in going but since it was such a nice day I went right after dinner. It was magnificent out—a good, fast-trotting pony, a clear sky and bright sun. We were there in no time in spite of the fact that the horse stepped through a hole and fell on his chin. I saw Max, had a cup of tea, and walked a good part of the salt ice back because it had gotten sticky. Arrived just in time for tea. Then to the Cottage for my usual loss at chess. The rest of my plan is to write this and go to bed. Waddell is not back and I sure wish he would come. The ice is breaking up off the point and he may well get stuck someplace.

Waddell rolled in at 12:30 just as I was turning in. He was in such a manic state after a fifty-mile round trip that he went right on to Tizzard's Harbor to see a neurotic, whose son had just returned from the woods and for whose attention she was making a bid.

March 19, '38. I realized with a start that in two days I'm supposed to leave for Washington to take the Public Health exams. The sun was bright and I hated to be indoors.

March 20, '38. Tried to clean up all the intravenous cases on the ward. Word came to be ready to leave by 9 A.M. At 6 A.M., it stormed worse than I had ever seen it. Blew a gale and snowed. I walked around the harbor paying bills. Saw the prisoner, drew $350.00 out of the bank. A party at night, not too successful. It was a buffet party with lots of rum. I took all my money along and "accidental like" scattered it on the floor for fun. Everybody grabbed for it and I thought it would wind up in a fight. I twisted Joyce's arm to get some of it back and she went crying upstairs, but returned. John got a chess bug so we played seven games. I won two. Waddell got sick and we all finally went to bed.

March 21, '38. Dawned dark and steamy. I finished off the treatments. They came up at 9 A.M. to get our luggage, which I frantically assembled. Marianne is going to the States too. We had two conveyances, a horse and cart, and a dog team and sled. We had lobster salad and apple pie and were off by 11:45 A.M. I started off with the dogs, which were in fine shape. At Bluff Head Cove, the Locke's warned us about distemper at Lewisporte. One of them was sitting on a frozen seal pelt. It looked like a great big pork chop, all one horse could pull. We took the ice at Gillard's Cove. Very good going. Both of us rode. I sat on the back and read my mail, walking only through the deeper drifts. It was not very cold but the sun was hidden. Sometimes we rode with the dogs, sometimes with the horse, and sometimes we walked. We crossed Trump Island and New World Island reaching Newstead by 4 P.M. Here we planned to spend the night. The Eveleigh House, where we usually stay, appeared deserted. Finally the lady of the house appeared, groaning and complaining, "When I'm sick, I can't do anything for anybody. I hate to see people when I'm sick. I can't get a girl to work for me that isn't sloppy. I've had two hemorrhages today." Complain, complain, complain. "What medicine are you taking?" ask I solicitously. "None," says she, and then, pointedly, "all I need is a little rest and quiet."

It seemed kind of pointless to ask if we could spend the night in the face of this. She did set out a fine tea for us and I set my socks on fire trying to dry them by the parlor stove. I kind of don't blame her. This house is a crossroads for winter travel. Everybody and his grandfather drops in here. The ten miles to Lewisporte were kind of dreary. We finally found ourselves well housed at the King George, miserable clapboard shack that it is. The linoleum felt like a Persian carpet.

CHAPTER IV

Journal from May 1938

May 9, '38. I have let my writing go shamefully and I'll never make it up tonight because I'm waiting only to have a cup of tea with Edith so that I can go to bed early. While bending over a patient tonight, I was suddenly taken with a monstrous pain in the back just to the right of the mid-dorsal spine. It seems to be muscular but of course tuberculosis of the spine presents itself as a possibility.

Today was quite a day. I was waked at 6:30 A.M. by Hazel. A lad had been sent in by Dr. Knapp, who said he should be operated on at once. I examined him, took a history, did a white count (6,000), and a urine (negative). His temperature was 100.4. His belly was hard and John said he could feel a mass. We opened him up and found an abscess with a rotten appendix lying on top. After waiting a while, we went in on Miss West and found her peritoneum an inch thick and typically studded with countless tubercules. We finally got her appendix out by slitting the casing and just sort of withdrawing it. Then I did two tonsils and adenoids and by that time it was 2:00.

I rushed through dinner and went to Purcell's Harbor, where a boat had been waiting since 9:00. We crossed the rough Main Tickle to Lobster Harbor and walked over the ridge to Indian Cove to see some pleurisy. The walk is a lovely one with a steep hill at both ends. I made five calls on the way back to the hospital. There I filled a few prescriptions, inspected and certified the death of a macerated fetus, and made rounds. After tea, I was doing some dressings on the ward when my great pain came on. I managed to cripple through an intravenous and do a bit of writing. After a cup of tea I'm going to bed.

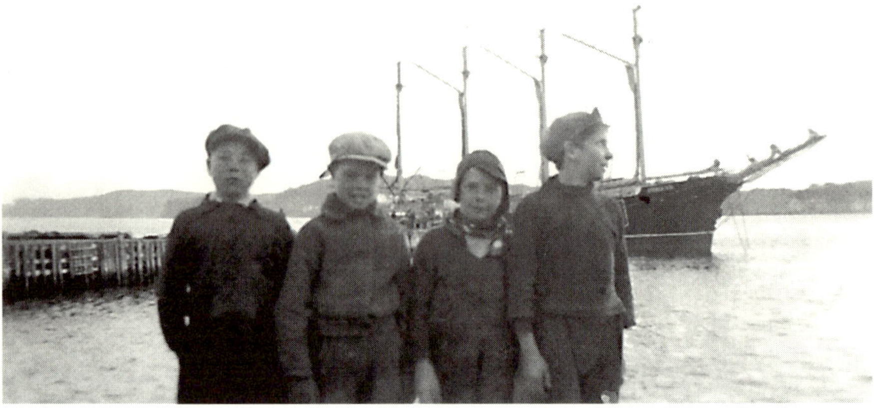

Young local stalwarts against the three-masted *Bessie Marie* broadside and an unknown schooner head on. Author's photograph.

May 10, '38. At 4 A.M., Hazel woke me to say that some men had come from Comfort Cove to get a doctor for a woman in labor. I should have loved to go but I couldn't raise my head from the pillow. By this time I had decided it was lumbago. They had asked for Dr. Olds but said Dr. Ecke would do. Then she asked if Dr. Wood would do and they said yes. When she called Dr. Wood on the phone, he thought it was kind of funny, because everybody knows where he lives.

I rose with great difficulty, did a cystoscopy and went over to Davis Cove for a very cold ride to open an axillary abscess in a nine-day-old babe and took the stitches out of mama. Mama was engaged six years ago and the wedding feast was all prepared at the groom's house in Black Duck Cove. When the bridegroom called for her in French Head her mother told him she couldn't come because she had just gone into labor. He went home and went to bed without even telling the guests and he never did marry her since it wasn't his baby. The veterinary stopped me on the way back to give me a clump of spring onions. He was in the very act of digging them as I passed his gate.

The day had turned as I left and become warm and beautiful. The afternoon was busy and I hurried down the Arm to a broken leg in a six-year-old. I brought him back in a splint to put him in overhead suspension. Rounds and tea. Four patients came in from Summerford, including a woman who had had a suspension. She was six months pregnant and having quite a lot of pain. Last year she aborted twins at six months. We had to send her home to bed. Then I put a new cast on John's sprained ankle and admitted a bad heart. It's a splendid night. You can hear a constant roar of surf and I wonder if the faint steady murmur, as of a distant train or city, can be the much-delayed northern ice coming in. Our own ice is all gone now, but we can expect the ice from the north anytime. This is the ice seals are born on. The moon is all but full.

May 16, '38. I am disgusted at my poor attempts at keeping a journal. The week has been the busiest of my whole life. We have seen twenty-five or so a day and have been glued to either the operating table or the OPD. We opened May West and her peritoneum was an inch thick with TB. We opened Bulgin Smith and he had an abscess. We opened Miss Purchase of Exploits and she was full of pus, with the worst appendix we've had in some time. It looked like a piece of rotten liver. We opened Mr. West to take out his badly infected kidney and he went into profound shock so that we couldn't do any kind of a job. I've been getting a lot of practice dissecting out veins to put in continuous drips. I can do it in fifteen minutes now. Today I did a tonsil and a hydrocele, a funny double one with a constriction in the center. The one I did on Decker is wasted, because he has developed tubercular meningitis and that means curtains.

Drover was down for three or four days and drank all our rum. He's a great guy though and it's always fun to have him visit us. Today it snowed a little and hailed a lot. Cold, nasty and wet. Today the *Clyde* comes. Sue Burnett sent me *Kennebec* with an inscription to me written by the author, R.P.T. Coffin. I wept. Those people are terribly important to me.

May 19, '38. As I write this, I wish I were out on the OB case that will materialize tonight. Edith went down with me an hour ago and prepared the patient. She was mad when she found that Kelly was going down with me later. Coming out from Yeat's, we went up that hill and the view was something. The dark blue of Burnt Island and Long Point framed a piece of peacock-blue sea. Against the lighter sky, a schooner was beating in with all sails set. It was as lovely a sight as I've ever seen. There's the bell.

I went down as fast as I could round up Kelly. The baby had already come, also the placenta. No tear, hard uterus, everything was fine. We fixed up the mother and the boy and left in half an hour. Armchair obstetrics I call it. I've had the OB bag down there for ten days and been dreading it. Today West looked better. I gave him lots of intravenous and I sort of feel that he has passed some kind of crisis and may even go on to get well. The mail was pretty good. Mother gave me hell for not writing and I've written her three letters. Tonight we had a grand tea. Just the three of us. All the lobster we could eat, good whiskey before tea, and a cigar after lemon pie.

May 20, '38. A rather busy day—I didn't draw a breath until 6:00 P.M. I was awakened at seven in the morning by the arrival of a girl in the throes of a bad appendix. John and I debated as to whether it was ruptured or not. She had been here before with other attacks and had been advised to come back and have it out. I opened her up and found a normal appendix. The second was an elegant perineal repair by John. There had been a bad laceration—gaped like an old barn door. He took a slip off the gluteus and tacked it across. Next I did a double vasectomy. Then in the OPD until 5:30. Among others I saw Mrs. Alf Warren—she was easily pacified. West is much better. Decker died tonight of his TB meningitis. It seems to me that sunsets here have a delicacy of color not gained anywhere else in the world.

I don't believe I've said enough about my trip to the States. We stayed at the King George and were a bit bored. Another party arrived from Twillingate escorting a patient to the insane asylum at St. John's. At 4:30 A.M. we caught the narrow gauge *Overland Express* at Notre Dame Junction to find Kay Kearney on the train. We were great friends in '34 when Mirick and I were summer students at the hospital, and now she was headed to a nursing job at Buchans. We talked furiously and had breakfast until we reached Badger. After a fruitless search for her camera, she got off without it. She has a sixty-mile dog team trip ahead of her. I then tried to sleep, but three loud guys were smoking bum cigars and drinking and playing Auction 45 in the section across the aisle. An important part of Auction 45 is hitting the table with your hand when you put a card down. The trip to Port Aux Basques was long and slow.

The *Caribou* couldn't leave that night but we slept aboard. The next day was spent in the ice. It's a fearful sound below deck, banging and crashing and heaving. Until you get used to it you think the ice is coming right into the stateroom. The ice got too thick for us and we spent ten hours drifting with it. Captain Tavenor looked very casual playing cribbage in the saloon. He didn't tell us until the next morning that we were being driven awfully close to a reef. There was nothing anybody could do about it and God knows, there was plenty of ice to get onto, if we started to sink. We spent all the time we were moving on the peak, watching the ice pans split up.

Marianne was so chummy with the customs officer at Sydney that I thought she knew him. The ride through the Maritimes was leisurely and pleasant. It seemed to go on forever. We were in good spirits and enjoyed the gifts of civilization.

I climbed out at Brunswick, Maine, at 3:30 A.M. and walked around town, had innumerable cups of coffee at all-night joints, read a whole paper at the Alpha Delt house and what not, until I saw the next door Burnett's newspaper had been taken in. Charles came to the door at 7:30 when I tried it and put his arms around me in a warm embrace. After breakfast, I saw Sue Burnett and was at home. I stayed there five days and then went to New York on the *State of Maine* with Jim Abramson and President Johnston of Colby. I had a joyous week at home, without going out at all.

The night before the exams, I hurried on to Washington by sleeper, arriving there in a bit of a stew. I hurried right over to the Public Health Office. They arranged immediately for my physical examination. I walked over to the other building and it was hot. The examination was accomplished with more dispatch than it was the last time, but my blood pressure was at 160. They didn't like it that high. They sent me out to lunch to calm down. I spent lunchtime looking for a bank and dying from the heat.. On my return, it was only a little better. I had called up Major General Birnie. I went over to a very enjoyable dinner and evening. At the Public Health Office in the morning Surgeon General Draper gave me very short shrift, in fact I was out of the running. I was a little annoyed but in a sense relieved. I left with a fellow rejectee who was bounced for his eyes. Though I had lived thirty miles away for six years, for the first time I saw the disappointing cherry blossoms. I returned to the General's for dinner again and then left for Baltimore to renew my Hopkins acquaintanceships. In Baltimore the powers indicated that they wanted me to work there next year on poliomyelitis. That was disconcerting. Another visit with my family, another stop at Brunswick, and soon I was back north again in the land of the lotus-eaters. The lotus' up here don't have enough vitamins in them.

May 26, '38. How can I gain the strength of character to keep a decent journal? This week has passed as rapidly as any in my remembrance. The weather has been perfect and I sit here now on a day unsurpassed—perhaps only by one with a little less breeze. The sky is a complete blue as is the sea.

We have been doing lots of appendices, circumcisions, tonsils, everything. This morning we explored a mildly obstructed man and found an adhesion to the large gut. We had demonstrated the exact spot by x-ray.

I've made a few trips to Indian Cove, Lobster Harbor, and Merritt's Harbor. The roads are all open now. West died this week, ten days after operation. He developed tetanus and floods of anti-toxin were useless. John was much upset. He had stayed up with him the last three nights. I had sat with him and planned a camping trip with him that I knew could never happen. He was to supply the dogs. I would supply the food. We were glad finally to find a chaperon to take Mrs. Watson to the insane asylum. Yesterday I drove down to Gillard's Cove to see a woman with a sacroiliac and just off Bluff Head is the biggest, whitest iceberg I've ever seen. I'd give a lot to get out to it and take some pictures but we're so damn busy it would be impossible.

It is swell with Waddell away. I have a great affection for him, but with him gone I can take a greater interest in the patients, and am consulted once in a while. John is an accomplished surgeon and a fine person, but he is modest and humble. He does not strut around as if every word he says is the latest medical discovery. I had a man in who wanted me to look at his knee. He didn't want to take off his clothes and I did not urge because I was busy and in a hurry. I looked at the knee and found nothing. He went to Beckwith, who did the same. He came back here, better, but not enough better. John made him undress and, by God, he had a full-blown tubercular hip.

Father Casey was here a couple of days from Fortune Harbor and we had a good game of poker at which the good father won, protesting all the time that he was new at the game. He's an affable soul and I enjoyed playing with him very much. John isn't well. I went over his chest and found nothing, but persuaded him to drink a bit of milk. Mail has been generous enough.

The afternoon was lovely. Dr. Wood held down the OPD while I went to Gillard's Cove on the cycle to see a baby's umbilicus. I strapped a half-dollar over it (my own) and fought with the mama to get her to put the baby out in the sun. We stopped at Bluff Head on the way back to see that magnificent iceberg. We walked up to the head to get a good look at it but within fifty yards the motorcycle gave one unmistakable pffft of a flat. It meant a long hot walk home. I got a splinter putting a picket through the call bag handles so that I could carry it home. As we arrived, they were looking for us to emerge on Jenny Bowen from whom we took the tubes and appendix. I don't know if emerge is a proper word. We used it at Hopkins to indicate an emergency unscheduled operation. The tubes were fiery

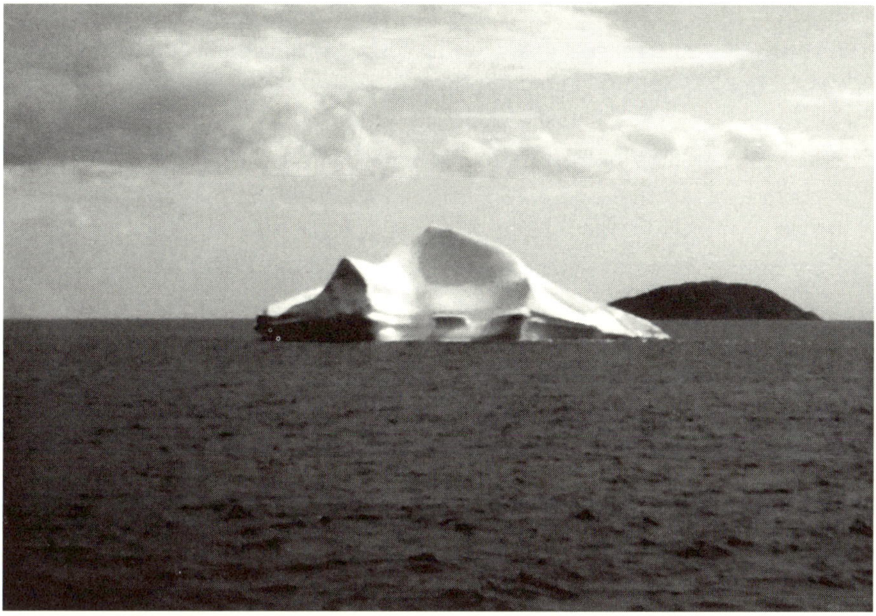

The iceberg. Author's photograph.

red and gelatinous. Then tea and off to Mamie Roberts for a pleasant evening of hearing about Twillingate Sterling and playing the organ. Twillingate Sterling was the daughter of Dr. Sterling and left here to become a world famous concert singer. She had a younger brother who fell into a rain barrel and drowned. She was also a favorite of H.M. Edward VII.

May 27, '38. Up at 1:00 to see one of our nursing staff, Nan, with a pain in her belly that must be adhesions. Her pain had moved from her gall bladder down to her appendix but thank God that's been out for years. Had to get up again at 5:00 to fool with Mr. Snellgrove. He has trouble passing his water. I couldn't pass a catheter and John suggested a silver one, which worked and relieved me more than it did Mr. Snellgrove. The silver catheter was over a hundred years old. I took it out of my collection of antique medical instruments gleaned from the estate of Dr. Sterling. Wildly busy the whole morning with OPD and a few casts. Dinner and we finally opened Snellgrove's bladder from above with good local anesthesia. After a busy afternoon in the OPD, I went to Bluff Head to tell a patient that it was all right for her to come to the hospital to have her baby. She followed me by a few hours.

Saul White is getting ready to go to the Labrador in his schooner for the summer cod fishery. I fixed him up a first aid box, a schooner box. I also did him the disservice of sending his best crewman, the fish splitter, home with the mumps. I told the Smiths to come for Selby Burt so he can die at home. I don't know exactly what that means because he has no home and no family. The day seemed extremely full and my feet hurt. John and I are both dead tired. He is worried about Nan, on whom he thinks he will have to operate, though he does not believe operation is justified on the basis of pain only, with no disturbance of physiology. Five people are dying: Snellgrove, Trowbridge with TB meningitis, Bartlett with TB hemorrhages, Selby Burt with TB everywhere, and Freak with pneumonia. Mrs. Adams and Janey are not at all well.

There is Hazel knocking at my chamber door. It is just midnight and she wants me to do something for Mr. Snellgrove. I will give him an intravenous and if that OB goes into labor I will scream.

June 1, '38. It seems to me that promises made to yourself are to be kept, as well as those made to others. That is if there is an absolute, and I think there is. Some things just are. A certain calm has finally come into our lives and things have not been so hectic recently, though on Saturday we did do Nan. All we found was a large adhesion involving the small and large intestines in the region of the middle ascending colon and she has been worse than Mrs. Adams ever since. When we had finished her, I was sent down to Manuel's Cove to see a Mrs. Gillard. The name didn't mean anything to me. I wandered down and it seems to me she has been pregnant for years. She has been in a kind of mild labor for three days. Doccy Wood has been watching her and wanted me to have a look-see. They must be the poorest people in Twillingate, but their house is the one where I would take a visitor to see a really lovely fisherman's home. Clean, neat, attractive garish wallpaper. Curtains of bleached flour bags with colorful bits of cloth appliquéd to make borders. The kitchen has lots of hooked rugs, a well-shined low stove, a few neat homemade chairs, and a good-looking sideboard, also homemade.

I didn't recognize Mrs. Gillard until I saw the missing leg. It was amputated four years ago for tuberculosis in the knee. She is a hard-working, honest woman. She lay there quietly in bed and told me how poor they were. No merchant will advance them food. There wasn't a crust of bread in the house. I examined her and the baby seemed to be huge. I felt we would never be able to do anything in the house. In fact, I was sure she would need a caesarean. I explained to her that she couldn't have a baby without an operation. There was none of the frequently encountered hysteria. She was silent for a moment while her eyes became moist. "All right, doctor," she said quietly, "do what you can to help me but remember, life is sweet." I was deeply stirred by this woman's plain faith in the world—in the face of the little it had done for her. I got out of the house quickly, so her husband wouldn't wonder why my eyes were wet.

John agreed that we should do a caesarean—out was dragged a hydrocephalic. The huge head made me wonder what would have happened if I had tried to deliver her at home. I told the nurses not to urge it to breathe but, of course, it came to life at once and thrives. I leaned over it in the nursery several times and wondered if I should pop a morphine tablet into its mouth. But it is not nursing too well, so I don't believe it will really survive.

Sunday was not very exciting, in fact I don't remember doing a damn thing—until yesterday evening. Just as Betty and Edith were going sailing a woman brought her seven-year-old boy into the OPD from Leading Tickle. He was bright and cute but had a hard belly with a mass in both lower quadrants. She was horrified when told his appendix had ruptured and she had kept him at home too long. She wrung her hands and said she would leave him for treatment, but she couldn't think of an operation. She was distraught all right, with much "save my poor child," and so forth. We told her she would be a murderess if she took him home. She said she would rather have him die at home than die here. My heart wasn't really in this argument because we felt he was hopeless. She changed her mind about four times while we said, "For God's sake, lady," and such. Finally she said she would leave him but she wanted to see what he thought about it. She then asked her seven-year-old if he wanted to stay. He said "No." And she said she didn't want him crying, so she would take him home. John grabbed her by the arm and I thought he would clonk her. She finally gave in and we found large abscesses and couldn't make any effort to get the appendix. He has been pretty good today, but he's been without eating and drinking so long that I have my doubts.

I've never seen anyone so mad as Joyce when we went for her to give the anesthetic. We caught her in her Girl Guide costume just as she was getting over Grenham's Hill to go for an evening with her troop. She threw a teacup on the rocks and broke it. Then wouldn't stir or say a word. I thought she would cry any minute. She didn't cool off for twenty-four hours.

Today I made seven calls and one of them was to the Clark family, where one old woman supports herself, the useless husband, two sons, their wives, and ever arriving children. Said wives refuse to bring their babies to the clinic. I had finally persuaded one, delivered by Dr. Wood four months ago, to take cod liver oil. Today the mother told me Wood had said a nursing baby didn't need cod liver oil so she stopped it. I was mad as hell. Before God, I make a promise to myself to write this journal at least five evenings a week.

June 2, '38. A bad day with John in a blood mood. In the first place, the Fogo doctor arrived in a pouring rain at 8:45 A.M. with a 13-year-old boy with "jaw-lock." To control the convulsions, he had been pouring chloroform on him all night in a perfect deluge and we will never know whether he died of chloroform poisoning or tetanus. I gave him 70 milligrams of avertin.

We went up to work on Ruby White who had an ovarian cyst and funny sclerosed tubes. I thought it was not the morning to assert myself, but John should have let me do it. I won't stay here if he doesn't let me operate a bit more. I am making no special progress and there is no need of my staying if I don't. I could go up to St. Anthony's and work for Sir Wilfred Grenfell's Mission I think.

After the operation, I cut down on the tetanus boy, who was out cold. Put a continuous drip near his ankle and had a tough time getting the apparatus to work. Meanwhile, John had his hands full operating on the old dame with a mass in her left side the size of a watermelon. I think it's a kidney cyst, but John thinks she has no kidney on that side because he couldn't find the ureter when he cystoscoped her.

I gave a transfusion to poor little Willy Hammond, who isn't doing very well. He's the seven-year-old whose mother we fought with. Then I put some air in Ruby Penney's chest. Dictated a few notes until dinnertime. In the afternoon I gave tetanus antitoxin to our boy from Fogo and just before rounds he had another convulsion. His chest filled up and his lungs got awfully wet. The right side of his heart apparently had failed. Willy Hammond died just after tea and his mother was very calm. She didn't know where she would get a coffin. She allowed almost any boat would come for the body from Leading Tickle. She hadn't been able to get one to bring her boy down while sick, though he had had a ruptured appendix for nine days. Now that he is dead, the population will fall all over themselves showing respect. I rigged up suction for the tetanus but I feel nothing can save him, though we have sent the family to Lewisporte to get more antitoxin.

John was getting a cold by 10:30, so I suppose he'll be worse than ever tomorrow. I don't care much, my own cold has me preoccupied enough. Now it's time for a cup of tea and to bed. I am continually cheered by the prospect of going to camp. I'm going to teach canoeing at Winona, in Maine, this summer. I know it will set me back months professionally. I also want to bring my sister back with me in the fall. She would enjoy it here and I would like having her. Her ability to amuse herself is rather well marked.

June 3, '38. Routed myself out at what I thought was an early hour. While taking a leisurely shave, I heard John announce that Arch Peyton, the custom inspector, was yelling for a doctor to go aboard a steamer loaded with pit props to be used down in the mines. I looked out the bathroom window and sure enough, there she was—flying her yellow quarantine flag. I hurried and walked down to Blanchard's Wharf. There was a launch tied up but neither of the blokes sitting on the deckhouse spoke to me. I then hurried to Ashbourne's Wharf, but not before I watched a fellow in the morning sun fixing a bit of rigging in a trim, forty-ton schooner. For a minute I daydreamed myself a trip to the Labrador. At Ashbourne's someone told me they were waiting for me back at the other wharf. I was sore at those two blokes for not speaking up. After all, they were there to fetch me and they knew me.

We were quickly at the ship, the 4,000-ton *Kirsten Maerkel.* The captain was a fine steady man with an amazing knowledge of English and a store of aquavit. I had some, smoked a few Turkish cigarettes, cleared the ship and invited him ashore. He brought a man into the hospital with a broken rib, well done up with a hot compress. There also came a crewman to have a tooth out. He stood quiet while I raped him practically. I've never had a tooth put up such a fight. The other lad was soon in bed and Bessie was making friends with him. How she does it without knowing any Danish is more than I can tell. He knows a little Polish. It might as well be Sanskrit.

The rest of the day was nothing much. Everyone was pretty good except Miss Trowbridge who is dying terribly slowly. She crawls out of her bed at night sometimes and scares Hazel to death coming down the dark hall on her hands and knees. She is a pretty healthy-looking girl but has the fatal TB bug in her brain. Nan had a great pain in her shoulder tonight. It's probably pleurisy. Over to Edith's to the regular late cup of tea.

They had gotten a pint of clotted Devonshire cream and a jar of bakeapples. The bakeapple is a funny-tasting local berry but sawdust would be good with Devonshire cream on it. The tetanus boy died at midnight last night. It could be straight tetanus and yet I don't know if pulmonary congestion on a cardiac basis could account for it. The father came hurrying back this morning with 3,000 units of antitoxin, all he could find in Lewisporte. The whole thing was a sad business.

My heart was again moved by seeing the ship leave this afternoon. I long for the snugness of a ship's cabin. It's an independent life. A ship is such a complete unit—so aloof, so proud. That empty piece of harbor shows no trace of a big boat with the midships pumped up with five feet of water as ballast. Even then the propeller stuck out two feet.

June 4, '38. Busy as hell most of the day. We didn't get around to break for tea until almost seven. Nan suddenly shot a temperature and has consolidation at the base of the right chest and pain in the left shoulder. God knows what it can be at this late date—too late for pneumonia—it must be an embolus. John is worried. Daphne has a pain in her right side. Miss Gillette has a pain all over her back. Miss Kelly has a pain in her knee. Sometimes I think I'll go crazy with all this ailing staff. I think if I ever run a hospital it'll be on a condition that the help go somewhere else with their troubles.

June 5, '38. A calm enough day. I sat in the sun until 10 A.M. and then boats came from Gander Bay, Herring Neck, and Change Island. People came from the Arm and from Carmanville. We treated until 6 P.M. then sent them to wherever they could go. These boats are busy fishing all week so Sunday is the day they come to the hospital. I took a long cutaneous horn from a boy's ear. I mooned around cursing the cold bath water and am on my way to bed.

June 6, '38. A busy morning. I took out an appendix and was sore as usual because John fished it out while I was washing my hands. Then I helped on a hernia, another appendix, and a cystoscopy. That was a bad one. The patient has TB in her right kidney and some nonspecific infection in her left. We can't do a thing. Then I took out the largest tonsil I've ever seen. In the afternoon I grew weary of doctoring the staff—Kelly with a knee, Locke with a nose, Gillette with a back, Wheeler with a side, Daphne with a side. And then there is always Nan Farrell's adhesions. The mail came with a letter from mother and dad.

A few nights back at midnight Dr. Wood sent for me to give chloroform for a home OB patient. She lay on her back in a most animal position, quite unclothed. Dr. Wood was cussing and fuming about how careless, slovenly, dirty and lazy the patient was—how she was carrying on. She herself was a condensed milk baby. Dr. LeDrew had delivered her mother. Nothing to work with; she was a lot of trouble; he would never come back; and so forth. The midwife agreed with him and I must confess there was only one diaper by way of a layette. She was on a piece of oilcloth Dr. Wood said he wouldn't put on his back porch. As a matter of fact the whole thing was quite unattractive. I poured some chloroform while he did a low forceps. He lost his sterile instruments in the bedclothes and poked around for them with his elbow.

June 7, '38. Up to do a graft with John, but I had to leave on an OB call to Louis Blake. I cannot describe the poverty and shiftlessness. The only place to sit in the kitchen is a box. Three teacups were visible by way of dishes. The boy with the knee I fixed a month ago was lying asleep on the floor with his head under the stove. The bed is falling down. A piece of firewood under one end. It seems to me someone could make a bench or some kind of couch for the kitchen. She wasn't doing much—I've been back to see her twice today. Daphne's pain got worse and we are about to operate.

June 9, '38. No time to turn around. Up early on a rainy day to help John take out a uterus. It was a great performance in a deep narrow pelvis. The patient has done well. The cutting of the vagina is a dreadfully blind business and I wouldn't have been surprised to see the leg drop off. I was called away to see Mrs. Cooper. She is doing nothing. Then I had trouble with a cystoscopy and had to call John. After a patient or two I had dinner, the first fresh rhubarb. After dinner, Mrs. Warren came in, desperate. I told her I might be able to help her but she would have to pay for the importing of expensive medicine—hormones. She asked what her trouble was. I said it wouldn't do any good to tell her it was in her glands—in her head, her ovaries, her neck and near her kidneys. She said she knew it all the time because she could feel every one of them. After tea it was raining torrents. I had to go out though to see a broken arm and I couldn't keep dry. I had just settled after that when another call came in. Mrs. Cooper again and it was another false alarm. I'd just gotten warm and dry when another OB call came. I took Bessie and went down to Froude's Hill. This was a strange woman, whom I thought at first to be insane. She lay quietly in a single bed that occupied three-fourths of the room. "Is this about the time you expected the baby?" I ask. "No," she says, "tomorrow." It came easily enough. I fixed it and her and left with neither good-bye nor thank you.

I was in bed two minutes when a man came from Exploits. I found a very tender belly. He'd had a stomach operation for ulcers fifteen years before in Toronto. The present pain was a day old. I opened him without advice and found a very red-hot appendix. It was 4 A.M. before I got to bed.

June 10, '38. This day was kind of fun. I did a million odd jobs including a skin graft on the Burt boy. He knocked his funny bone against the door-jamb and fainted, falling with his bare feet against the hot stove. His mother fanned him and tried to bring him to, but did nothing about the toasting feet. The afternoon was spent on tripe of various sorts. A patient from the *S.S. Northern Ranger* kept me up until 2:30 A.M. She either can't or won't swallow. I had to feed her intravenously.

June 11, '38. I was being very busy in the morning when Arch Peyton, the customs man, called for a doctor to clear a steamer, the *Hans Maersk*, 2,300 tons, A.C. Christianson, Skipper. While Arch was pettifogging about a three-ton discrepancy in the registration, the sergeant and I had quite a bout of aquavit, scotch, and ale. I had been a long time since eating and could scarcely get down the gangplank. I got to dinner by about 3:00 and spilled a glass of water on my lap. It made for a bad afternoon. I hate to work without sleep and hungover. There was a chance to lie in the sun on the flagpole curbing for a half-hour until the laundryman's wife found me to pull some teeth. I paid for it. When Hazel woke me at 2 A.M. for a delivery upstairs, I was paralyzed with lumbago, worse than the time before. Then the pain was near the sternum, but now it's in my back and killing me. This delivery was no fun. I had to prop myself up. I lay on the stretcher until she delivered and it took a lot of codeine to get me to bed.

June 12, '38. Up about 8 A.M. and I crippled to the Cottage to steal a cup of coffee and chat a while with Dr. Patten. He is a surgeon on his way to St. Anthony with his wife. I liked him very much. Business soon picked up. Another OB was cooking and I planned to let it go until after dinner but

John changed my mind. He and Dr. Patten came down to watch me do a low forceps. It went smoothly but dinner was late. Then hundreds came in from everywhere. Squadron Commander Pattison was here from the Botwood Seaplane Base. He took the boys out in his tender, which will do 34 miles per hour. After a cup of tea at Edith's, I'm going to bed and I hope to God nothing happens tonight.

June 17, '38. Somewhere I've lost a week. It passed with no special event, except that on Monday after an extremely busy day, Tommy announced it was her birthday. This was just before tea and would we like a nip. It would have to be quick because Dr. and Mrs. Patten were waiting at the Cottage for us to join them. John and I went over for the nip. Things moved rapidly and in half an hour we were for letting tea go. We sent a note to Betty telling her to leave her guests and come down for a drink. She came down all right and gave us hell and made us all troop up to the Cottage. I wore Tommy's glasses and an ice cap and carried a bottle of rum under my shirt. In a short time, we were all very merry. I did some yoga and was being a great success when Joyce put my shoes in the fire because she didn't like them and someone cut the belt of my pants again, my favorite blue dungarees. We started to have tea but I left in the middle and the rest was silence until 4 A.M. when Hazel announced a patient in the OPD. I didn't think fate could be that cruel. I've never felt worse in my life. And here was a ruptured appendix from Fogo and we had to operate. I lived fifty years doing that operation and even had to cut down on a vein to start a drip. I was only a little better at 9:00 when John did a repair and I felt all gone the whole week. Every morning has been hell to get started and we have been very busy. We are fretting for the Hopkins students to arrive. We heard that they will be here tomorrow but now it is raining and blowing a gale.

I was lying down when a call came to see Mrs. Lewis White. By the time I figured it must be Mrs. Lewis Blake, it was too late, but I arrived in time to tie the cord and she was glad to see me. She is actually charming and has handsome friendly children, though the whole setup is grotesquely poor. I want to give them at least a chair but I'm told it will have to be of iron or they will burn it. The ride down to that house was a wild wet one. I blew a tire and had to walk most of the way back with the heavy OB bag. A good mail, including a letter from Aunt Dob. I'm eager to be off to camp, but won't get there until the second day because Waddell is slow in getting back from his trip home to Virginia.

I've been doing a lot of operating—boldly slashed a lip to take out a cancer when it would have terrified me only shortly since. I believe that I am beginning to get a feeling for surgery and will try almost anything.

June 18, '38. Hazel came in at 2 A.M. to tell me that Mrs. Burdin was going at it strongly. I couldn't believe my ears but there she was, only two hours along and about to have her baby. I thought I must be dreaming but I watched her with a doze here and there and at 5:30 she delivered. It was a forceps—just a matter of lifting the head over the perineum. That early start made the day seem long and it rained furiously most of the day. A little after 2:00 the students came and we had rounds.

Solomon Coles was here and a more obnoxious person I can't imagine—all the time whining about the death of his wife here with her broken leg. He says he lifted a bedstead at her funeral and strained himself. He also wanted a hat of hers that had disappeared. There is a rumor that he didn't get his wife's body at all, but Mrs. Osmond's or some girl from Gander Bay. His wife had a relative who went to Australia and made millions. He came home poorly dressed and lived with his relatives as if he were broke. He then left his money to them according to how they treated him. Mrs. Coles got quite a bit and it certainly ruined Solomon. If I could have blotted him out today, I would have. He drives me crazy with his story of something gathering inside of him and bursting— "like flesh." We had a few drinks at the Cottage and went to bed early.

June 19, '38. Hazel was after me at 7:30 to see the Bridger girl. I took my time for I have a belief that if the baby comes before I can get there they didn't need a doctor at all. I took Hazel and was there by 8:00. I sat around until 11:30 and she wasn't getting anywhere. I read a dull book—don't remember the title of it but it had a cockroach pressed between the leaves. I listened to the tale of woe from the mother complaining about her daughter's not having a husband. I took Hazel home and brought one of the students back with me getting there just in time. There weren't any sutures in the OB bag and I had to dash all the way back to get some. There was quite a lot of interest in the baby. It weighed eight and one-half pounds and had to be an eight-month baby to make the right one guilty. He certainly looked mature for that age.

After tea I still had seven calls to make. I took the other student and after the calls I showed him my favorite Codjack Cove. The crannies are filled with moss flowers and white violets. The sky and sea were blue and

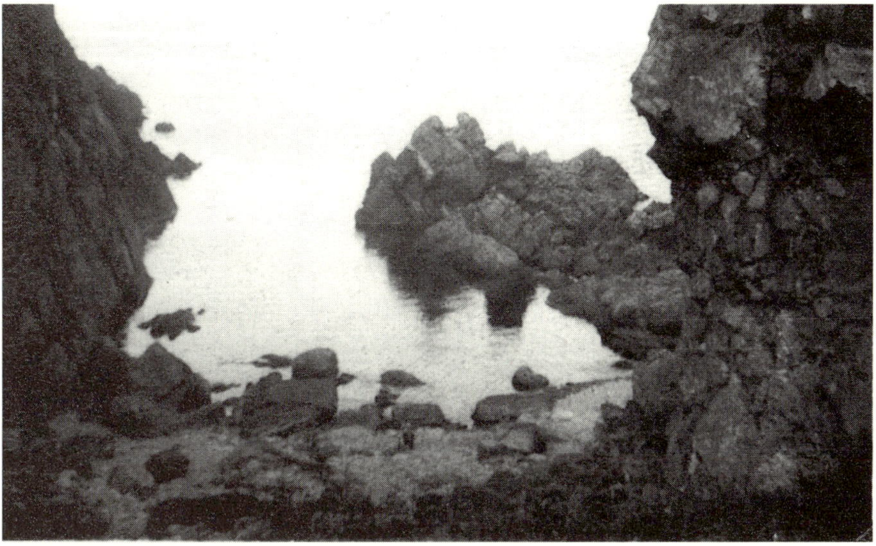

Codjacks Cove. Author's photograph.

the air soft and sweet. From the cliff we saw a steamer coming in so I hurried back because I thought it was the Swedish ship with the good scotch. Just as I got back Mrs. Boone had some kind of a fit and I thought she would need a tracheotomy. John came down to diagnose it hysteria. Then I went out to the steamer which was a beauty. It had a funny, shore-like quality with curtains at the portholes and pots of flowers and a checkered tablecloth in the saloon. That's because the captain and his two mates have their wives along with them. This time I was threatening to go ashore before I got a drink. The captain confessed he hadn't offered it because he didn't know whether or not I would be offended. Offended indeed!

June 20, '38. My God what a night! I was in bed twenty minutes when Dr. Wood brought in an OB, a strange young girl. She had had a pain in her belly and her father couldn't cure it so he brought her down to see if Dr. Wood couldn't find out why she couldn't dig potatoes. Dr. Wood was disconcerted to find a head on the perineum—he was scared to death she would deliver in his surgery. He rushed her down to the hospital and harried me while I delivered her. Everything seemed to go wrong and with one thing or another, the night wore on. This time, I was in bed a half-hour when a woman came in from Fogo with some abdominal pain. Her story was typical of appendicitis but she had had it out four years before.

I got Olds up about 5 A.M. and he couldn't make much of it either.

By 8:30 A.M. I was busy in the OPD. Canning came in with his bad foot. He'd been sitting around with it two months but made only three or four efforts to walk. I did several cystoscopies and sewed up a long laceration of the face. After dinner John decided to do that belly and we found a cheesy, rotten adhesion about the appendix scar and a mildly obstructed abdomen full of tuberculosis. The end of the ileum showed many dark purple spots that we were afraid to leave in because we thought they would perforate. We resected three feet of gut, which was quite a formidable procedure. I then showed the boys how to start a drip by cutting down a vein and it was teatime.

We had a party for the sergeant who is suddenly being shifted to St. Anthony. There was more fresh lobster than seven of us could eat. To bed at 12 A.M. and up at 3 A.M. to fix the drip. He's doing fine.

June 21, '38. Up too late to catch the *Clyde* and I had promised to get the boys' mail on it. I did an appendectomy with one of the students. It was my first operation of any account by myself. It went beautifully. Then I hurried over to catch Colbourne to send the mail but he had left. There were lots of odd jobs and they filled the rest of the day. I opened another mastoid abscess—that's the second, but I've never seen an acute one. It is only a week until I will be in Lewisporte on my way to Maine. I'm having a wonderful time being professor to these children but I know it will not last when Waddell comes back. In a way I wish I were going to be here. I do think it might be a decent summer, but there are going to be plenty of doctors and I wouldn't shine as I do now. My paper on Newfoundland came out in the *Bowdoin Alumnus* and I like it. I make everybody read it. Must do something to keep myself from getting too rusty at medicine this summer.

June 24, '38. This has been a busy and important few days for me. I finally got the mail off by rushing to Colbourne's the first thing in the morning. A double hernia was awaiting me on my return, no sac but all the same it was fun to operate as the boss. The rest of the morning was full of cystoscopies. I've done about six the last three days. I did two appendices this morning; on Tuesday that girl who kept me up Sunday night started to have pains about four in the—O God, I am getting old—what day is this? Well, anyhow she's doing beautifully.

CHAPTER V

Year the Second in Twillingate

September, 1938

Here I am starting a second year in this place. There is the summer to record, and the journey back. The day back in June I finally got off for Maine, Drover was hanging about, a little drunk. A month earlier, I got him to play poker with crafty Ralph Smith who still owes me $2.40 from last year. Bert Pardy and George Hawkins were in that game. Drover had put his feet on the table and insulted all of them. This was a little annoying since I felt sort of responsible for the game. Now as I was trying to pack, there was Drover in the room. John was there and the students were there. Everything was in a terrible mess and as a result I didn't assemble most of the things I wanted to take with me. The hospital had been going to send me to the medical meeting at St. John's. John was going to go at first so I would have had to wait until Waddell got back which would have made me quite late for camp. Two days before though, Cody, the bank manager, revealed that he was obstructed and John was afraid to leave him, had him on a preoperative regime, in fact, and was about to work on him the next day.

I planned to go to town but the board met on Saturday. The upshot of their deliberations was a decision not to send anyone to the medical meeting; too short sighted to see that the rest of Newfoundland regards us as high-hat and that a bit of intercourse would be good public relations for the hospital.

Eventually I took off for Lewisporte, sitting in the rain all the way. We passed right beside a beautiful iceberg. I just caught the train, after telling the characters at the station that they had made a mistake on my ticket. They denied it, then came running out on the platform to refund the $18.00 they had overcharged. Determined to go cheap I had got an upper, but after that I couldn't hold out, so I ate well and enjoyed the ride. The *Caribou* trip was smooth as glass. With a few hours in North Sydney I had a meal with the wonderful McKenzies and caught the train. On it I made friends with a professional baseball player farmed up here by the Yankees. I also took care of a kid, a six-year-old boy who had a four-year-old sister and a distraught mother with him. Before long they were both in my hair with butterscotch and what not.

Arrived uneventfully in Brunswick at 4 A.M., but on the way heard a good story in Truro where I fell in with Mr. Keile of Montreal who took me to breakfast. Keile owns the movies in St. John's and he told me of a trip he took on the *Florazel* in 1916 on New Year's Day out of St. John's to get films in Halifax. There was a lot of drinking and one thing and another and a roaring gale with thick snow. They rounded Cape Race only to run smack into the shore, having turned too early. He helped a terrified stewardess but she died of fright and the cold in a bunk, while he stood knee deep in ice water in his locker trying to keep himself warm by his breath.

He got on deck finally to find 30 survivors in the radio room but the heat and the smell were too much for him. The *Portia*, or some such ship, got boats to them at last. They gave him ginger ale afterwards on the rescue ship, for which he was given a bill for 20 cents. He started out the next day and got through. It was during the war and because of radio censorship his wire was the only one that made it through, "I was one of the lucky ones." All of St. John's besieged his wife for news of relatives. Over 100 had perished.

Perhaps the less said about the summer the better. The bright aspect of it was the time spent in Brunswick with the Burnetts. I was with them three days on my way to camp during which my arm was growing tender; becoming so painful during the drive to camp that I reported in at the infirmary, stayed there four days, went to Portland, had it operated on for an abscess and spent ten days in the hospital waiting for my temperature to come down. After four or five days in Brunswick recuperating, I went back to camp at which point mother and father came up to visit me for a week. The day they left my arm got sore again and I went through my routine—infirmary, hospital, Brunswick. By this time, the summer was over and I had done precious little canoeing.

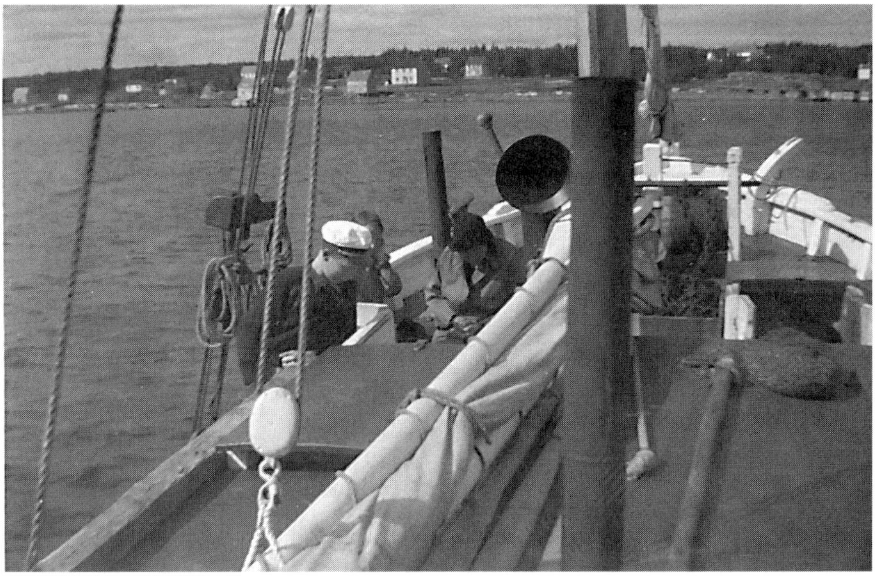

Patients at the clinic hatch, hospital boat *Bonnie Nell.* Author's photograph.

The Burnetts sent along a companion for the trip back to Twillingate—a big, prize Irish Setter, Dudley Sean O'Connor by name, probably the most beautiful specimen that elegant breed ever produced.

September 11, '38. Well I seem to be back in Twillingate. I arrived two days ago and have done little but get settled. There's not much sense in getting involved because in two days I take the *Bonnie Nell* out to the north side of the bay. I've decided to take the dog, Dudley, with me. I'm afraid if I leave him behind he won't know me when I come back.

September 12, '38. Left Twillingate after sixteen false starts for the north side of the bay run. In true Newfoundland manner, though the *Bonnie Nell* has been laid up for five days, they found the bearings were bad just as we were ready to take off. Confusion reigned. The students were leaving by *Clyde* and trying to get last-minute pictures of everybody. They even made Suzie get dressed in her red dress and hat. They also made me get the motorcycle out to pose in calling costume. I went back and forth from the wharf for fifty forgotten things. No watch with a second hand, no alcohol lamp, at least we didn't find one until I had gotten another. The stickem paper was all stuck together. Before we really left I took Dudley up

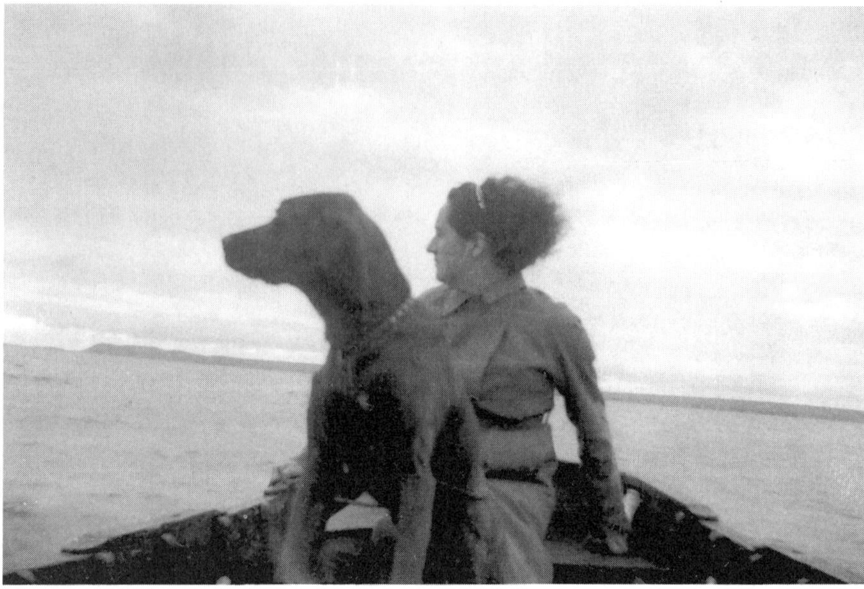

Doris and Dudley—profiles in auburn. Author's photograph.

to the Cottage for a bit of food. We finally pulled out of the harbor at 12:30 for Black Island.

I put on shorts and took off my shirt, then fought with Dudley for a place on the mat on deck. It was warm for an hour or two. The boat is a good one, 25 tons, 50 feet long, 13 in the beam. There's a large saloon midships, with two small cabins—mine and Doris Downer's, whom I didn't know by name before she signed up for this jaunt. I have to go through her room to get to the john, which is entered through a doorway four feet high, but you can stand up once you get inside. It has another entrance from the engine room. The saloon could be swell but is piled with boxes of medicine and boxes of food—enough for an army for a year. If proper lockers were made, it would be nice, but it's good enough and in this country, anything that's good enough is plenty good enough and not to be fooled with. The wheelhouse is aft as is the engine room and then a large wasted space. It fairly eats gas. She carries the usual canvas—a big jib, a gaff-rigged mizzen, but a Marconi mainsail.

We made the funny little channel between the islands and put out the grapple. All we did there was pull a few teeth and we sent word to Carter's Cove but no one came. We don't expect much business from these places

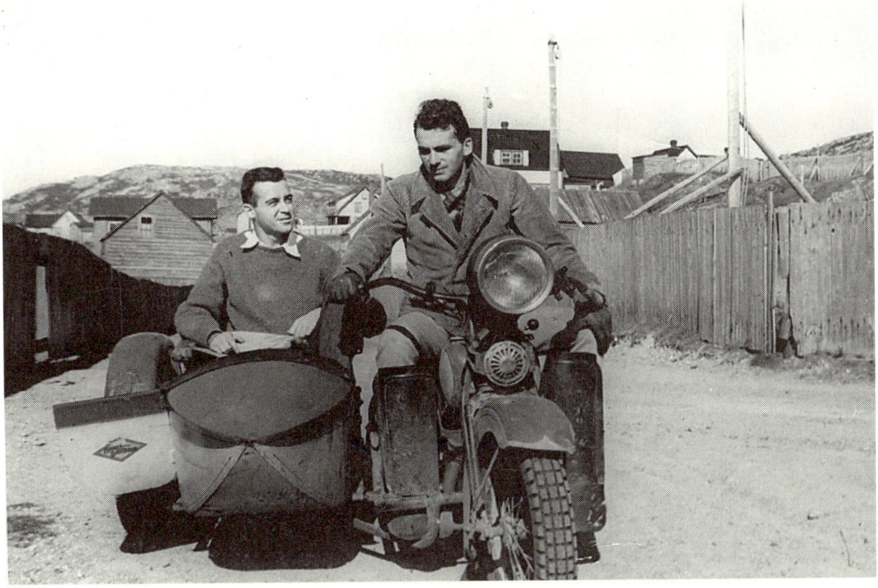

Dr. Ecke and Hopkins student Finney on the hospital motorcycle with sidecar. Author's photograph.

that are so near the hospital. It is only a few minutes to Samson's Island where we also landed in a tickle, and the story was the same—meaning no business. One old codger came way over to us in a motor boat to ask if I was a government doctor. When told no, I was from the hospital, he allowed as how he wouldn't see me because it would cost. He didn't even give us a chance to bargain. Then on over through the run, straight into the setting sun and Exploits Island.

We arrived at 7:00 and after a long wait pulled a tooth and made a shore visit to a one-room house where a seventy-six-year-old pair are eking out the end of their days, both fairly strong, but she with a shaking paralysis and he with a bad heart and quite irrational. I could only josh them a bit and give them a little false hope. The son is solicitous enough. The old man gets up on the table thinking he is still running his schooner. He says his feet are as cold as clay. Dudley is not much trouble. He can't get up and down the companionway and he won't mess on the boat. I am afraid he will run amuck the first time he sees sheep. Well, it is night and I am to bed after a fair day, the first of what should be a pleasant month.

September 13, '38. We didn't leave Exploits till eleven, because there was a little work to do, nothing special, we didn't hang around long after the last one. It was raining and rather cold, but little wind. We stopped at Charles Brook, two hours from Exploits. An ancient couple came aboard. The lady wanted a tooth out. It was an old snag in the lower front that had worked around until it pointed outwards. He said she had poor nerve—all smooth-water people had poor nerve. By way of telling me he was a farmer he said he "scroped" the ground for a living, and ar'a bit of work made his waters stop. The median lobe of his prostate was the size of a watermelon, but Dr. Smith had never happened on it. Two hours along to Botwood.

The mate cooked some meat that was so tough Dudley could hardly handle it. The reception was slow here. We hung about for an hour before anybody much came—they were all home bathing and powdering because there was plenty of evidence of both on examination. Then from 8:00 to 11:00, I saw ten people. I had to talk to Mr. Gate House, the head of the hospital contract committee. He wants me to meet the committee. I said I would if I were here tomorrow and I'll break a leg not to be here. As we entered this harbor, we passed one of Ashbourne's old schooners. She was beating against the wind, making a very lovely picture. She had a load of limestone from Chaulker's.

Saw ten patients who had very little wrong with them, except one who had adhesions and one who had a painful cervical stump.

September 14, '38. We spent the whole day at Botwood. I worked like a little beaver from 9 A.M. until 11 P.M. We pulled very few teeth. I made several shore calls and we didn't see much of interest really. No end of bad backs, sides, and stomachs. I don't compare very favorably with the local doc. He can examine them through their clothes and tell them from the door what's wrong with them. He also gives much larger bottles of medicine. The Steamer *Geraldine Mary* came in but I didn't get a chance to see her. She's one of Lord Northcliff's boats. A German boat came in after lying to all night waiting for news from Germany, afraid of being interned. I was dizzy by night. We had our usual cup of cocoa before turning in.

September 15, '38. This day was exactly the same as yesterday. We pulled in $40.00. I saw very few seriously ill—oh, yes—one terrible job on a broken femur from Bishop's Falls. It was healed fibrously at an angle of about 45 degrees. The day was a tough one. The committeeman Mr. Gate House talked for 20 minutes while the people waited.

September 16, '38. A beautiful day. We pulled away about 7:00 so no patients could stop us and I was glad to go because I didn't want to see that cyst I dug out yesterday. We tied up at Norris Arm—where I took a swim. Doris stayed below so it was all right. We spent the whole day there and worked until 11:00 again. The water was cold and brackish. I just jumped in and out climbing up the rope ladder.

September 17, '38. Sunday. We are still having beautiful weather. Worked until about noon. I had another swim from the boat and went to see the circumcision we did yesterday. They hadn't had the heart to take the little bandage off. This kid was a wonderful patient. He was only seven and didn't say a word though I did it under local. The mother was nervous for everybody. About 3 P.M., I walked along the shore with Dudley and Lidge and had another swim. Lidge enjoys the dog. Lidge would hide from Dudley behind a tree. The dog misses him and goes crazy looking for him. He even tried to climb a birch tree after the skipper. The dog is more and more of a pleasure. He can't climb up out of the saloon, which is a good thing. He is very dependent upon company and won't leave us for a minute.

About 4 P.M., we slipped our mooring for Botwood because Northern Arm is no place to spend the night. I started to put flea powder on the dog on the Botwood wharf but it looked so foolish to the Sunday promenaders that I quit. Perry, the minister, came down to see me and we chatted until he said he had to go for tea. I had been making up reasons to refuse to go with him but wasn't invited.

We had our own tea, and I wore my corduroy and bush jacket and we went for a walk, the three of us, Dalley, Doris, and I, strolling down to the airport. A guy showed us a gate through the back fence and in we went furtively to look around. It was quite impressive, with the great concrete runway for hauling out the flying boats. There were huge rubber floats to moor the boats and all sorts of things. When a man came toward us we were getting ready to run for it but recognized Commander Pattison. I couldn't introduce Doris because I forgot her name. Pattison was very hospitable, and took us back to his house where we met his little, lonely British wife. They had a very tiny dog that was amusing—by standing on his hind feet he could just reach Dudley's neck.

The commander took Lidge and me to a chart room and talked an hour on navigation. The Rhumb Line cuts all the parallels of latitude at the same angle. The Great Circle route is 60 miles shorter to London. Weather bulked large in the conversation and he said he would take us up to the meteorol-

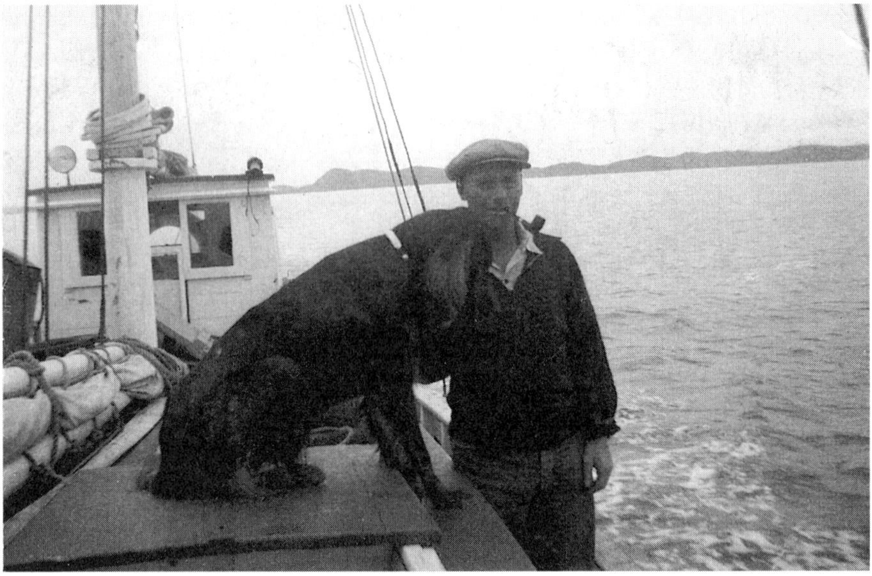

Dudley and Lidge. Author's photograph.

ogy station. First we went upstairs and saw what I considered a very fancy setup for guiding planes into the station. He laughed at my innocence. Then we walked across the field into what I suppose is a typical British station. The boys were sitting around in tweeds consuming Scotch and soda. There was an especially pink-cheeked weather expert who is going to help me with a wind determinator. I played darts and won. The walls were covered with silhouettes of famous aviators. We stayed there until 10:30 and then went a considerable distance to the weather station. They make the most complete weather map in the world. Three shifts of 12 radio operators each do nothing but collect weather reports. The radio masts are 600 feet high. From there we went back to Pattison's quarters for cakes and Scotch.

September 18, '38. I was amazed to find our bow in the mud. The *Clyde* had come in at 5:00 and found us at her berth. I hadn't heard us being moved. We worked a bit in spite of a hangover and managed to get away by 11:00. As we passed the airport, Pattison came out in the fast little tender and ran circles around us in farewell. Then on to Northern Arm, where we tied up at a broken-down wharf and did quite a lot of business. We were afraid to stay the night and drew away at 7:00 to land at Lawrenceton—where I saw two patients before going to bed.

September 19, '38. We worked hard all day and managed to get away by 7:30. The weather is still good. We left in a beautiful twilight and came down to the strange Porterville.

In the dark we had a bit of trouble warping around to the lee side of the wharf, where we are now. Dudley tackled a big husky, leading with his neck. He will be chewed up yet. It was fun having trouble getting into the berth. I put some clothes to soak in a bucket of seawater. I don't think we'll be busy here. We have collected $175.00 so far. I've never seen such weak nerves—women who tremble so I can't get near their teeth—mothers who get faint and have to sit down while I examine their children. Dudley fell overboard at Norris Arm and I had to fish him out with a gaff.

September 20, '38. A little work at Porterville in the morning and then on for a quick run to Little Burnt Bay.

There an old bird, who said he was 93, came for me to see his woman, who had given her leg a hell of a scald. She had dressed it in sulfur and castor oil and done a fair job of healing it. But two small places remained. I left instructions on how to fix it. I knocked 50 cents off the bill and our elderly friend gave us a mess of codheads and a couple of nice fish. Fish were plentiful he said, but he hadn't been able to get any salt anywhere. He said he hadn't exerted himself to get any but had sort of just sat around. He spit anywhere, even on the hearth under the stove. The poor cat had to keep on the move. He had a sort of humor and joked about losing all the women he brought on board to be examined. We left there about 4:00 and at 6:00 drew into Campbellton.

We made arrangements to have our laundry done. Dudley misbehaved, chased children, sheep, and chickens. I saw six women before going to bed and I thought I would scream if there were one more story of a weak back and a "giddy haid."

September 21, '38. Left about 11:30 because we had to wait for our laundry to dry. I was annoyed to find that the drawers I washed had blown away. Bad luck with the sea water washing. Nothing came clean and my red socks dyed everything. It was a nice run down to Newstead.

We thought we wouldn't have any business here but $8.00 was waiting for us on the wharf. We had a hell of a time getting a berth because Earl's tub was in here. I handled the stern lines. We left about 5:30 and it was so hot in the fo'c'sle that I lost my appetite. So I lay down in the saloon with Dudley and had a little snooze beating against the wind to the perfectly landlocked harbor of Loon Bay.

No one came aboard except a kid who gave us a few smelts and some flat fish. There is no wharf here so we are at anchor for the first time. It is a deadly dark night with quite a breeze but no sea. The halyards slap against the mast and the anchor chain is rattling against the side. We added a little rum to our usual cocoa in the fo'c'sle and the men got talking about their trips to the Labrador. Lidge, who is no fisherman, made three trips in an 80-ton schooner, and there is stuff in his stories. Once they were in an open cove when a storm beat in on them and they thought she was going to sink at her anchor. They abandoned her in blinding rain and wind and escaped ashore to spend the night in an Eskimo tent with 30 others. An old squaw beckoned him in. She was leaning against the pole and he sat the whole night propped against her knees. He said he couldn't look at her or he'd be sick. But tears came to me when I thought of that meager but generous hospitality. The schooner did not go aground, so they boarded her again in the morning, a little sheepishly.

Every spring there was a pretty sanguine competition among the schooner captains to stake out the prime fishing berths as soon as the ice was gone. He told of the races through the ice and fog and dark, six or seven schooners at a time with their lights out so they couldn't be followed. They couldn't see Tom White's schooner, but they could hear them swearing on deck. He told of how they had run into an iceberg in the dead of night. The boom was caught in the berg and snatched away and then jammed back against the mast with a shock that threw them all to the deck. They beat around all night to keep clear of the bergs that couldn't see. They were racing along before a stiff wind and were quiet below deck when the top half of the main mast came down and hung in the rigging. They wallowed along all night before the gale. When they shot off some guns it turned out the nearest schooner was skippered by Jim Gillette, lifelong enemy of their skipper.

He stood by them and dropped a line back as soon as it was light and towed them into the wind until the weather slackened. The drag on the rescue ship put her stern under at every swell. They made a harbor and Gillette came aboard. Both skippers embraced and cried and then opened some rum. (I cried too.) They stayed together nine days while they fitted a new spar. He recounted dashes ahead in a motor boat or rowing 20 miles with blistered palms under the cliffs in a calm to grab a good fishing berth.

Lidge went on to speak of the time when 200 schooners were tied up side to side in Icy Tickle, icebound. You could step from one to the other for a mile. There were rough goings on with the kind of girls that would be making that trip. He spoke of the tenderness of salt-rotted hands splitting fish until 2 A.M. and going fishing again at 4 A.M. There was a time when 50-pound kegs of gold were shipped for the herring fishermen. Now they don't sell any. The cod is split and packed in salt to be taken home and dried for sale to merchants. Herring could be sold for gold to buyers who followed the fleet. American saloons served pickled herring at the famous free lunches. Prohibition had killed that market and the taste for herring never returned.

September 22, '38. I didn't mention that I saw those two Cooper children at Newstead whom I had visited last winter. Both are bedridden now. One with a rotten heart and one with amyotrophic lateral sclerosis. We did a bit of business in Loon Bay in the morning and were late getting to Birchy Bay.

It is a lovely large harbor but too shallow at the sides for a wharf. French runs a mill here. The Evangelists on his side of the harbor have given up their hospital contract. We had a couple of patients and I went ashore to do an OB examination and to see a post partem who couldn't pee. I also saw a tremendous, five month, 25-pound baby, who was so fat he couldn't breath.

We needed a pilot to take us through The Reach. Though we had put a flag in the rigging as a signal, the pilot was busy in the bay and didn't turn up until dark. He was loath to start then because there was no moon. We settled down after dropping the hook, to a quiet evening but a fellow came aboard with a sebaceous cyst of the cheek. I took it out with a little interference from Dudley and I must say it was a neat job. By then it was time for our evening cocoa party. It was another night at anchor which was hard on Dudley. He had gone all day without going to the john so I got out with him three times and he finally was persuaded to do his stuff way back in the corner on the quarter deck. Fine weather the whole trip, not a wave. The sun hasn't been out much, but it has been warm and smooth.

September 23, '38. We upped anchor at 7:00 and started on the beautiful trip through The Reach inside of Chapel Island Reservation. On the other side of the island it is called Dildo Run. It was a quick trip and the pilot had a four-hour row back for his $2.00.

At Boyd's Cove we got our work done and waited for our cake and bread that came along with a set of sweet rolls, all for 40 cents. I'm going to school this winter to learn navigation. I wanted to give a patient some tonic so she went ashore to look for a bottle. The skipper started the boat up and we had to turn around again to make delivery.

Port Albert is a rock bathtub with no wharf. Here we pulled no end of teeth and made a little money. Then on before dark to Horwood.

I was much pleased when Hodinott took us aboard his craft, the *Miss Horwood*, which he wants to sell—and he gave us a drink of rum. I went up to his house to hear the news and was relieved to find that the hurricane had not wiped out New York, as had been rumored. Our layer cake was good. It is a starlit night with a fresh new breeze and cool. We're on the outside now and may get a wave on our jaunt to Gander Bay.

September 24, '38. Sunday promised nice but with a gale of wind and I was awakened at 6 A.M. by much ado above. The men were shifting the boat so it would face the wind. The engine was not reliable or strong, so there was much manual heaving. I settled back into my bunk for an hour and then after someone dropped a crowbar over my head for the third time, I got up. The rest of the day was kind of odd. We pulled a few teeth and did see the Salvation Army captain, female, who planned marriage and had to have a health certificate. She had a lousy heart. It seems that one officer must marry another or quit. I went for a walk with Dudley, which is always fun. He is reluctantly learning not to chase sheep. I was going to throw a rock at a church bell I hit last year, and was wondering what would happen if I missed and it went through the window when the door suddenly opened and a dozen people came out. I slept the afternoon away and opened a breast abscess in the evening and pulled some more teeth. The wind has shifted around to the north and it is much colder. I had to put the funnel on the top of the chimney to make it draw properly. Now I am writing this and after a few letters and a cup of cocoa will crawl in under the deck to my bed. If it weren't for the diuretic quality of cocoa I would consider it a super evening drink. There . . . I just stopped to pull two hard teeth on a young fellow who fishes for smelt and salmon. He looked liked Lew Ayres and, dressed, would be acceptable anywhere. He certainly is a desert bloom. But soon you saw his blunt red hands and he spoke the dialect. "We does well some days and some not ar'a fish." He fainted twice. He had nerve though.

Horwood of the Horwood Lumber Company appeared on deck when I went up. He was staying with the Hodinotts and invited me to hear the news. Doris didn't want to go, but they sent for her again and she came up. Mrs. Hodinott took her into the kitchen because she said there were too many men. God knows how they amused themselves out there. Horwood is an interesting sort of guy—black moustache, stocky and rather British. He talks very affably in a knowing way. All the time I find myself being friendly and even liking people whose methods I question. He treats his workers with a minimum of empathy. The news was very disturbing—all about the German politics. We stayed until almost midnight and had a feed.

September 25, '38. Victoria Cove. It hailed large hailstones while we were here and the "governor general," old John Oakes, who has the welfare of all at heart, came aboard and as usual showed me his varicose ulcers. He also asked me to see a baby with a prolapsed rectum at Clarke's Head. We anchored in one fathom of water and were busy in a minor way all afternoon and evening. The people seemed very loath to pay for anything. We did scrounge some bread. I went up the bay in a light motorboat, to see an influenza. Lidge went along to give the dog a run. It was a grand fall evening, blustering and cold with a rich red sky. It gives me nostalgia. I love autumn. The Gander Bay is a funny shallow place. No one can build a wharf to withstand the ice. The sebaceous cyst I took off for a protested $2.00 broke, and I had a little time with it.

September 26, '38. A lovelier, crisper day than yesterday though blowing a gale. The lop is not to be sneezed at either. I had to get up early to see a large congenital inguinal hernia and it was nice to be out in a skiff. Gillingham, his knee stiff from an old ax wound, took us over to the south side where Lidge and the dog and I walked a pleasant two miles on a pine-lined road to visit our two-year-old patient. She was walking about in a room and a half—a hovel. She did have a large rectal prolapse, out two months but in fair shape, very little ulceration. I tried to reduce it, but she will need ether and a week in the hospital on her stomach, so I ordered her to go down to Twillingate.

Back to the ship in very rough water. Then we moved over to Main Point. The lop was rolling in there for fair but a few braved it so I pulled a lot of teeth. These men have money. They were working for French and he treats them right. He conducts a cash business with moderate prices and pays his men in money. We had heaved in most of the anchor again, but it tripped and before we knew it we were driving for the shore. It was only by quick work that we got the patients off and started up our useless engine. We just got away from that place, deciding that we couldn't risk Main Point any longer, so we put out for Frederickton.

Lots came aboard, including a poor wretch much scared because he had had contact with Mary Dole and everyone in Newfoundland knows she is in Twillingate for venereal infection. I couldn't see anything but told him to go down for a blood test. One stinker with plenty of money came aboard and filled my hours with talk about himself and then announced that he wasn't going to pay me. I hated him for it. When I think of the many who can ill-afford to peel off their hard-earned cash and he calmly ignores the problem, I get sick. I feel that the doctor must never discuss money with his patient. It spoils the relationship. Poor Dudley is a little low today from rolling in that lop, particularly when we went broadside to miss a broken log boom, it kind of put him off his feed. The northern lights tonight were striking—deep rich blood-red and dark cherry. "Long may your big jib draw," said one man to me when I told him he didn't have diabetes.

September 27, '38. What a day. I heard them getting off at the crack of dawn and slipped on a pair of pants to help them wind up that goddam anchor. It seems to weigh six tons at times. I hopped back into bed expecting to get right back up again for Carmanville, but I fell asleep and was rudely awakened to be told we were approaching "Aspey" (Aspen) Cove. It was such a good day the skipper thought we should seize the chance to do the straight shore. We did a land-office business in teeth for an hour or so, while we tossed at anchor in a ripping offshore breeze. Then we got out of there after another soul-wrenching crank at the anchor and went around the small cape to Ladle Cove on "the Straight Shore."

There we anchored way out from the houses because it was such a poor harbor. Every once in a while we would grunt and the anchor would slip a fathom or so and catch with an awful jerk. We were going out to sea, so it was all right, but it was no easy task for the people to get out to us. One man couldn't pay, so he brought us a dollar's worth of potatoes. He was bent on making half a barrel be a dollar and a half so he could get money out of us, but the skipper was firm. We got away from there about 3:00 and started up the coast to Carmanville. The breeze freshened all the while but we made fair time until we were outside the point which marks the entrance to Alder Harbor. From there, it is a wide indraft to Carmanville and we couldn't do a thing against that wind.

The quick water from the propeller drifted ahead of us, a clear demonstration that we were going backwards. This made the skipper sore and with a mild curse, he spun the wheel around to beat it across Sir Charles Hamilton Sound with the wind behind us. We put all our canvas on, wing and wing, and headed for Seldom Come By. If there had been no land in that direction, we would have had to go anyway. The sound was full of porpoises. Their curved symmetry played all around us in that ominous green swell. She rode beautifully, though Dudley got seasick when he came into the fo'c'sle where I was holding the kettle down trying to make a cup of tea. Seldom Come By was a dream. It is a fine sensation to get out of a storm into smooth water. There were 12 schooners in this little harbor out of the wind. The *Bessie Marie* was here and another big one—a 130-tonner. When the wind dropped, that one pulled out to get a berth at the mouth of the harbor so as to be off first in the morning.

I went ashore to see a dame with pleurisy. Thc man said shc had water trouble too. When I asked her how long she had this water trouble, "Let me see," said she. "Gerald is 23 years old. I've had it 23 years." Then I opened an abscess on the neck of a ten-month old. You never saw such parents. They trembled and kissed the baby and cried and sweated. I finally cleared them all out and got the skipper to hold the baby. Meantime, schooners kept leaving the harbor, though it's a dark night with the wind freshening again. If I hadn't brought the wrong size film, I could get a swell picture.

September 28, '38. Woke to find the harbor mysteriously clear of all the schooners except the one moored at the end of our wharf. We soon had to change berths with her so they could put her on the outside and haul her down to scrape her filthy bottom. She must have had six inches of seaweed and all kinds of nautical junk on her. We did a great business in the morning, of teeth and what not. Then had started off when we remembered a cake plate we should have returned. We nosed back to the schooner and a man ran out on the bowsprit to get the plate. By 4:30, we reached Indian Island. Everybody was off to a funeral. I urged the skipper to get up anchor and make for Carmanville whereupon a call came for me to go ashore. The people had a $10.00 hospital contract so I made only 50 cents and almost froze. Some teeth finally showed up and it was too dark by then to leave. About 10 P.M., a pitch-black nightwrack came up and the halyards beat out that monotonous, frantic message on the mast, "You got what ya got—ya got what ya got—ya got what ya got—ya got what ya got." Finally the skipper went aloft and lashed them down. It rained and blew all night.

September 29, '38. What a day! I upped at dawn to help wind up that miserable anchor and then back to bed until the start of work at 9:30 A.M. in Carmanville.

We were moored to that high government wharf, which lets the waves through. There was also the dratted east wind beating right on us and my stomach turns now to recall that terrible heaving. The patients had to get into the rigging to get down to the boat and we were hoisting them up and down all day. We made $30.00. It was dreadful working down in the saloon with the patients sliding from side to side. I had to go ashore every once in a while to get my stomach back. While there, I made two shore calls, one to West with beriberi and a bad heart—had to talk an hour to get him to go to the hospital. I opened a face for an abscessed tooth and then to a kid with impetigo and itch and then pulled two teeth at home on a strange cripple with hands and feet in contracted knots. Her tongue wouldn't work. She handed me 50 cents when I was done. I had intended to charge more, but in view of her twenty-one years of cripplehood, I stopped.

There were 20 waiting on the boat when I got back at 10 P.M. We shooed them off except two: Mrs. Tulk whom I shipped right off to the hospital to have her appendix out, and the widow Hicks, who was not really ill, but had brought us a fine cake for which I allowed her 75 cents. After a bit of cocoa I am ready to turn in. My room smells lovely since Dudley rolled in cow manure and slept on my bed all day.

September 30, '38. I woke as usual at daybreak when they started the motor. I didn't notice the weather but was soon lulled off to sleep by the uncertain faltering of what passes for our engine. She becomes worse and worse and stalls at the slightest strain. It is a quaint sensation to lie in bed and hear them put it into neutral and then grind into reverse and stall. You

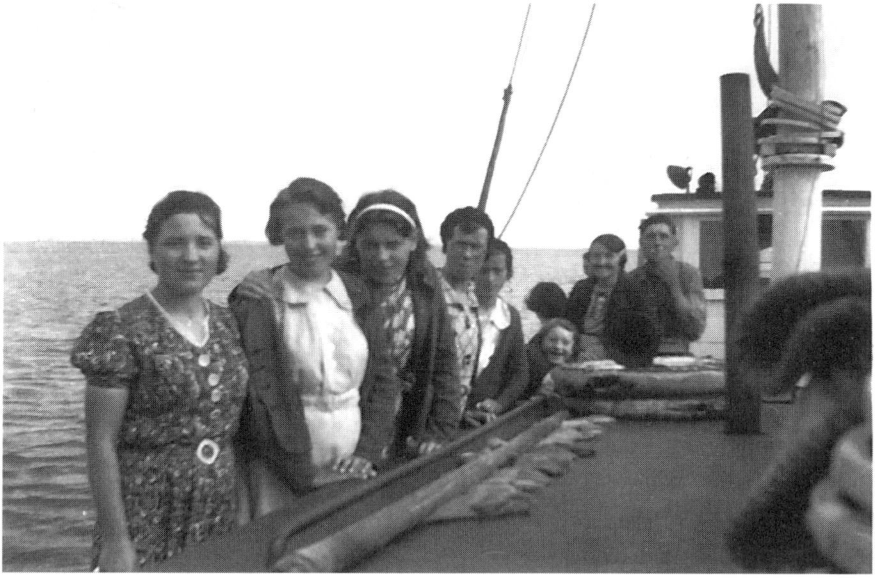

The waiting room on the *Bonnie Nell.* Author's photograph.

don't use reverse unless you need it, and the interval, until you strike what you were planning to miss, is a long one. Well, I woke as it idled and waited a tense moment, but was surprised to hear it slide up against the wharf. I puzzled a while and finally concluded that we were back at the same place; such proved to be the case.

There is such a sea on that we have turned back. The day was a mess. More rain and wind. Plenty of patients came aboard however, and just as it cleared a little, we moved over to Green's wharf at 4:00 where we had one of our incidents and went sailing right into it. Jim Green was in bed with most of his clothes on and all curled up with his finger in his ear. He cried and asked me not to torment him. I hauled him out of bed and tried to get him to the door, but he got surly and squared off, offering to sock me. He came only to my chest, though he is fatter and stronger than he looked that day in the hospital when we thought he was going to die of too much paraldehyde. His full-bearded old father told me about taking him to the Labrador in one of these moods. He would salt fish in the hold all day and never look up or say a word. They tried putting him on lookout. He would stand in the bow and never sing out when he saw something, but would let the schooner run into a pan of ice first. I went over the hill to see a man. I had only a thermometer, but it seems to me he has typhoid. Back to the boat and on to a very precarious wharf at Noggin Cove.

We left the wharf to take a berth in midstream with a strong west wind blowing off the shore. We took a woman with us who had been overcome by some kind of a reaction while we were pulling teeth and like to died. She lay about the ship for three hours, fainting to the left and to the right. We finally put her in Doris' bed. Her friends all laughed and said she saw fit to have these attacks when most inconvenient for others. She was bad enough off though, because I could feel her get hot and she looked pale. I don't know how much control people have over functions of that sort.

October 1, '38. A nice looking day in the beginning, but it turned out badly. It clouded up and blew around the compass until it was right in. I was worried and woke the skipper from his afternoon nap to tell him, but he didn't think it would be much. The biscuits I made for tea tasted from the smoked salmon cooked in that tin yesterday. We could eat only the tops. We did only a bit of work today so I had time to finish *With Malice Towards Some* and found it one of the finest. The day finally passed and there was a rainbow. I could see a ship through it only twenty yards away, so *we* must have been at the end of the rainbow. But R.P.T. Coffin says the *State of Maine* is at the rainbow's end.

October 2, '38. Up at dawn to crank the big anchor and I strained every fiber of my carcass. While breakfasting we entered White Point.

It was a fine blue morning with a fresh west wind and a hangover sea coming in from the east, so we rolled a bit. I lolled in the fo'c'sle daydreaming and thinking I should write a book. I'm afraid I would be consciously saying smart things like in *With Malice Towards Some.* I tapped a hydrocele, saw a rotten lung—a mass in the upper left quadrant—and pulled lots of teeth and everyone had definite trouble. The weather looked so good that we went on to Musgrave. Did a few dollars worth including a cold tuberculous abscess, called a cyst by Dr. Diamond who is going to carve it out when it gets ripe, so he thinks.

As we passed Alder Harbor this morning Ted's boat hove to and put a note aboard inviting us back there for the night. We said we would come, but when we got through at Musgrave, the skipper was unwilling to turn back. I sent our regrets by wire and we were glad to get out of that wretched berth behind a rock with the surf breaking on it at Musgrave.

We put on all canvas and soon had Musgrave off our stern. This must be a weird craft under sail, with her funny high bluff nose, her foresail, her mizzen which is a decent size and has a gaff, and her main, which is short, being above the pilot house and Marconi rigged in a droopy way. The general effect must be that of a Chinese junk. We tore along and everything that was loose and some things that weren't spilled about on the saloon floor. I took the wheel as we rounded Cape Fogo and approached Tilting.

On a beautiful evening with a good cold wind we wove in and out of buoys into this snug but tricky harbor. We put down the anchor though we knew it was pretty shallow water. A man came aboard to tell us we were on Mercury Rock, and would strike at low water. With much finoogeling and stalling we knocked a few planks out of Earl's rickety wharf and tied up. A cutaneous horn came aboard but shied at the knife. I pulled one tooth on a demoralized papist, who called on her deity and vowed in a loud clear voice that she had to suffer in this world. She screamed so that I let go once to make sure that I didn't have her by the cerebellum. It couldn't have hurt that much—I had cocained it well.

A party, after reading *Mill on the Floss*, and now to bed if I can get there before Dudley takes the best mooring, otherwise it's like sleeping around a post in a hotel lobby.

October 3, '38. Some little work here this morning. Dudley distinguished himself when he was chased by some sheep. This is unique in Newfoundland dogdom. We left a little too early for a disappointed patient who had gone into the shop first (India relish, 40 cents for a small jar) and came to the wharf just as we got into the channel. They had hours and hours to get to us. Part of it may be that we are on a peculiar time of our own, some one hour and a half ahead of everyone else. We sailed quickly and beautifully to Joe Batt's Arm where we did no business at all. During the confusion of docking, Dudley sneaked into the fo'c'sle and ate the skipper's dinner. He also ate all the rabbit in the pan in the oven. He was smart enough to leap for shore the minute we touched and disappear behind the houses. On my search for eggs, a total stranger greeted me by name and ushered me into the parlor and gave me eggs and milk for free. She was an old patient.

At Barr'd Island we anchored while I made a famous spider corn cake, like my sister-in-law Esther's, except that mine was flat and wet and hard. They ate it loyally. I proved myself very nautical, noticing that all the anchor chain wasn't out when the skipper thought it was. There wasn't enough tide or wind to pull it all out. While we were at tea, it suddenly went all out and he leapt on deck thinking we had been rammed. We left there without seeing a patient and went on to Fogo through a grand twilight trip into Easter Tickle. It got colder as the sun went down. Fogo Harbor is a good one, large and surrounded by very high headlands. It has three entrances—Easter Tickle, Wester Tickle, and Seal Cove Tickle. On a calm day, in the Easter you can see the top of a Swedish steamer. Instead of waiting for a pilot, the skipper of said steamer allowed a passenger to bring the ship into the harbor. They got only as far as that rock in the tickle. Once the *Segona* didn't know where she was in a fog and a passenger said, "Here's a good place to anchor." They let go of the right bower and she went with 200 fathom of chain and was never seen again. "Drowning your anchor," they call it.

We tied up at the export wharf and I waited until a decent hour to call on Dr. Beckwith and his wife. About 7:00, the manager's son took us over in a boat. I found them at home and was interested to see how the bit of good silver they had with them shone out in the simple furnishings. Mrs. Beckwith has done well, bakes well, preserves and all that. But her hubby is pretty ineffectual, though she's fond of him I suppose. I was not sorry when a call came for him to go to Indian Island. I stayed and talked to Mrs. Beckwith until 12:30. She made a salad out of their one cucumber, which we had with a lot of tea and layer cake and sherry.

October 4, '38. We woke in Change Island and were unable to get to Billy Earl's wharf until they moved his schooner. Meanwhile, I was called out to see a congenital idiot with contraction and athetoid movements of the hands. He is going a little uremic. Went back thinking we could get away, but two patients were on the wharf. One bothered us no end by having me pull teeth, see her daughter, and talk to her—all on a $10.00 contract, which made it for free.

Midafternoon I was called to the north end again to see a woman who had fallen dead. Such proved to be the case. Aunt Lucey, a local spirit, had died, probably of apoplexy. Then back and still more. We seemed to be clear by 6:00 but the day was too bad to go home so Billy had us up to tea for a can of duck and one of lobster. The house was beautiful, called Four Winds, open on all sides and set high on a hill. Billy showed me around it; he is a simple, honest man. After tea I pulled more teeth. The day showed 30 patients, 60 or 75 teeth, and about $30.00.

October 5, '38. Billy is going to the hospital with us and I think it's a good idea to get board members on the *Bonnie Nell* so they can see what a rotten boat it is. There was a bitch of a sea on and we rolled to it. When Billy came on board, I got up though I would have given anything to have stayed flat in bed. I made an attempt at breakfast. Four times we had to stop the motor to drain water out of the gas. Without the motor going, she really pitched. Everything came loose. I was happy to coast into Twillingate Harbor and get off.

After a parting cup of tea on the boat, I saw Stan Hardy as we got up to the hospital. Stan is John's age, about four years my senior. His wife, Annette, is a Hopkins nurse. They are joining the staff. Marianne arrived about a week ago.

October 11, '38. There is little to say about the elapsed time. At moments I am annoyed to distraction. Socially, Waddell is more charming than ever. He is generosity and kindness itself. Nothing is too much for him to do for you, but professionally he is, to me, unbearable. He thinks and acts as if he were the only doctor here, being the first to any bed. He crowds all over the place and breaks his neck to get to the order book. He tells you what. He grabs all the patients. He breaks into the middle of your giving an order and gives one himself. He tells even John what to do during an operation. I did take a male breast off this morning, but it surprised me, as I don't usually scrub if the case is interesting since someone else's hands are usually on it already. I am the 12th wheel on the wagon. You would never dream that John and I had run the hospital alone last spring. I won't stand it much longer; may even threaten to leave.

Stan thought a typhoid was perforated tonight. I wasn't even spoken to. Stan says, "I'll tell John." "O, I'll tell him," says Waddell and beats it like hell for the Cottage. If he's in the bathtub with the door shut and someone knocks on the outside door and there are five people in the room, he takes it upon himself to say "come in."

The other night Kelly came in for an order to get some codeine. I heard her as soon as she opened the door, but she talked and talked to Waddell trying to get sense out of his sleepiness. I finally spoke up and gave her the order. Then she sent someone down to tell Waddell that Mrs. Canning had delivered, the patient he had induced earlier in the day. He lay in bed without a sound. I waited five minutes and got up, sore as hell. I thought someone ought to see her. I was so mad it wasn't possible to go back to sleep. Is it that I am to have chores to do that no one else wants?

However, he is so efficient and greedy that he does even the dirty work. Today I read two whole detective books. If things don't pick up, I'll have to manufacture something to do.

November 6, '38. What has happened since October 11th ought not to be written in the frame of mind in which I find myself at the moment. I've never felt lower in spite of a Benzedrine. It is all due to the sudden realization that I am wasting my life. If you're not getting anywhere professionally, at least you ought to be having one hell of a good time, and I'm certainly not doing that. I could go from morn to night and not say a word to a soul. I wish to God I could see through Waddell. He, at times, makes me feel so well disposed towards him that I go around taking back all the things I have thought and said about him. Then I am surprised when Annette tells me that I never said anything against him. He shows such consideration and is so careful and friendly that I don't know what to do. Then he ups and kicks my behind. I think that I will have to come to a decision soon and either accept him and forget the insults or reject him and not ever speak to him again.

Today I spent moping. It was a nice dreary day, which I spent in Stan's room writing and listening to the radio. Marianne sat with me. The Olds, the Hardys, Konopka, the new dentist, and Edith went to the Tilt and got very drunk and went swimming and what not. I mooded and brooded all day. After tea, Marianne and I went for a walk down along the Arm. It was a strange, moonlit, misty night. Steamy is the word. The whole world had an unreal, deserted, wrecked appearance. As if it had gone off its axis and everyone had been killed by poison gas and we drifted on in constant gloom. Dudley came along for a touch of reality and now I am going over for a cup of tea and then will sulk until bedtime. Some things have to happen 50 times. I've made up my mind to tackle John and tomorrow if I don't get to do any of the cystoscopies or scrubbing, I'll get out of here, I swear. I don't know where I will go. I think it will be north.

November 7, '38. This was a quiet day. I did a bit in the operating room. Waddell did a spinal fusion, which is really not much of a procedure. I think I could do one all right. Then I did a cystoscopy but couldn't get the machine in and had to send for Waddell. He pushed like hell and got it in. Neither of us could see much through it. Then he did one on that staghorn kidney stone. By that time it was dinner and oh, yes, he scraped an osteo and I took off a toenail. In the afternoon I cut a tongue-tie and took off another toenail. I was feeling much better. The evening disappeared easily. Suzie had us up to tea.

November 8, '38. I tried to maintain the dumps but felt pretty well. I helped John do a simple appendectomy, where he cut the skin crosswise. I kept my scrub, but when I went back into the operating room, John and Waddell were getting ready to cauterize a cervix and do a possible abdominal operation. I threw down my gloves and gown and left in high dudgeon. Waddell came in afterwards to sort of soften me by saying they hadn't done anything after all. Meanwhile, he was putting on his coat to go on an OB call that should have been turned over to me. He got there too late, however, though he did shoot 12 bull birds. The afternoon went quickly, as all afternoons do.

November 9, '38. Well, I lost $1.90 in the poker game last night but had a fair time of it. I did speak to John about the situation and he was very good, saying I might take out that prostate. I wasn't much excited at that prospect but I suppose I'll have a try. Waddell put it very succinctly when I griped to him— "What you do, I don't." However, on this day I did an appendix. The next thing was that Waddell went on a call to Bluff Head that I had said I would go on. With some trepidation, I saddled Jack and went off on him, but he behaved beautifully though he is the devil to mount. It was a lovely ride through the rain, way down to Jenkins Cove and back around the Arm to the Pond's where there is a boy much sicker than he ought to be.

November 10, '38. This was a fair day; I helped on a gastro-enterostomy and then did two tonsils. I had to yell for John for I thought I had tapped the abdominal aorta. There was a terrific gush of blood but I finally stopped it by quilting the whole throat on the twenty-year-old girl. I lost quite a bit of perspiration over that. Then I did another tonsil and after dinner took out another appendix.

Got Jack out again and went over to the north side where it was really blowing a gale. The waves behind the telegraph office were throwing spray and spume 25 feet and more behind the rocks. Jack was feeling his oats and tried to stop me from remounting. He stepped on my foot. The evening went quickly with tea at the Cottage and a long talk with John afterwards. He gave me *One Life, One Kopeck* to read. They put up the doors up again between the living room and the porch. It was quite a ceremony—just like last year.

November 11, '38. Tonsils and things in the morning and I took out another appendix. Tonsils—tonsils—I wish I had never heard the word. The first tonsillectomy I ever saw gave me the creeps and that was being done by a world authority. I never got over the feeling, even when I would be doing six in the course of a morning. The most exciting tonsil operation I did was as an intern—but the excitement was rather of extraneous nature. Tuesday was our tonsil day at the Baltimore City Hospitals. Monday night meant an overwhelming influx of prospective sore throats. Once a little boy was given his examination and taken to the operating room. His tonsils and adenoids yielded gracefully and the recovery from surgery and anesthesia was without event. The excitement came when his mother arrived and wanted to know if we had repaired his rupture. This was accomplished somewhat later but relations with the family had been irrevocably distorted.

During the summer after my third year of medical school, I suddenly found myself in a position where I had to take out a set of tonsils or admit that I was scared of them. I removed said tonsils and found it an unpleasant occupation. I didn't like the idea of working blind in a deep hole trying to outwit capricious bleeders. For the rest of the season I saw fit to hide in the linen closet when unassigned tonsils started for the operating room. The experience of internship and later at Twillingate did make me more and more comfortable tromping around in the back of somebody's throat, but I never lost my respect for tonsillectomy. The surgeon experiences few discomforts like that of having to take a tonsil patient back to the table to sew a bleeding vessel that has continued to ooze after the patient is returned to bed and awake. After that has happened to you, you become very conservative with the pharynx.

The veterans gathered to give the wreath and sing *God Save the King*. We gathered to be amused but I found myself wet-eyed to see those serious, and a little abashed, middle-aged men; one of them with a wooden leg. The rest of the day was nothing. It rained and blew. The wind was from the northeast so they moved the *Bessie Marie* out from the other side of the harbor. They apparently have learned their lesson with her. Tonight they are going to fry some chicken over in Edith's room. This evening, Pat

Cody taught Tommy and me to play cribbage; it's a good game and puts to use the antique inlaid board that I got over at the Sterlings.

November 24, '38. The Lord only knows why my character is so weak, why I can't do a little writing each night. The conditions have not been good anyway; no proper place to write. But now that's all fixed with a large table and a good light.

A lot has happened in the past two weeks. The Olds have gone on their first vacation in six or seven years leaving young David, their son, in the care of Marianne, a maid, and Annette. Dr. Stan Hardy is to be director meantime. I've accomplished my first prostatectomy—with some difficulty—superpubic. It certainly is important to know how much energy you can put into dissection. I find you can be pretty vigorous if you keep away from the ureters. There was also a strangely free, discrete ovary I took out of the Steele girl, which turned out to be an abscess. She is doing well. I've been doing a lot of appendices, two of them a little difficult and very good, for me. Appendicitis we have always with us. The so-called surgical belly or the abdomen in need of surgical interference will be appendicitis more often than it will be anything else. I heard a well-known, expert, introvertive surgeon say that if he sat at the front door of Johns Hopkins and wrote down "appendicitis" every time a patient came in clutching his abdomen, he would be right in his preoperative diagnosis more often than the surgeon who examined the patient and opened the belly. Persistent critics of surgery must not seize on this admission and eagerly shake their collective heads and say "I told you so." The surgeon who says an emergency patient has a ruptured ovarian pregnancy before operation and then finds a ruptured ovarian cyst in a patient two months pregnant has, to be sure, been wrong in his diagnosis. Actually it has made no difference at all. The belly had to be opened, it was opened in the right place and the guilty organ had been indicted.

I was brought up in the school where the time to operate for appendicitis was when you made the diagnosis. I still cleave to that belief, but we had to make concessions at Twillingate. We became a little liberal on that score. Many of our patients lived on outlying islands and exposed parts of the rocky coast where in the winter or because of storm they would not be able to reach us for weeks at a time. If one such gave a story of an appendix-like attack during the winter before, even though there might be a minimum of trouble at the moment we were inclined to remove the appendix. As a matter of fact, given no rupture, I figured out that one of the safest places you could be was on our operating table with a diagnosis of appendicitis. One aspect of this problem used to give me to wonder: It was not unusual during the summer when patients could get to us easily, to have emergency operations—sometimes two or three a day—when we would remove hot appendices; on the other hand, we hardly ever seem to hear of people dying from what was probably appendicitis during the long storm-bound or ice-bound winter months. Sometimes when I see a situation that seems unwilling to resolve itself, I get a sort of cold flush and a feeling that I am absolutely in a field I never should have tried. My surgery is an intellectual persuasion, I am convinced. The arts or literature or civil engineering is where I should have worked yet it is cheering to find that, regardless of the skill or unskill of my manual activity, the patients do like me and I am getting a very good obstetrical name.

One night last week I was up at 2:30 A.M. to go see Mrs. Hull, who rocks from side to side and talks of gas. I have seen her before; she was all right but distressed. Just as I had gotten back into bed, Kelly came in again for me. I made out I was asleep already and Waddell had to go out to deliver twins while I slipped down into the blankets and blessed my happy lot. Then at 5 A.M., Kelly was back, for me to go way over to Back Harbor where I arrived and sat until 11 A.M. before delivering the woman. Worked all the day and was nonplussed when Doccy Wood came for me at 2 A.M. to help him with Mrs. White's delivery. He put the forceps on again and again, saying it was transverse and that he had to rotate the fetus posterior, because it wouldn't come anterior. Finally I had one foot against the wall and helped him push. He had told her he was going for help, that he couldn't do anything alone. I poured chloroform, then ether until it was all gone, and shifted back to chloroform. She had been in labor too long to produce a live baby. The report came in later, by the grapevine, of the patient's impressions of the proceedings: she had been left in labor until I came down and took charge of things and then everything had been all right. While it was far from the truth, I was pleased.

Except in the case of outside calls, Waddell has been very good; he started off on an OB call that should have been mine on Sunday. He tried to hitch up the dogs but they got away, so in desperation, he hitched the dog sled up to Mack, the truck horse. In the midst of this, a call came to go to Herring Neck. It was a nice day and he preferred to go to Herring Neck since the child was probably born by then anyway. I took the dogsled on the OB call. It was very small and lacked a shaft, just hitched with loose traces so it kept running under the horse. I rode him a while, but the bells were right where I wanted to sit and when he broke into his infrequent trot, I got them where it hurt. We waited two hours for the woman to do something in the second stage of labor, but she wouldn't. It had been nine years since she had had a baby. We put her to sleep and with the forceps drew out a very blue small baby. The mother flooded rather briskly and worried me, but soon hardened down.

I've been deep in the dumps at times. With Hardy as the new director, things are a little strange. Waddell is so overpowering that resistance seems useless. Nurses ask me where Waddell is when they want to ask a simple question that I could answer myself. I am willing to admit that in the presence of a strong personality—sure of itself, my attitude may not inspire great confidence. I ask too many questions of people who don't know any more than I do. When alone, with no one else to ask, I'm fine.

It has been blowing great guns for three days. Went over to Back Harbor today with the horse and slide. We had to hold the slide down on the Tickle Bridge. The bight was throwing spray 50 yards over the land. Men went out from the Arm to their herring nets this morning and this afternoon. Saul White is getting his steamer into shape to go out and look for them. He thinks they have made Burnt Island, but I think that if they are on Burnt Island they could easily make the fact known to people along the tickle.

Ted Drover was here all week and made two drawings of me. The one he did of Stan Hardy, he tore up. Dudley has been a source of pain and pleasure. Marianne and I took him for a long walk over the mish on Sunday. He snatched a stick out of my hand and ran just ahead of me to tease. I ran like hell down a hill to catch him, he keeping two feet beyond me and when I was at top speed, he stopped suddenly. Not since I played football against Wesleyan in the fall rain have I taken such a flyer in the mud. I went head over heels, end for end. Dudley wasn't touched but acted as if his feelings were hurt.

I had a terrific run-in with the dentist who objects to the dog eating out of table dishes. He's afraid of germs. I repaired the situation but we had another tiff when this dentist thought I was still offending. He said if it continued there would be one less dog. I leapt to my feet in the crowded dining room and said if anything funny happened, there would be one less dentist. I was a little ashamed afterwards. But he is crude. A handsome type every inch the dentist; what smattering of information they get seems to qualify them to stand up against any doctor in the world. He has a foul mouth and decent conversation is impossible for more than four minutes. I feel that once rapport has cracked as badly as this, it can never be re-established. I'm sorry he's so big. It gives pause since during his "education," Temple kept him employed as a football player and heavyweight boxer.

Today Dudley was beset suddenly by Sport and Jake and a few hairs were torn out. He fainted and was carried upstairs inert by the frightened Marianne. He was on his feet when I got there but now he is too scared to go out.

Tonsils have been giving me the devil; three now have had to be put back on the table for bleeding.

While in the midst of a hectic OPD, I got a wire last Monday telling me of P.H. Cobb's death. He was killed by an automobile at Governor Dummer Academy. Camp Winona will find it difficult to get another such director. I couldn't go off by myself and mourn my dead but had to fuss around with bad backs and giddy heads. I can ill afford to lose P.H.; he believed in me and was very important to me. He represented an era in my life and I'm afraid it will come to an end with his going. That makes a very high mortality rate among my friends—P.H. Cobb, Bob Barrows, Chuck Sommers, Jean, Dr. Cram: all people I needed.

November 28, '38. A quiet lunch which left me in an introspective mood. I sat in my room looking out the window and wondering what the hell. There are sudden flashes of futility. You don't have to be drowning to have your life, from some strange impulse, be suddenly reviewed. A.E. Houseman had a solution for it but that's too easy. Into this gloomy moment Hazel burst to tell me that Ethel Crockett had sent a call in for me. She was said to be in labor. "It can't be much of a labor," I protested, having seen her only five weeks ago and she didn't look pregnant then. Ethel had worked for us at the hospital and had been vaguely complaining to the housekeeper. That worthy had sent her down to the OPD for examination. Ethel had refused examination and stalked out of the hospital. Probably I'd only be prescribing for a miscarriage, I thought, eyeing the heavy snow that was falling, and estimating I'd be back for tea.

It was four slow miles to Ethel's house during which there was time to get back into my Russian mood. The house didn't raise my spirits any, nor did the patient. In the first place, the shed door was completely off its hinges. You had to pick it up like a box cover and pull it into the frame behind you when you had got inside. The door to the kitchen wasn't much better. The panels were loose and stood right out in the breeze and there was lots of breeze. The kitchen was dark, cold, and dismal. The wallboards had all rotted near the floor and you could see right through them into the cove. Little piles of snow were gathering about the edges of the room. A few wet sticks smoldered in the broken stove. The tearful thin old mother wrung her hands and complained silently with her red-rimmed eyes. Two cats sat right on the stove. Beside the stove, in her overcoat and with a scarf tied over her head, sat a husky neighbor in one of the two rickety kitchen chairs. She was knitting furiously and acidly commenting on the patient's family. "With two girls working they have more money than anyone in the Cove. You'd think they could manage to get a bit of wood or coal. There's no kerosene for the lamp and it doesn't even have a chimney. You'd think they'd get these walls patched up. I'll get my death of cold. I never saw such shiftless hopeless people. I'd be ashamed, etc., etc." She seemed a pretty accurate observer to me.

The bedroom was in much the same style as the rest of the house. It was too short for the old iron bed. The sidepieces were driven into the wall. The springs sagged to the floor and way down in the gulch was my patient. Not only was she in obvious labor, but she was two weeks overdue. She hadn't come to the hospital because she didn't want any of us to know about the baby. She won't be married until her man comes back from the woods. She wouldn't have sent for the doctor and didn't want to see me now. She had been in labor 24 hours and the relatives had gotten frightened.

I examined her and couldn't feel a bit of cervix. The head was way down and it seemed to me that she ought to produce, at the most, in another hour. I waited in misery for two hours and then decided to bring her into the kitchen and see what the trouble was. The friend sent up to her own house for a few sticks of wood and a drop of kerosene. We never did get a chimney for the lamp. In the gloom and cold, I got her on the kitchen table and cleaned up and spread my sterile equipment on the floor. The old mother was terror-stricken when I asked her to give the chloroform, but our lusty neighbor took the bottle avidly and seemed to get a perverse pleasure out of putting Ethel to sleep.

I did a rectal and to my consternation, found that because of peculiar anatomy, the head had been able to descend fully without opening the cervix at all. In other words, I couldn't take the baby now. I hated the thought of her waking up and finding that nothing had happened. At this moment the cats started a game and before I could shoo them away walked all over my sterile stuff. Then I knew I couldn't do anything in the house. I persuaded the mother that the best thing to do was bundle the patient into a sled before she woke up and take her to the hospital. I figured we could just make it. They soon had her hidden under a pile of blankets and coats. Our helpful neighbor sent her husband for his sled and pony. I strained my back lifting Ethel and all the blankets into the box on the sled. I knew she would never go to the hospital if she were conscious. When the air hit her she started to have hard pains and to vomit and to proclaim that the baby was about to arrive. This didn't add to my comfort any more than it did to hers. Finally we were ready to start. We had to go up a little bank to reach the road. It was dark and snowing harder. "Giddap," said the driver and snapped his whip. The horse made a lunge, there was an ominous snap in the harness and off went the horse onto the road without us. While they caught it and made with baling wire, I really felt frustrated. The patient alternately groaned and was sick. I couldn't do a thing for her. She was completely buried in that mountain of coverings. I thought distractedly, that if she does have the baby, it'll take me ten minutes to find it in that mess. Our slow cavalcade finally was reorganized. A man walked ahead of us so that we would know where the road was. I eyed the dim light of each house we passed wondering what the dwellers would say if we suddenly appeared and asked permission to have a baby on their kitchen floor.

We made it though. Waddell supported me when we reached the hospital. He thought she was at the moment of delivering. When she finally came to, two hours later, we saw that her condition was such that any doctor would have had justification to think as we had. I felt sorry for her and hated to have her face the hospital staff. She lay the whole ten days with her head turned towards the wall, not saying a word and frequently weeping.

November 29, '38. Cold, snowy, and lots of drifts through which I walked down to Mrs. Blake whom everyone has had a look at. All she does is languish in bed and have pains and smartings in her feet, legs, arms, belly, and what not. I told her I would try to get her into the hospital. Marianne and I walked back over the inside of the island, which was fun and a foretaste of winter. Not so good without skis.

My last tonsil looked awful and I'm ashamed of it. There are lots of tags so I'll have her come back. I admitted a deformed, pregnant woman with a funny thick neck and high shoulders from a childhood injury. She also has a flat pelvis and will need a caesarean section that I trust I will be allowed to do.

Lots of aides are laid up with sore throats and until they are better, we won't do any more elective surgery because throat culture shows that it is beta strep. I had only a few. Won $2.60 up at the Cottage, $4.00 last Saturday, also at poker, and twice before that, $1.00. My outlook on life has taken a turn for the better.

November 30, '38. In the morning I snatched a quick appendix. The most definite operating I've done. It went well. Then I was having a quiet cup of tea with Edith when there was a call for me. The little girl whom I had taken out of a TB back cast the other day had a pain in her side. I moaned a bit and got ready to go right away but found Waddell almost all dressed to go. At that I protested that the call was for me. The old tendency is cropping up again so I went along. We walked down the lane together because it was too bad for a horse and we didn't know where the dogs were. It was tough out and the road wasn't packed a bit. The wind fought us the whole way so we arrived pooped. It was an even harder push back and dark then. We hurried up to the Cottage for tea and played crossword games. Dudley is still so scared to go out that he made his water on the ward.

A few days ago, I did a nice delivery; the woman came in the morning already in labor. I examined her and thought she was little dilated. While I was dressing some burns, along came Waddell to butt in saying he couldn't feel any cervix. I couldn't either, I admit, and rushed her into the operating room. There we urged the poor woman to push and little happened. I was prepared to put the forceps on but did a vaginal first and found the cervix would only admit a fingertip. She had fooled me just the way Ethel Crockett had. I put her back to bed. Waddell and Stan and the nurses were all eager to get the baby away from me. But an hour later I moved her into the operating room just in time and with a little paraldehyde and chloroform and an episiotomy, got the babe, which was a swell one. A good repair was made and all is well. If I had been left alone, I might have timed her case more accurately. I believe I have no place in such a racket where decisions are so important.

December 11, '38. I did that caesarean section. The operation was fun though the blood certainly appeared in profusion when I had to plow through the placenta, which was anterior. She stood it and is doing pretty well except that she's a little distended. She had a Wagensteen suction apparatus put in last night. I know that no one can demand respect in this business but one can demand courtesy. I suppose they meant well but the director calls Waddell away from a poker game to whisper to him in the hall and soon it was apparent they were cooking up a drainage for my patient and here I wasn't even told that she was vomiting. I was so mad that I didn't even mind losing at cards.

The *Clyde* came in unexpectedly at 5 A.M. on a special trip to bring an OB patient from the north. She had been in labor four days and brought a letter from her local doctor, a poor old conscientious duffer a little out of his depth. The woman had been in labor some time before he could get to her. He said, further, he had tried forceps many times and then version. Nothing had availed and he was sending her to us to see what could be done. She couldn't pay, but he would underwrite her. We found the woman in poor shape; she went to sleep on an eighth of morphine. The baby was obviously dead, the head was high. We rested her and gave her intravenous support then I put on the forceps and withdrew a baby with only moderate effort. The foul smell indicated advanced infection. She went into moderate shock in the operating room and was pulseless. Waddell belched loudly in the operating room and her last words were, "Who vomited here?" We transfused her, gave her a continuous intravenous and all the supportive drugs. She rallied from her shock but the temperature soared. We gave her sulfa—the new king—and this morning, just after I gave her 50% glucose, she vomited, drew a deep breath, and died right in my face. I put adrenaline into the heart, but she was gone and the wonder is that she endured so much.

This morning Waddell went all the way to Friday Bay to thrust poor, hunchbacked Selby Burt on to his unwilling father. Discharged moribund a year ago, by some trickery he turned up again at the hospital. We couldn't help him and we can't use our beds to board the Bay indigents. We kept Mackey, another patient, for four months when he came down on the last ship from the Labrador in the fall. He only had a small fistula, but the burden of his song was "I got n'ara father nor a mother to take care of me. I'm a poor orphant." He was 45 years old.

December 18, '38. This week I became a patient. What seemed to be an insignificant infection was breeding on my wrist. It didn't look like much, but Saturday night in the midst of a poker game I couldn't go on. I was winning too. I divided my chips among the contestants and staggered up to the Ashbourne Ward, our private room. Marianne specialed me for week, while Dudley spent all his time on the foot of my bed. Waddell took good care of me.

Being sick, I missed the wreck of the *Corsair.* I could have watched it from the hospital window if I had I been in room #10. She was a one-hundred-ton American-built oak schooner. When it breezed up she was anchored near the north side. The *Bessie Marie*, outside of her, fouled an anchor and started to drift down to her. The *Corsair's* skipper had to get out of the way. Behind him were the Bedlamer Rocks. He slipped his anchor, started his auxiliary and came full steam toward this shore planning to turn into the wind and find a berth in the lee of Carter's Head. At the turn she didn't answer the helm. The masts came out as she struck the shore and in 15 minutes the seas washed her deck up onto the beach. Waddell helped put a line aboard to get the crew off.

January 1, 1939. As the days roll along, there are many pregnant moments, intense at the time, which soon fade, so I will try for current comment when there isn't the time for ripened retrospect.

A screwier Christmas I never spent. It wasn't as bad as the Christmas I missed here though, with Joe White dressing up and playing Santa Claus on the ward. Doing a few dance steps to amuse the patients, by some misadventure, he ruptured his Achilles tendon. I like the thought of Santa Claus breaking his leg—it's kind of Russian. It's getting bad again, not his leg but my arm; today I compressed it all day. There was a plan for me to go to Fogo tomorrow but it has started to snow powerfully so probably the trip will be off. I am glad because my arm is not well and there's a trick in the situation. By having a trip now I can't complain when Waddell goes to Lewisporte to meet John and Betty in February. I am still feuding with the dentist; he doesn't like dogs and I don't like dentists. What I want to do is go to the Tilt alone for two or three days this week. That's it for current comment because Hazel has come to put hot compresses on my arm.

January 3, '39. An old snorter of a day; blew so hard that it was impossible, almost, to go over to the nurses' home. An OB call came in early in the morning. Waddell went off without a murmur, nor did he wear a hat. Whether this is bravado and a bid for local comment, I don't know. Anyhow it irritates us who wear hats. They asked about my arm over in Crow

Head. The implication being that they would have called me if they hadn't thought I was sick. I tottered around all day, and in the evening a call came in for Hardy from one of my OB patients. I offered to go but Stan insisted, braving the weather.

January 4, '39. Snowing even harder today during which we did nothing but read. By evening, Stan, Annette and the dentist and I got ourselves together and went over to the Ranger's to play bridge with him and his wife. They are well housed in the jail and very civilized. With them is a small dog they brought down from the Labrador, an Indian hunting dog named Lakamush, which means small dog. It is. Every time it came near the dentist the dentist would secretly pinch it or bat it in the head to make it stay away. Waddell came for us just before midnight and we had a great trip back through drifts ten feet high. The horse wallowed in the lovely soft snow while I hung on behind on skis.

January 5, '39. The best time I ever had in the snow today. Hitched Dudley up with Sport and it worked perfectly. All the dogs came along but the two in harness pulled like the devil up and down hill, over anything. I just followed them and we went way into the interior of the island. It was beautiful and lonely with all the hills looking alike as the sun went down. I was having such a good time that I went on to the Arm trail, over to the Little Harbor path and back by the road. It is thrilling to be hauled over the bushes and through the drifts.

I got home for rounds, hot and wet. I was dead tired after a tub and tea at the Cottage. At 2:00, they came for me to go to Bluff Head Cove where the whale washed ashore yesterday with a harpoon in him. They have been cutting it up all day for the dogs. The team of five was no good. I ran most of the way; sometimes I jumped on for a minute. Once I was running and helping the dogs when the two men were riding. "Pretty bad," says one, "when you have to push we." On a call the men are supposed to provide transportation even if they have to pull the sled themselves.

The moon was so bright you could tell bright colors by it. With a bit of wind behind us we hurried along the winter trail, met halfway by someone who urged us to put on more speed. I was unable to conceive of any obstetrical emergency, except bleeding, and if she were bleeding like that a minute would be her death. We did put on a burst and found the house in an uproar. "Something is coming out!" shouted the midwife. I looked and sure enough, something was. I thought for a moment it was a prolapsed uterus, but after getting some pituitrin and ergotoxin ready, and putting on some gloves, I saw it was a fetus held in by the cord around its neck. I unwound it and withdrew the offender alive and quickly after it the placenta. It was about six months. No bleeding but didn't think all the membranes were out so I left a long course of ergot.

Only one man came back with me, running the whole way. He had been down on the arm mummering and had come half way to meet us. Here he was again, with no pain in the side though I had done a double hernia on him last spring. I'm sure that he's no drinker because he can't afford it. I brought him into my room when I got back and handed him a tumbler and a bottle of rum. It was startling to see him fill the glass right up to the top and drain it off like rootbeer. I hope he got home all right. There was no mention of pay though they are not on the Center.

We had a good party Christmas Eve. I took Benzedrine and drank very little. My tuxedo looked swell. The girls were all dressed up. Marianne was particularly beautiful in a new, black velvet, off-the-shoulder business. There was a lot of lipstick spread around. I left early and couldn't sleep. Just at dawn on Christmas, an OB call came in and I sent for Marianne. We arrived at the house an hour after the woman had delivered. Her first intimation of pregnancy had been the night before, while milking the cow. It's 18 years since her last baby. "She's fine," said the midwife. I found her in shock. Pale, weak pulse, the bed full of blood, the uterus up to her chin and a bad, second-degree tear. There were strings tied around her thighs "to prevent flooding." I gave lots of Petrussin and massaged out the clots and sewed her up and fixed the baby and collected $10.00.

Joe Gillard said he could get us home in an hour. It wasn't cold but squally with dense snow that blotted everything out. The water was thick and oily with cold. We hurried and just as we got near the narrow tickle saw a big boat with a stretcher on it and a lot of people looking like Christmas trouble for the hospital. To the right of us, there was a string of five boats of wood being towed in. We shouldn't have tried, but we put on steam and pushed the boat of patients, happily recognized as Mr. Boyd coming for his TB wife, well over toward the concrete marker. We then crowded the string of towboats the other way, toward the shoals. We just skinned both of them and were home in one hour and one minute.

Up at the hospital, my depression returned. Waddell was just finishing his Santa Claus act on the ward and was pretty tight. Eggnogs were flowing so that I had two—then a so-so dinner. Stan Hardy volunteered to be the non-drinker and had to take care of our usual Christmas emergency—a cystoscopy—this time for pyelitis. Santa Claus meandered into the apartment and was snoring in three minutes. Tommy came in and we sat on the couch a long time. I read her my friend's letter (Charles Burnett) that wound up with both of us in tears agreeing that the world was a terrible place. With this thought, Tommy fell asleep and Waddell was still asleep so I worked in the OPD. When Waddell woke up I told him that socially I liked him very much, but professionally I hated his guts. He changed his tune completely and now doesn't do a single thing without telling me about it first. Christmas night we had tea at the Cottage and all is forgiven.

At this moment we are all good friends. There is no feud or grudge afoot. Everyone is speaking to everyone but to this inquiring eye reservations are apparent. This state of affairs interests me because it makes me wonder about my concept of "rapport." I have always contended that, no matter how well founded, there is a point in any rapport at which it can be shattered and once the buttons are off the foils there's no putting them back. This I know involves the philosophy of repression and restraint. Good friendship is a strong solid thing and of course can withstand storms. Love is probably better defended. While it may or may not have the reasoning background that friendship has, love does have that extra defense provided by the all-powerful but irrational glands of internal secretion. If one partner allows himself to lash out with the bitter unvarnished malicious truth, then I say he has held neither love nor friendship for the target of that attack. Literature, both good and poor, depends for its very life on the universal appeal of the patched-up lovers' quarrel. This yearning of the public soul for proof that love is not killed by an unbridled tongue is in itself the proof that such has not been the general experience. It is a matter of record that many a married couple living in the realm of bliss come to sudden acrimony but soon afterwards are seen soaring again in that same ethereal atmosphere. How much reality was there in the first excursion and how much auto-suggestion and compromise in the second? Every one of us here at various times has revealed rather ugly sentiments to any of three or four others. Yet there is no doubt that it is necessary of course that we all be friends. Our group is small and we are in desperate need of one another yet it would be hard to detect any false note in the present relationships.

January 6, '39. In harness, Dudley and Sport pulled me on skis for miles back on the island, dragging me up over anything and tearing along so you're unable to look where you're going. I really felt all right although tired when I got back, until Doccy Wood told me I oughtn't to be out when I was sick. I protested that I was well and he said I didn't look it.

January 9, '39. Too warm for skiing. A lazy day until we had a few sniffs of Highland Cream before tea. Then I went to the Harbor View Hotel for a tight five hours of bridge and didn't get home till toward dawn.

January 10, '39. A promise of enough freeze in the air to make it worthwhile hitching up the dogs this afternoon. This morning, a patient, Lucy Bridge, slightly toxic and much unmarried, went into mild labor. I didn't hurry upstairs because I knew all was well. Waddell went up and did a rectal. In the mid-morning, I was up a second time and found he had examined her again and ordered an enema. I was sore and asked him what good two sets of examinations were and why he hadn't recommended the enema to me—I was open to suggestion. He said I got sore over nothing and it hadn't looked as if I were paying much attention to her. That's an old trouble I've had with other people. They don't realize I have methods of my own, and while they may seem, and more than seem, to involve a certain amount of procrastination, I do get things done. He quickly shifted to another conversation and obviously doesn't want an open break. Nor do I.

It seems that I was right in saying that Hazel, the over-wrought night nurse, had paroxysmal tachycardia. Her heart slowed when pressure was applied to the carotids. She frets and stews in bed with her sore throat. I told her it was mostly in her head and talked rough to her, which was what she needed. I was too tired to go out in the afternoon and I couldn't go to Wyn's for tea because my patient was coming along. I had tea here instead and she broke her membranes about seven. I got her into the room where Waddell gave her a few sniffs and she was neatly delivered—a nice girl, no bleeding. Waddell told me, "Take the horse, Mack, over to Wyn's to get the people who had gone for tea." I said I would, but walked over rather than tell him I wouldn't do what he suggested. I got lost on the way and started for Crow Head. On eventually arriving, I was taken aback to find they had saved some dinner for me, so I consumed a large plate of chicken and pie and turnip, etc. We stayed until eleven. The walk home was fun. One's stay in any house is governed by the capacity of one's bladder. Arrangements are sometimes too mysterious to go into.

January 11, '39. Misty and warm again; this will ruin the skiing. At night we had tea at the Cottage and played Lexicon. I enjoyed Stan very much. His training and ideas were good. The lights weren't working well. He wandered around all night trying to get them to work—they were on a new engine. It seems that they defy all rational thought and the more you turn on, the brighter they get. He looked as if he were arranging the lighting for the Versailles Conference.

January 12, '39. It's much colder, with a nice breeze from the northwest. I examined Mrs. Woolfrey, a red-faced pleasant woman, who had a kidney out here seven years ago, and was toxemic with a baby two years ago. "You know, doctor, the fits." Now, she is about to have more offspring.

Out on the pond with skis this afternoon, I had no trouble at all being blown clear across, but it was plenty of trouble coming back over a sheet of glass. I assayed a single slide down the spot where we had the jump last year, but it was too fast for me. I had planned to take the dogs, but just as I was leaving I thought that I ought to tell Waddell I was going out so I said, "I'm going out for a minute." " So am I," said he. "Are you taking the dogs?" I inquired. "Yep," without any hesitation. So I didn't take them. He hates to have anyone tell him anything. If you say, I don't suppose you've seen such and such or done thus and so, he is bound to have seen and done it. If you say you haven't seen or done something, he has. If he belches, and someone remarks that sounded pretty sour, he'll say it was a very sweet one. It must be work to maintain that attitude. Tea at the Cottage was a respite. I lay on the floor with Dudley and listened to the BBC Symphony.

January 13, '39. A call came at 3 A.M. and the man who was supposed to come for me said there were no horses at Back Harbor. It was blowing and snowing to make up for lost time. I got Stanley out and he harnessed Mack, then we got Marianne and off we went, after repairing the harness, into a bitter night. I don't blame Doccy Wood for not answering the phone. We found a lady having very little pain. A slovenly hired girl sat and knitted, and wouldn't do a damn thing. I sat behind the stove on the floor and waited a while. The patient was having such poor pains that we gave her a bit of pituitrin, and she went right to work. After waiting only three hours, I had only time to put on one glove. Her uterus was slow to harden, so I hung around for an hour and a half. Having lost a mitt on our trip over the night before, I had everybody in Crow Head looking for it. The rest of the day was slow and lazy, what there was of it.

January 15, '39. Waxed my skis.

January 16, '39. Didn't get to use the skis.

January 17, '39. Drove back to Crow Head. It is a long way and cold. I visited a man with a bit of grippe, and his insane daughter. She is a great big fat thing with a TB knee and whiskers. Mack, the horse, is so slow we were all day driving back. I found my mitt. Hodges had it. Burty Hodge says he wants to cross swords with me again on the chessboard.

January 18, '39. Snowed like hell all day. I stayed in until night, then walked down to Burt Pardy's to play cards. Dudley wouldn't go with me.

January 19, '39. I did a caesarian section the first thing this morning and it went beautifully. Mrs. Jones has a flat pelvis—only 22 cms. Then I went out with the dogs and Waddell and Marianne. The day was perfect with bright blue sky, sunshine, and great snow.

Perhaps the most dramatic surgical caper is the caesarean section. There is a quiet period of preparation. In the classical type of section the uterus is carefully exposed through the abdominal incision and packed off to prevent contamination of the abdomen. Then there is the moment when the knife is poised and a check made that the team is all prepared for its respective roles. Then the tempo changes. The uterus is opened rapidly, there is a great surge of amniotic fluid, a quick grope for the baby's feet, the speedy extraction of the babe, the tying and cutting of the cord, the handing of the baby to the nurse, the medication by injection to help stop the bleeding from the uterus. In opening the uterus one has to cut through the large vessels that nourish the baby. A calm comes again when the uterus firms up to stop the bleeding and one can then suture the incisions with less indication of bustle. The sewing takes place in a better frame of mind if it is to the music of the wailing newborn. Usually there is no trouble on this score but caesarean babies do breathe a little more reluctantly than the natural ones due to the mother's anesthetic, though their heads may be more nicely rounded.

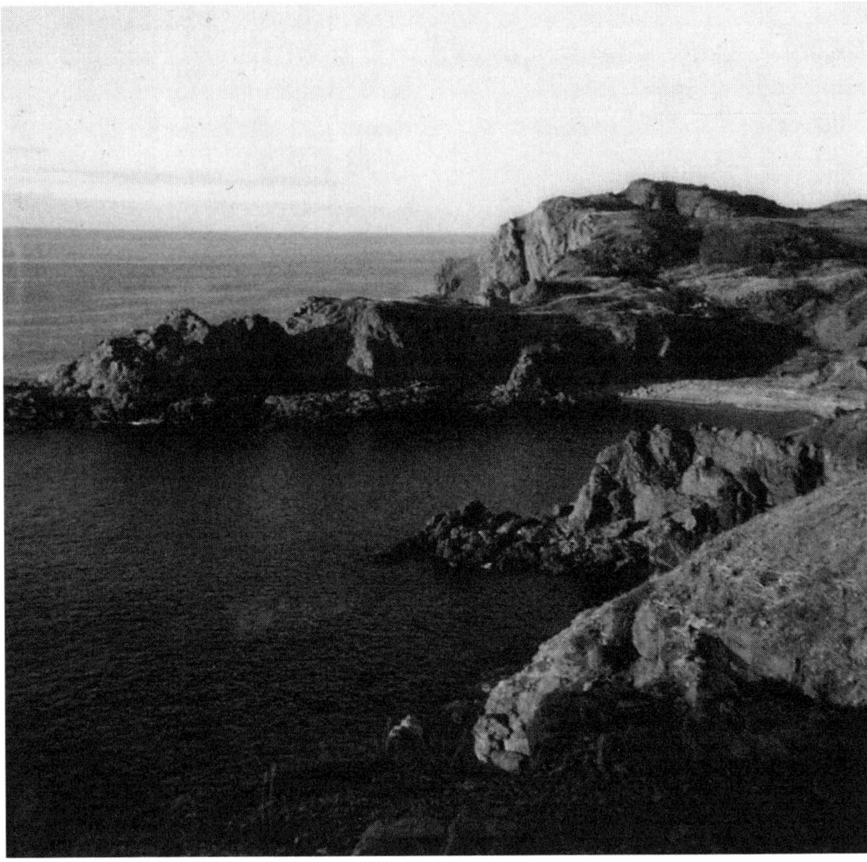

Sleepy Cove as seen from Crow Head. Author's photograph.

January 20, '39. Some goings on. I started out in all innocence by wanting to go skiing. Dudley was there but I couldn't find the others. I went up in back and slid down the hill by the pond and fell, knocking the living stuffings out of me. My ski pole went ahead and I fell on it, wrenching my shoulder and striking my head. Then I found the dogs. I hitched Sport up and Dudley ran away. While I was chasing him, Sport broke away and beat it. I swatted Dudley a few times in a pet, and went to dinner. After dinner all the dogs were gone. Then I got a call and tried again. The dogs had come back. I hitched up Sport and Dudley but they were possessed. I've hardly ever been so exasperated. Sport lay in the snow and wouldn't move without Jake, and I couldn't catch Jake. After mature consideration, I used the ski pole on him, but he wouldn't move. I dragged him until my shoulder got too sore. I yelled till my eyeballs ached. It was a stiff fight, but we finally got going—down to the Arm, only to find that Dr. Wood had beat me to all three cases. I called on Mrs. Blake just for the fun of it. She was lying down. "I can't walk. I smurt and burn and ache all over my hands, my feet, my side, my back, my stomach. I ain't quite numb." I told her to wean the babe two months ago and she hasn't done it. I told her to come to the hospital and she won't. I don't know what's the matter with her but she's no damn good to anyone and she makes me tired. Finally I got home, sore and tired out. Turrs for tea at the Cottage.

With my shoulder aching and my neck stiff, I fell into bed and slumber at the same time, but not for long. I was much annoyed to be summoned at 3 A.M. by Hazel, who said that Austin Roberts, whose wife I had delivered the night David was born to the Olds, was here again for the same purpose. He'd been here a month ago to say that his wife was about to deliver and had gotten into some trouble with the business manager because he hadn't paid for the first one and he wasn't even on the Center now. I got Marianne and off went all of us on a little frame sled you could lift with one hand. The miniature horse trotted all the way. We found they lived in their own house, which made it easier to straighten out the generations. The father has a sister only one year older than his own child. His mother is young looking and has two batches of children of five each, one batch his age and one batch his children's age. Besides that, the old generation is still around. It's the most confused four generations I ever saw. The only ones you can be reasonably sure of are the great-grandparents. They do seem to be a little older than anybody else in the house.

We had to wait nine hours to effect delivery—more time than was strictly necessary to sort out the family. She went to work after a while and when she started to complain that no one would or was helping her, I knew she was getting along. With a few drops of chloroform and an episiotomy, we got a nice girl. I knitted the toe of a homespun sock while waiting. It was not smooth. It tapered off like a Byzantine steeple but it passed inspection and a lot of time. Finally I fell asleep behind the stove and it did little to ease my shoulder and neck. We got back for tea, toast and pumpkin marmalade at the early sitting that morning. I felt not especially well but saw some patients in the OPD and gave the syphilis treatment. A tub before tea and then some poker and I consider myself lucky to get off winning twenty cents. Before that I was all ready to quit the game for good because I'm tired of passing out money to the local townspeople.

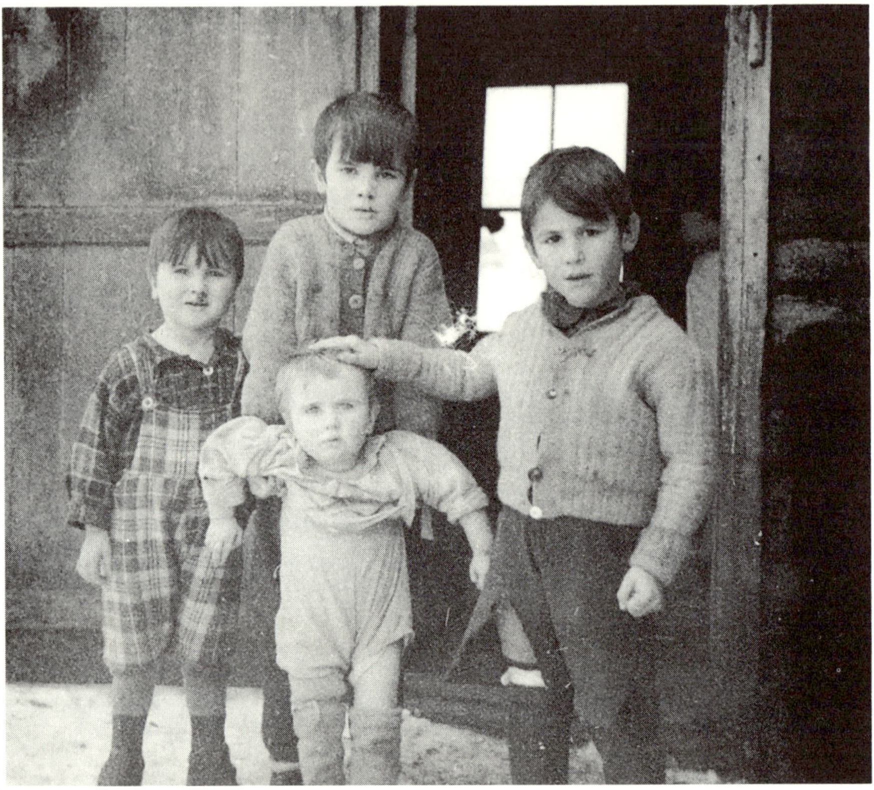

On the Arm at Blow-Me-Down, near Carter's Head, the Dalley brood faces the camera. Author's photograph.

January 22, '39. A regular Sunday, nothing but a patient or two in the morning. Lucy Bridge has a temperature of 104 and I can't find a thing. There is a tender spot in the breast, but it's not enough. Lungs, liver, and uterus are clear. Sulfa seems to bring the temperature down.

January 23, '39. Somehow the morning disappeared easily with a hernia under local and very little after it. In the afternoon I sat around until three, then went up and told Marianne I was going skiing. She said she was interested and might follow along if I went up to the pond. I hitched Dudley and Sport and with Jake running ahead as a volunteer pilot, we crossed the pond and got mixed up a little in the back country. Sport would not go an inch in any direction away from Jake. I followed him then until we were suddenly on Minty's farm. I recognized it by the disused piggery or "Hardy's Folly." They will never use it because pigs fed on fish taste like fish and fish is the only food you can get cheap. I thought we were making for the road but found myself on the top of a cliff by the sea. Jake was down on the shore and Sport was intent on dragging me down to him. I held out and we finally got to the top of a high hill. After numerous tumbles, we reached the junction of the road and the Arm trail. I started up the trail then cut inside to get to the hospital. It was getting dark and I wanted to get home. Sport suddenly refused to go in the direction that I wanted. A dog in heat had crossed the trail ahead of us. I broke my bamboo ski pole on him but it made no difference. I was as mad as I've ever been and really tried to hurt him. I fought as hard as I could and then gave up. I started off with Dudley in harness and Sport's harness over my arm, now really worried about getting back. I plodded along for what seemed like a long time and to my horror found myself on the Little Harbor Road again, only further away from the hospital than when I first started home. I had gone in a complete circle and crossed the Arm Trail without knowing it. Jake appeared from somewhere and I hitched him up and we hit the hospital by the dam. I was played out. I know that Jake is in terrible shape, thin as a rail. We had tea at the Cottage and instead of laughing at my being lost, which I had expected, they all were concerned because it shows how easy it is even on a clear day, to get lost. After all, I am better acquainted with the interior of the island than any of the others.

After tea we listened to the reception for the survivors of the *S. S. Cavalier* torpedoing. Then I went down to Burt Pardy's and we played bridge until 1:30 and I won sixty cents. Mrs. Pardy provided a very good soup. Burt got me interested in a trip that would take three or four months and cost about six hundred dollars. The idea is to catch the Hudson's Bay supply ship *Nascopi* in St. John's or catch up with it on the Labrador and go to Fort Churchill, then to Saskatoon by rail and on to McMurray. From there we'd drive a car to McKay and then a boat across the Great Slave Lake and down the MacKenzie River (2,500 miles) to Aklavik on the Arctic Ocean. You can reach Fort Yukon by dog team, then Fairbanks and out through Alaska to Hollywood. It would be 4,000 miles all told. I don't know—there are a million things to be considered.

January 24, '39. Still talking about the trip, we hugged the fire most of the day due to the cold, zero and a stiff northwest wind with a bit of snow in it. I fell asleep after tea and slept until midnight. Then got up and went to bed. This is a bad habit recently grown worse.

January 25, '39. A very devil of a day with snow and a gale from the southeast. A plaster cast or two. When Reverend Bitt came in for the director's meeting, he said the widow of Obadiah Young needed a doctor, she wasn't on the Center, would anyone go. Braving the tempest I went down. She allowed as how she didn't need a doctor and was much better, after a fall ten days before.

I went up on the pond with Dudley to try the weather. It was stern stuff. The wind drove a sleety snow so hard in the face you couldn't look ahead at all. I sat in the lee of a hummock with Dudley curled down beside me. We had a long silent conversation.

In the evening there was an extremely dull hospital association meeting. The records show an earning for this year of about $1,200 dollars. Afterwards we had a quick round of poker and *mirabile dictu*, I won $2.70 and so did Cody. The worms have turned. This was a lot more interesting than the meeting. I spoke some more to Burt about the cross-Canada trip. He said it would be easier to go down the Porcupine River in the fall before it froze. That way would be quicker and cheaper.

January 26, '39. Alas and alack, woe is me. This has been a sad day for I got a job, or at least the assurance of one. Dad wired me that a Dr. Hirschorn had phoned saying he was forwarding application blanks for a job in New York—practically assured. I don't know what kind of work or where—I don't care much. That would put off my Arctic trek for a year or two for I know as sure as I am alive that I will make it some day. There I was all set for a leisurely period of squandering the thousands of dollars I will have and now it seems I will have to do something that will pay my current expenses. It's possible, and I pray so, that the job doesn't start until the winter or fall and I will be pleased if it holds off until July or August. In that case I will go as far as Churchill, at least.

In the morning I helped Waddell do a complete hysterectomy on Mrs. Saul White. We advised her to go to the States for radium, but we could not drive it out of Saul's head that he would have to buy the radium. The operation was tough. She was deep and full of cancer, but she stood it well. I was about to go to bed, after midnight, when I heard Dr. Wood's ring on the party line so I eavesdropped on Mr. Sid Boyd urging the doctor to come down and see his wife who, he thought, might be in labor. Dr. Wood didn't see the sense in going out on an evil night just to tell her to come to the hospital. He said, "Bring her in." Dr. Wood then rang the hospital and after a decent interval, I answered. He told us he was sending a patient. I went to bed and sort of waited, but she didn't come in after all.

January 27, '39. This morning Mrs. Boyd came in about 11 A.M. The afternoon brought no one and went quickly doing nothing. I finished *Turning Wheels* and started *The Great American Novel.* At rounds, Mrs. Woodford said she had had one OB pain, very slight.

At tea, only three-quarters of an hour later, Marianne asked me to go look at her and I found the head on the perineum. She said she was going to howl and I should forgive her. I hustled her into the operating room and she did howl. She also squirmed, gasped, and shouted, "Kill me, kill me." In record time she was delivered of a good-sized boy. After tea I read a bit, had a nap, and went to bed expecting to be called, but nothing happened during the night except that my blanket blew off and I almost froze. The G.A. novel makes me self-conscious about keeping a journal. It's a skillful book.

The morning was uneventful within but not outside. I took the dogs and skis and started out, soon repenting. It was cold as hell and a fierce northwest wind at work. The recent thaw with following freeze had the ground as slick as grease. The dogs could gallop as fast as ever they wanted and I followed as best I might. I never went so fast on anything without an engine in it. By the pond, little sharp stones stuck through the ice like a nutmeg grater. Stopping short I went sprawling on them and thought my right arm broke. The elbow came out of my leather windbreaker and the skin came off my arm and shin. It hurt so much I was sick to my stomach. My hands were frozen and numb and there was no turning back because my pilot dog was way ahead. They dragged me after I had fallen. I fell again and again and finally got so cold and sick and felt so bad that I was frightened. I wanted to come home. By that time we were way down on the Arm near Ralph Smith's. The trail was too slippery and Jake, who is a smart dog, finally saw what I was driving at and led us to the right of the trail. Dudley certainly pulled. When I get into trouble he comes back to lick my face and he stands over me when I fall as if to keep Sport away from me. I wonder if he would fight for me. Sport has plenty of reason to bite me. Soon I went over an abrupt drop of about four feet. In this sheer white you can't see sudden rises or falls until it is almost too late, or too late. The dogs stopped short but I sailed ahead of them. While I was still in the air, the trace tautened and I landed in, shall I say, a sitting position.

Sport, ninety pounds of him, was jerked into the air like a tooth tied to a doorknob. He hit the back of my neck with a very human-like grunt. I arrived home frozen, stiff, and bruised. My pet jacket may be beyond repair. Tonight is poker and I'm going to win—see if I don't. At any rate, if I lose, Waddell owes me $2.70, so I'll only be out thirty cents. I sat and contemplated our room. It is pleasing from every angle. The three big windows facing the harbor are covered with reddish, tomato-colored woolen curtains, just far enough off the red to be gentle. The walls are a decent light corn. Between the windows hangs a white sealskin that makes a good contrast. The kerosene lamp gives a good soft light. One big wall panel holds a clever sketch of a strange medieval ship. The big bookcase is full of books and on it my elegant big clock against a taupe silk hanging. I won twenty-five cents.

January 29, '39. The ice is gone as far as the breakwater this morning. I wonder if it will ever freeze over. Without ice around the island, the snow will never get deep enough for good skiing. It blows into the water. If there is ice, it blows onto the island as well as off and the drift is equalized.

Coffee this afternoon in Edith's room, then we are all invited for dinner to the Cottage where Suzie has promised us Yorkshire Pudding. This means very little to me as I hate the stuff. But meals are fun. I always enjoy them. I like the people I eat with and on the whole I enjoy what we are served. The Olds are very generous about inviting us to eat with them and so are the Hardys. These meals always have the quality of a party or a celebration about them. A small libation before the meal tends to help the conversation. I always try to dress up a bit and we maintain a little formality. I look forward to these evening occasions. Ward rounds at the end of the afternoon usually find us dragging with weariness. It is not unusual to gather then in one apartment or the other to sample the latest shipment of government rum. The girls join us in this and we are very social. John and Stan and Rube, Marianne and Betty Olds and Annette Hardy all have wide interests and there is much to talk about. I have never felt that our intellectual or emotional stimulation were any more narrow than our cosmopolitan cousins enjoying the advantages of the cultural centers of home. Our meals are of all sorts. Sometimes it is a full-dress imported business where the company and the decor and the dishes would not be out of place in Bucks County. They grade down then through simple meals of moose hamburger, sea birds, and lobster or rabbit or dried cod or turbot or salmon or seal to canned corned beef. Little imported things liven our eating—a Virginia ham or some of Annette's Pennsylvania parched corn.

When we gather around the table talking gaily and eating well I often have a feeling of isolation—the small tight feeling of a small group against the world. It is then that I feel like the proverbial empire builder besieged in an African wilderness.

Fortunately I like dried fish. Fish and brewis is the national dish. Fish is boiled dried cod and brewis is boiled hard biscuit. Over all is poured tried-out pork fat and scraps. I can do without the brewis, but if you substitute good firm hot boiled potatoes I will take that combination any time. In fact I hold it to be a delicately flavored and altogether superior comestible. I am sure my friend Robert P.T. Coffin would back me in that. I don't know what he would think about the way we eat lobsters. He speaks of "A lobster." I only see that delicious creature as whole platters full of the meat. We even find it necessary to leave some on the platter. It is a tribute to the animal that even in very generous supply it loses its charm not at all.

Fish we concluded is good food. We like it smoked, we like it salted, we like it roasted or boiled or fried. There is one form of it however which meets with unanimous condemnation. We DO NOT like fish when it comes disguised as chicken or pork and it is unbearable when it assumes the form of hens' eggs. Food in general is so hard to come by that fish is fed to chickens and pigs. This is all right up to a certain critical percentage—then these animals and their products take on a piscine essence and for some mysterious reason, thus transmitted, that naturally subtle savor becomes just short of nauseating. The pedigree of eggs is carefully watched. All hens' eggs are numbered with pencil so the seller can be traced. One fishy egg in the Christmas eggnog does it no good at all.

February 7, '39. Anyone who invites me anywhere knows that Dudley will show up too. When I go to the Cottage he starts out with me but leaves half way to commune with nature. After I am inside for a few minutes he barks, and scratches at the door nearest where I am sitting. Tonight he left me as usual and when he didn't come to the door within ten minutes, I knew something must be wrong. I called and whistled and looked around the barn and pond but no Dudley. Since he hasn't done this before I am worried.

After tea I distinguished myself. On returning to my room, rather preoccupied, I sat in the big chair. After a while I shifted and the chair moved a bit and as it did so, I heard the tinkle of broken glass. I looked down at the concrete floor and saw a broken rum bottle and near it a little puddle of rum. What I didn't know was that it had been a full 40-ounce bottle of high proof Hudson's Bay Best Procurable, belonging to whom I never found out. Abstractedly after lighting a cigarette, I dropped the match into the puddle and whoosh went the whole end of the room. The curtains started to blaze merrily as did the wallboard. I threw a hooked rug on the blaze, but it was only added fuel. I have a favorite fire extinguisher, by the dining room door, that I always use when the laboratory catches on fire. I ran and seized it and with several well-directed squirts, out went the fire. Those carbon-tetrachloride fumes sure stink in a closed room. No one was amused.

February 14, '39. We are in the midst of examining schoolchildren, with about 250 more to do. We take thirty at a clip and have the clinic well organized for business. We find surprisingly little pathology, mostly of tooth and tonsil, but did spot two children with TB, brothers in the deplorable Lambert family. We had Mrs. Lambert in the hospital, rotten in TB to use the vernacular. Her husband came and took her home because he missed her. The Salvation Army children are obviously in poorer health than the others. The best nutrition is in the Church of England children.

By long telegram, Dean Chesney of Johns Hopkins has offered me a research fellowship at the Children's Hospital School in muscle degeneration. Then the letter came from Hirschorn offering me a surgical job on a rotating service. I couldn't understand that and sent two wires, but no answer. If it's an internship I won't take it, but will be condemned to another year in Baltimore. That wouldn't be too bad—I was happy enough there before and I would organize it differently this time.

Waddell has been behaving pretty well. I think he doesn't realize that he isn't fooling me. I made a trip to Herring Neck, but only after he had turned it down. Whether this was because he had made one and wanted me to have a turn, or whether it was because it was a dreadful day, I don't know. Anyhow, we started with eight dogs from three different teams collected for the occasion. They were no good and I walked every step. I wanted one of the men to stay behind. One was willing, but the other, brother to the patient and owner of four of the dogs, wanted three men along. It was a cold, blowing, snowing day and it seemed a long way to

Brassy's Harbor, then across the ice to Indian Cove, down Goshen's Arm and over to Two Good Arm.

There I found a woman getting over typhoid and a little girl, very sick from what may be typhoid but looked more like TB pneumonia. I had some bread and tea there, in spite of all the germs, but was hungry as hell and it was two o'clock. Two men brought me back but travel was slow and it was dark and dirty when we reached the far side of our island. I decided to stop at the Tilt because the men could never cross the island with me and get home that night. I left the bag by the Tilt, sent the men back and walked the quarter mile to the Warr's, who sort of keep an eye on the Tilt for us. They were loquaciously nice. She urged me to take half a dozen fresh eggs, but I compromised on four. I took a bun of bread and struggled back to the Tilt, refusing to stay for tea. It was hard going and that maneuver was the most tiring of the whole trip. I soon had a fire going, trying to thaw out some of the food. I put butter and peanut butter into the oven. I found coffee and put some on.

There were sardines (no good because of freezing), toast, coffee, eggs, and peanut butter. All this tasted fine. I found a carton of cigarettes, alcohol and lime juice, which I didn't drink, John's flannel pajamas, writing paper, detective stories and some bars of chocolate. After pulling the bed over by the stove I was supremely happy and comfortable and snug, lying there by the fire, reading and writing and smoking and thinking. Just as I blew out the lamp near eleven, I was surprised to hear above the sleet on the roof and the roar of the wind and fire, some voices very near. In the morning it turned out that some people were going by to see where the fire was—a house burned down in Virgin Arm at Hellgrade. Mr. Warr came up early in the morning because he was worried about me. He hadn't told me not to go out on the ice and he thought I might have drowned. There is always a swatch just off Indian Cove where several have met chilly ends in the past few years. His son came part of the way back over the winter road in the morning. It had gotten even colder. The borrowed snowshoes wore out. It felt good to get home and wash and shave and bathe and go to a good dinner at the Cottage.

Still no news of Dudley since the week ago tonight he disappeared. The rumors are all kinds—of his following someone to Burnt Cove, to Kettle Cove, to Chapel Cove, all in the same general direction. Also that various people have him tied up to breed him. The ranger investigated one and offended Reggie Reed to no end. When he came up to me furious, I told him I had heard nothing concerning him, not realizing at the moment that he was the one I had heard about. I have offered a reward and hope rather than expect anything out of it.

February 23, ’39. A week has passed of activity, very pleasant and of indecision that is racking. The people in New York are as poor about making up their minds as I am. Hirschorn answered that the offer was an internship. He says the residency would follow, but I’m afraid of eighteen months in a hospital which is not in especially good professional standing. I’m inclined to go to Baltimore. Though I waste lots of time here and I know I will there, still it’s a better place to do it. There is no great hurry though it is firm in my mind that I must learn to operate and I get no younger.

Well, I got back from the Tilt and enjoyed a quiet day. Then on Tuesday night two boys came in at five o’clock and wanted a doctor to go to Cobbs Arm, where “everybody is sick.” They wanted, what is more, to start at once. Waddell was all for going without further ado. I told him quietly that I would go the next morning and there was no sense in him trying to go then and going to Lewisporte the next day. I got in the tub and he came in to say that he had arranged it and one of the men was to stay in Twillingate. I was up early enough, but my man didn’t show up and I was not surprised because it was very dirty out. They arrived about ten. The one who had agreed to stay here was sick and insisted on coming with us. It was poor going. We met the mail over near Brassy’s Harbor. It took us an hour and a half to get to the tickle, the sick man lagging behind. At Indian Cove two teams were waiting to relay me. My man stayed behind to wait for the straggler, but that character went round the other way through Lobster Harbor and we never did meet up. The two new teams were no good either and I still had to walk. We went through Goshen’s Arm, inside Gut Arm and crossed over to Two Good Arm at Herring Neck and into Pike’s Arm to Cobbs Arm. By that time another team had picked me up and I visited all the hell around Cobbs Arm. Everybody had the flu. The one who had sent for me was not very sick but was being taken care of by her husband, who was much sicker. There were very few well people in that place, but not one would go to bed. At each house, they sat around crowded into the one warm room, coughing into each other’s faces. There were several on the Center, but the one who sent for me was not and had to pay ten dollars. If any of the Center members had called, I would have come for nothing—poor team work.

I walked a mile back around the point to George Chaulkers, owner of the quarry there, who lives in a small well-furnished cabin, even boasting a portable ship's washstand with a letdown basin and a place to drain the water. They fed me well. Mrs. Chaulkers had a bad cold but not the flu. I never tasted anything better than that drink of dollar fifty per bottle rum. I stayed only the half-hour to rest, then two teams came just after mid-afternoon to bring me home. Both teams were rotten, and I walked the whole way back, stopping at Indian Cove to make two calls. My men arranged for a tea there on their way back. They were strangers in the place so I had to guide them. I led them way around the swatch at Indian Cove Rock and we made shore just at dark and it was really dirty going. I showed them the trail back over the island so they could avoid the sea ice. The evening got darker and dirtier until the only way you could tell the trail was by the comparative hardness of it. The island was covered with water. By the time we got to Rocky Pond, it was pitch black. The trails could hardly be smelled out and I noticed we never seemed to climb a hill. When we passed under the wires, I knew we were on the Arm Trail—which would add about three miles to the trip, but I was afraid to strike off over the hills to the hospital. We got to the Arm and backtracked up the road and I was ready to die. I stopped at Pardy's to leave my bag for I felt I could never carry it the 200 yards up the lane to the hospital. Mrs. Pardy offered to feed me and her tea saved my life. I dissuaded the men from starting right back, though one of them was very anxious to be in the Orange Parade the next day.

In the morning I was a rag, with a bad blister on my right heel. Those cotton socks get hard when wet. There was a call to see old John Gillard so I went wanly down with the horse and slide. It wasn't raining, but the westerly wind had piled a lot of water up on the shore and because the snow was so bad on the land, we went over the water-covered ice. It got deeper and deeper, until I was standing on the seat holding the bag on my shoulder. We couldn't see the sled at all and only half of the horse. There even were waves.

John Gillard had pleurisy. This developed later into lobar pneumonia and was given up by Stan Hardy, but he recovered later—much to our amazement and his amusement. He's a nice old guy. I am treating his wife for a broken wrist. They are old-school Newfoundlanders. They eschew the dole and have worked hard all of their 75 years. His son is in difficulty for earning a little money while he's on the dole. To pay his fine, John Olds bought a sheep from him for five dollars. I had refused to help him because I thought staying out of jail was a luxury he couldn't afford.

Well, before Waddell came back from Lewisporte with John and Betty, a wire came from Father Casey saying, "Married woman, 44, frequent, severe abdominal pain, gastritis, stubborn bowels." I replied that it sounded like intestinal obstruction and little could be done at home. "Advise come hospital." His counter reply was, "Please send doctor." All the next day we tried to get a horse or dogs, and only late in the evening did we locate one Ray Roberts who had a good little pony but he wanted dogs to come too, because no one had any idea how the ice was, or if we could get anywhere near Fortune Harbor, which is almost halfway across the bay. When Reggie Reed came out of the bay at night, we engaged him to come along with his dogs. He agreed to call for me at five in the morning so we could get off our island by daylight. He fed his dogs salt herring that night, including his two favorites, whom he never used in the bay for work, but only for trips. He locked them up without water, I suppose so as to be sure to be able to find them in the morning. In the morning the two favorites were dead. I imagine from too much salt. One more gave out before we left the hospital. I was ready to go at five. I waited until six, and found him outside where he had been waiting an hour. It seemed like a poor start. Three dogs gone and him so "stun." We started off and it was cold. My overcoat fell off the dogsled five times before he tied it on. At Bluff Head Cove we picked up Roberts, and I got on the horse slide. We started across the bight at Gillard's Cove, the cold wind searching us. We met a few teams, including the manic Chum Grenham, who danced about and shouted. His horse was dragging his dogs and a cold disconsolate child who sat on the dogsled, obstinately trying to keep warm by retreating within himself. Our dogs, by this time, were way behind us. We asked Chum to come with us, and we would send Reed back. He said he couldn't because he hadn't been warned and he couldn't buy dog food. The last was true and we concluded that being on the dole, he couldn't afford to make any money. We decided to cut into Chance Port and cross the neck to Bridgeport, when Reed caught up with us and we stepped into Dove's house to get a warm. When I came out I slipped down the hill onto the Cove, must have gone thirty feet. The neck was only recently frozen after the mild and the going was bad. Everybody told us we couldn't possibly get to Fortune Harbor and I would have to go way into Lewisporte for the train to Badger and then out 60 miles by dog to Fortune Harbor. We kept on through. In Bridgeport I met Rideout, whose giant-cell tumor I had gouged off the nose. He thought we might be able to get to Black Island which is out in the Ships' Run on the line for Fortune Harbor. We tied the dogs to the back of the horse slide and set straight across the Run. We cleared Cottle's Island and reached Black Island in an hour. It was so cold I didn't know where I was. There is a fair settlement on Black Island. We picked the largest house and went in. The big, fat wife was very cordial and slipped into another room to change her dress. The old man told us about his bad stomach while she got some tea and bread and butter ready. We opened our own food and ate a little of theirs. I left some oranges for them. They had a large family and great numbers of guns around the room. Our host recognized Ray Roberts. What a story came out of that. Some years before, Roberts had been passing the island with his passenger boat when it started to leak around the propeller shaft. He had landed his twenty passengers and collected ten men from the shore and the thirty of them had stood on our host's wharf to pull the boat out so it could be repaired. The wharf collapsed, throwing all of them into the water. Roberts turned to see how the owner of the wharf was taking this sabotage and found him laughing so hard he couldn't stand up. All he said was that if he ever wanted to go to Lewisporte, Roberts would have to take him free. I was struck with the touch and go and give and take, the affection between these isolated island people. It was much different from the Twillingater, who has been spoiled a little by the near civilization we have there.

On we went another hour to Swan Island. During this leg we met several skaters incredibly gliding on strange homemade skates, Turkishly curled up in front. They were mere pieces of iron, fixed into large wooden blocks, and strapped to the shoes with ends of twine. They reported the ice was good enough. We didn't stop at Swan Island for more than a minute. We did see the man who lives there alone with his wife and son and another stuttering child. We wanted to borrow a pot, but he said he had "neither." We left the dogs there and made our dash across the Run with the horse to Norther Harbor. Our Swan Island man had said he supposed we could get across the Ships' Run with the horse, but no one had done it that winter. In fact, no horse had ever been known to have made this course from Twillingate—not in the last twenty years at any rate.

It was only an hour or so to Norther Harbor, over the sea. A squall obscured it for a while but we had no trouble and found it a lovely place if I've ever seen one. A narrow neck of beach separates a salt pond from the Run. Over to the left a jagged head guards the harbor which communicates with the pond. Thick woods ring it all around and high hills watch over it. There are several stilted houses but no "liveyere's." All are gone to Botwood to work in the mines. There is a camp there where Harry Pinn was staying when the stove exploded and he was so badly burned—almost all over. His friends had raced to Fortune Harbor and had a boat come from Exploits. They got him back to the hospital where, by some miracle, he lost only a finger and lived to play bridge with me every Monday night. We broke into the cabin and found a rusty kettle and boiled a bit of water and made some tea. We had cake and toast with it. We rested a while, being days ahead of schedule. Then we made our way the four miles through soft, deep snow. No horse had been through this year. I beat the trail out ahead and lay down at Pine Pond until they caught up with me. We hurried on through the lovely valley to Fortune Harbor where we met a man with an ox, the first I'd seen in Newfoundland. It's a good form of beast, works for you and there is no prejudice against eating it. The Fortune Harbor people impressed me at once. They are independent and industrious. There was no one on the dole here for years and now there are only a few. It's an all-Roman Catholic community except for the principal businessman, who is a favorite here. These people consider each other with politeness and respect.

We soon met up with Father Casey, who took me to the Fowlows' where the woman seemed to be having a mild gall bladder attack and a small *crise de nerf.* Then I made a call or two elsewhere and retired to the parsonage where I was well received. Though the place was a little junky, with the system of a bachelor, there was a good bed. We talked until midnight. He asked if I wanted a cooked supper, of course I politely said no. He stepped to the door and shouted, "Never mind cooking anything!" I had a good tea nevertheless, though the tea we drank was the strongest I've ever encountered. He amazed me by knowing so much about his parishioners. I asked when so-and-so expected her baby. "Let me see," says he, "she had her last regular period in November, a little spotting in December, none in January, and then in February she spotted a little," and so forth. I was being very careful about phrasing and editing when he came out with, "Doctor, what do you think about sexual intercourse when the woman is pregnant?"

The morning was bright but full of "dwys." Afraid of the weather, the men didn't come for me until eight. I borrowed a loaf of bread from Casey who had risen at five to eat with me, and off we went leaving what is said to be the best harbor in the world. It would hold the whole British Navy, is infinitely better than St. John's, and that's a famous harbor. Fortune Harbor has only one rock and plenty of deep water protected from all winds by high bluffs. It looks like the Hudson River. A ship is often piloted in at night and has no idea of how to get out in the morning.

There was a lot of local talk about secret submarine bases and possible enemy attack.

We followed our own trail back with a fine wind blowing, rested a moment at the camp, then tackled the Ships' Run. We turned back when a thick squall blinded us. Then started again with the wind behind us—otherwise we couldn't have made it. The breeze was phenomenal—Ray let go of the slide and he literally blew away. He couldn't get to his feet. He scratched at the little snowy places but couldn't move. He tumbled nearer and nearer to the edge. We had to go and get him with the horse.

The ice cracked during the night, but it was twelve inches thick. We got to Swan Island to the surprise of Mr. and Mrs. Wills who had never thought to see us again. They put our horse in their little barn, making room for it by chasing a goose out. There were chickens, cows, and sheep—all piled in the shelter like eels in a basket. Mrs. Wills was combing her hair in the kitchen and continued to do so until she was through. Then she set out all she had, including cake. We had a nice visit. I gave the boy my compass. There was much joking and a nice regard between the married couple that was new to me. Mr. Wills showed me a boat he was building. He said he couldn't build them fast enough, everybody wanted one. He bemoaned that his sons were not interested, but only wanted to go to the mines and woods and work their guts out for the quick, poor pay—no love of craftsmanship.

He didn't know who would make the boats when he was gone. These people are completely isolated. They have to go all the way to Exploits just to get their mail. We left the Wills for another hour at the ice to Black Island where, again, we were received as risen from the dead. This time we had pie. As I finished, the large family, a whole crowd of grown men and girls came in from church. The teacher lived with them and seemed to be the object of a lot of good-natured mauling. They said grace and sat down to pack away great piles of spareribs and codfish. We kept on for Cottle's Island Tickle, inside of Bridgeport, because we thought that this wind would be breaking up the ice. The horse insisted on going back the way he had come. We had quite a job persuading him to take the new unmarked trail. I was glad to reach the tickle, to get protection from the wind. It blew through my overcoat and leather jacket as if they were chiffon.

The ice, too, was behaving peculiarly. At first I thought it was my eyes, but when we stopped to look, we noticed waves about twelve feet from crest to crest, passing slowly and almost imperceptibly through the ice. It was a strange, weird feeling—a sort of frozen slow motion. The horse would suddenly, and by some unknown force, be on a hill in front of us, and then in a valley, yet everything was smooth and flat. The ice was groaning, especially along the shore. We were scared and stayed close to the island. I couldn't ride anymore and to sit a minute was to freeze. We emboldened and struck out to sea for Bridgeport, though discretion would have kept us into Summerford, deeper in the bay, to get better ice. The ice got worse. The driver said he didn't know anybody that would go out on ice like that and he certainly never would again. I got blown away here and they had to come and get me. Bridgeport Run seemed ten miles deep as we drove in right before the wind. I got colder and colder as it blew harder and harder.

At three o'clock we got over the neck and stopped at Skipper George Doves'. The men wanted to spend the night there, but it didn't look like a likely spot. Dave is eighty and so is his wife. They got tea for us at once. I offered to pull his teeth for him for nothing because they put on a terribly poor mouth. Skipper claims he hasn't been the same since he fell twenty feet off the school building and landed on his head. Has a bit of the rheumatics too. I told him he was lucky to be alive and to stop talking about it but he was one to speak his mind. Had lots to say about how little the doctors worked and how much they made. But I enjoyed him, and his wife was charming. We ate all there was, and, reluctantly, set out.

Landing on Trump Island, just at five we had some trouble. The horse went through to his belly where the ice was broken at the shore. A team was just leaving for Twillingate, only three miles away. We asked if it was safe to go on, and the other team, Lewis Legge, said it must be for they had left Twillingate only two hours before. It looked doubtful to us. Right where we were, the ice was groaning and moving and beginning to break up. Besides that, we couldn't see land and it was getting thicker. The other Twillingate team started out boldly. We followed hesitantly. In half a mile the ice got terrifying. It swelled and heaved like something was alive under us, nor could we see even fifty feet ahead. In the dark I stepped on an ice pan only as big as a wash boiler. If the horse had stepped on it, we would have been lost. We quit and went back, getting onto Trump Island only with great difficulty. Legge had disappeared into the gloom, we thought forever.

A boisterous, talkative, complaining Mrs. Smith gave us welcome and we didn't even have to ask if we could spend the night. Their house holds three ordinarily. I was worried when I saw that besides her husband, she had two daughters-in-law and their four children staying with them. One daughter was there because her husband was in the hospital with a slashed foot. I had sewed it up only a few days before. This daughter was a cripple. She talked in a strange, high theatrical voice. "You'll naver see your daddy again. You will call for him in vain," she shouted to an imbecilic-looking baby who squalled and bawled. Then she would heave it one breast, then she would feed it out of a cup, then some bread and milk, then spoon after spoon of molasses. Then she would heave it the other breast. About then Legge and his party staggered in, and that made thirteen of us. I just sat dumbly beside him. We had his son, crazy, in the hospital. He himself had been on trial once for incest. He turned out to be a pleasant, good-natured companion. I was afraid to give up my seat on the couch, for I planned to lie on it if bedtime ever came. We were fed after the children. Our hostess was crippled with lumbago or would have provided better than loaf and tea—if she could have moved. We had loaf and tea with a vengeance. I could not stay awake. She kept asking me why I didn't go to bed but that didn't seem possible while three men were sitting on the couch I had claimed. About midnight she struggled to her feet and said, "Come, if you are bashful I will put you to bed." To my pleasant confoundment, there was a nice, clean bed in the next room. To be sure, each slat is carved forever on my back, but I slept well, even took off my clothes. None of that second-hand flavor to this bed, but I know what a job it is to wash blankets in this country.

The morning was clear and bright. After more loaf and tea we took off. I bought a hooked rug before that. Fortunately, the cold had hardened the ice so the trip to Gillard's Cove was nothing. At the Cove they told us that no man could have landed the night before and we might easily have died trying. I was happy to pay the men and turn the twenty-five dollars over to the hospital.

The first person I saw at the hospital was John Olds, returned, with Betty, from their longish holiday. There was a restrained greeting, we have never reached a backslapping stage and I suppose one never does with him. He is constructed much like myself, I think, only less lazy and more intelligent. He has the same fears, except physical ones—he has none of those. We do have the same emotional approach. The account of their trip back from Lewisporte to Twillingate is a lesson in temperance. Their route was inside mine all the time, on better ice and with better weather but they were beset by every trouble that one can find in this world, almost. They apparently started in good enough time, but had a great deal of trouble getting loaded. The stuff kept falling off the sled. One horse fell and broke up the rig. At one difficult point, John fell under the horse and Betty closed her eyes because she thought he was going to be killed. The barrel of flour fell off and hit Harry Osmond on the head. Betty said she was more unhappy than she has been on any trip in her life. They had taken the land at Chanceport and cut up over the marsh to Moreton's Harbor. It was on the marsh where most of the trouble arose.

John was back only a few days when he somehow got us talking about Waddell's prospects for getting married. Waddell is about to join the seal fishery as doctor on one of the steamers. The hunt starts soon from St. John's. Tommy is going on her holiday to her home in St. John's. I said matrimony was ridiculous because I'd been seeing Waddell about twenty-six hours a day and knew there was no affair with anybody. I bet John ten dollars Waddell would never get hitched in Newfoundland. Edith was so sure he wouldn't that she bet twenty-five. But they were leaving for St. John's together.

Harry Osmond came up to Twillingate for a party the night before the Lewisporte expedition was to set forth, which he would skipper. We had a bit of rum, not any great quantity. Marianne came in late, off duty at eleven, but she refused a drink. On going into the Olds' bedroom with a lamp in her hands, she stumbled, dropped the lamp and broke the chimney. She cut her hand and there was much to-do, but no fire was started.

Next morning there was a grand departure. After repeated thumpings on the barometer, Stan and Annette decided to go along for the trip. Waddell was loaded down with gear for the ice and Tommy was all excited about her holiday. Waddell took the lead, then the Hardys, and Tommy was the last one we saw disappearing down the hospital lane. She looked very chic in her sealskin boots and fur hat.

It seemed very quiet, for a while, when they had all gone. I was busy enough finishing up a few odd jobs in the OPD, then sat down to dinner

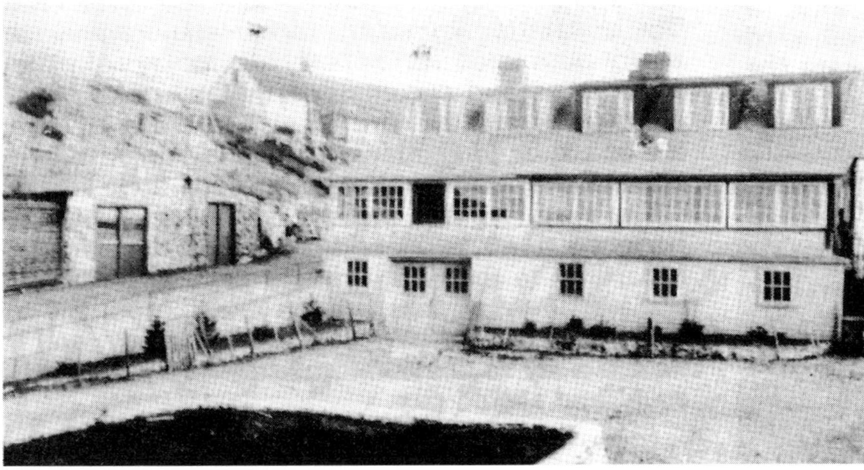

The Cottage. Author's photograph.

at one o'clock—meat pie. I was just putting a forkful in my mouth when Wyn stuck his head through the doorway and said something about getting to the Cottage. I didn't hear him very well, but I thought he told me that I was invited to the Cottage for dinner. I started a long speech about people who didn't invite you on time, and who did they think they were and I wasn't going to stop in the middle of a meal—intending to go right on with my dinner. At a rhetorical pause, I noticed the people around me looking rather peculiar, as if something had been said that hadn't registered. Suddenly David's nurse ran in through the back door with David naked in her arms. She said the Cottage was on fire. I grabbed my favorite fire extinguisher and rushed up. John and Betty and ten men or so were standing out in front. There was a nasty, loud crackling and flames were visible at the living room window. I tried to get in at all the doors but it was impossible to do a thing. We couldn't breath or even see. Black clouds rolled out of the windows. I confess I didn't think of any particular mission; it didn't occur to me at once that something ought to be saved. The fire gained rapidly. Mabel and a few of the women started to grab water to put it out, but there wasn't any sense to it. In two minutes the upper part of the house was a solid flame. I went into the cellar with some of the men and wheeled the motorcycle out. The doors were hard to move against the ice. We fooled around the porch window trying to get the radio. George Hawkins climbed into the porch but we hung onto him and begged him to come out. He has a wooden leg.

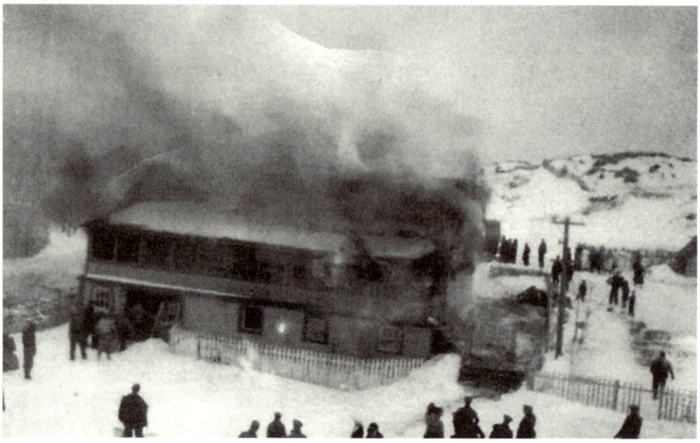

The Cottage—going . . .

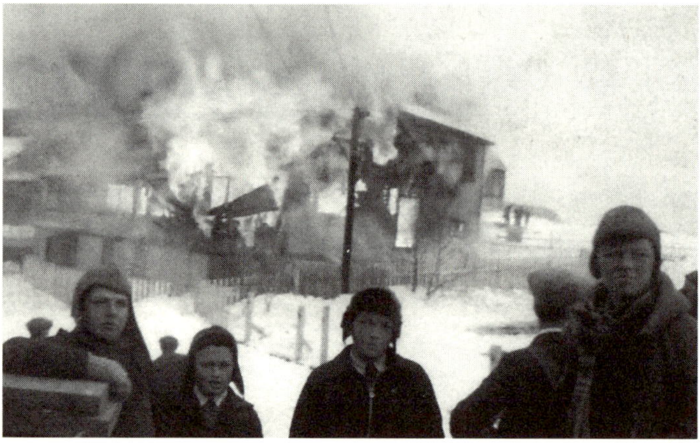

going . . .

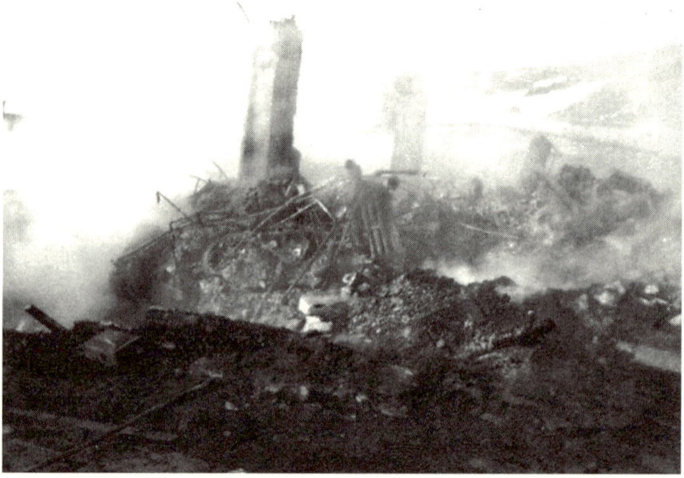

gone. Author's photographs.

The windows were difficult to break. The hard wood bars were like iron. Someone had been right in the kitchen when the fire was discovered and had emptied John's closet which communicated from the bedroom to the back hall. The Olds had been at the dining room table when they heard a crackling noise in the cellar. They had gone down to the cellar to investigate and had seen nothing. When they came upstairs, the room next to the dining room was in flames and as they left the dining room, the floor burst into flames behind them. Betty had gone out of the front door and John to the back to shout up to David's nurse and the sleeping night nurses, Marianne and Hazel. By the time they had grabbed coats, it was hard to get downstairs. David and his nurse only just made it. Suzie lived in a basement room. Men were able to get into her room through a window and save her possessions. The hospital windows got hot, but no damage was done there.

When the last wall had fallen, they counted losses. Marianne and Hazel and Betty possessed only what they stood in. For Marianne and Hazel that meant slippers, nightgown, and coat. Betty didn't even have a coat. She was in a dollar-and-a-half utility dress. She had lost the first new clothes she had bought in six years. David was naked. Books, maps, silver, beautiful English furniture from the Sterling estate, furs, guns—all gone. They were pretty brave. We assembled makeshift costumes for them and we all had a drink in my apartment. I had fortunately borrowed John's raccoon coat so Betty had that at least to wear. Here John took the opportunity to announce that Waddell and Tommy had been married at New Year's. These two shocks in one day made it seem a very full one. Bets were not collected because he had known all the time. The Hardys were certainly surprised to find the Cottage gone when they got back. They were also a little miffed at having gone on the Waddell honeymoon without knowing they had been married.

CHAPTER VI

New York, April '39

Lo, verily, I am caught in some kind of a sink, not knowing if the work will be useful or completely useless. Details can be saved for a time when I am not feeling the load of a continuous jump since leaving Newfoundland a fortnight since. I've never wished I were back in my icy fastness more than I do today.

Nothing could be more remote from our esoteric and almost monastic medicine than this skullduggery and malpractice. And this I say without exchanging a word with anyone, that is, with anyone on the outside service. All the attending interns say that the outside MDs are punks, that they don't know a goddamn thing and I'm beginning to believe it. The resident, one Brady, is a believer in Father Coughlin and Hague of Jersey City. The interns have no relationship with the outside men. Apparently the patients are kind of dumped on us and we never know whether to leave an order or not. They're not our patients and that's a prize gripe. I'm far from determined to stay here much more than my six months. Since the resident is the most unpresuming guy and will turn over anything at all to me, I don't believe the residency will be anymore advanced than my present assistant residency. What I don't see is how a great marble palace, equipped like a castle, can house such cheapness and fakery. This place has lower standards than Hitler.

April 23, '39. Well, how can I give a correct picture of this place? It started as a university hospital but was vacated when the medical centers coalesced uptown, except Bellevue. With McKim, Meade and White grandeur—marble, bronze and all the fixings. Somehow it got into the clutches of the Randall family. It was said that he had a million dollars behind him for the start. It is tall and well furnished and handsome with high ceilings. Randall has a great big suite downstairs—a whole fleet of rooms 30 by 30 with 30-foot ceilings, dim lights and Persian rugs. He sits at the head of it, but it has been confided to me that he doesn't know a thing. He dabbles with a form of pediatrics.

We are quartered on the fourth floor like servants, in hygienic but deadly surroundings. My room has a high ceiling too, tile floor on which my watch breaks, no rug, a hospital bed, no curtains for the high narrow windows looking out on a dim court.

They say it is cool in summer, but I will never test it. We are shepherded by a chief of intern service, one Herman Trueman, an old Army man, who was kindness itself. Furthermore, he is very straight and will back you to the limit; he will also give you hell without a murmur. He says we will sign a contract for six months, and later would discuss the staying longer. No contract will hold me the first six months. The trouble with my job is that I have nothing to do but spell the resident when he goes out. I never see him. The housemen take good enough care of the patients and the attending visit so much that they follow their own cases quite closely. I have to make a superhuman effort to know any of the patients, but that effort will have to be made soon, for one outside M.D. called me up tonight and gave me hell for not being on to a patient with whom we had had trouble when the intravenous was hard to start. He wanted to know just what my job was and one thing and another. I don't get scared for I don't care what anyone wants to say about me. For that reason I sign in and out as I please and I don't have to toady one bit.

We are fed way up the back stairs, very much like menials, but the meals are good enough, though the boys raise hell all the time about them. The meat is inclined to be racy and for that reason rather overspiced. I like most of the interns, especially soft, little Feitel with his pleasant full face. The interns seem respectful enough to me except Bruno, who knows it all but is really over-inflated and very independent. Some of outside staff are fair, a few are good and most of them are lousy. They plow around. The OB people are especially bad; they all do vaginals at the drop of a hat. They give Morphia at any old time and are unable to tell anything from a rectal examination. The medical service I don't know very much about for I don't see those patients. A lot of my time is spent in the surgical service. Dr. Schwartz, a big, round, beefy, slack-faced type with a scoop mouth and widely separated teeth, does a fast, sort of rough, surgery. He keeps the seventh floor full and does about 1,200 operations a year, ten minutes to a hernia, and the boys are afraid of him. He doesn't wear a mask and noisily sucks air through his teeth.

My first night on duty a man came in who was posted for 8:30 in the morning. I examined him and thought he ought to be done at once (11 PM). He had a hot belly, high temperature and a high white blood count. He was an Alpha Delt from Brown. I told the lad on Schwartz's service to call him and ask him if he knew the belly was so hot. The lad said he wouldn't call him for anything in the world, so I called him. "Listen, Doc," says he, "I know this patient (he had never seen him, it was a fee splitting referral) and I posted him for morning, and I don't thank anyone for butting in." He apparently couldn't go back to sleep though, for he showed up in a couple of hours and took out a gangrenous appendix that certainly would not have gone till morning. He ate a hell of a lot of crow and has been nice to me ever since. He sort of instructs as he goes along and is really genial. (Father has a client who knows him, says Schwartz is a bastard and was thrown out of a community hospital. My Father months later told me that Schwartz was in Sing-Sing for insurance fraud.) Jacobs is a professor at the University and has a certain style. What gets me are the sycophants, the Warren Brothers, who bring their work to him. They spread the goo over each other until I don't know what to do. Jacobs is a fair surgeon, though inept and slow. He listens to me and will let me help him. When I told an intern that I was pleased when a OB man let me do a forceps he laughed and said the doctor didn't know how to do it. I enjoyed assisting a nose and throat man on a mastoid, but beforehand the doctor got my goat by saying there was no sense in doing work cheap. He said, "Soak them and they'll think you're better." I can't repeat all his statements, but I've never heard such a commercial aspect put on medicine. As a matter of fact, when the surgeons get together in the Green Room after scrubbing, instead of exchanging ideas, they talk about collections and fees. Their knowledge is safe with them, like trade secrets.

I am on a job to find out what is happening to the morphine, which is disappearing. I have no idea yet, for one of the suspected nurses has cleared out. I'll keep this record better and do my Yoga and hope for the best. I must get hold of Hirschorn soon and have an understanding.

My stay at this place was lightened by an acquaintance I made through the night nurse supervisor, one of the people here that I really liked. She called me on the phone one night about nine to tell me there was a British doctor downstairs who had been a short time in New York and wanted to look at the plant, would I show him around? I hastened to comply, and was introduced to Captain Romney, late of His Majesty's Hundred and Something Royal Hussars, a good-looking gent about my own age, on his way to England from Malaya. As he chatted with me in his tweeds, he kept leaning on his tightly furled umbrella, which, as he leaned, kept slipping on the marble floor. This convinced me he was English. I was further convinced of his Englishness when he commented uncomplimentarily on everything he saw: "D'ya mean to say this is your x-ray room?" "You have to live in this gutter?" "Is this the best operating room you have?" Since I didn't like the place, either, this common bond of destructive criticism cemented our friendship. As he borrowed my tobacco, he told me how he used a special English blend, which he aged with rum, and offered to send me some to try. When he found I didn't like most of my colleagues, he asked where they were and then sauntered along into the room where they were playing pinochle and reported back in five minutes that he had told them what an awful place this was and how dreadful it must be to work here.

My interest in the North stirred him—by Jove, he knew Sir Hubert Wilkins, and it would be a good idea if I went with him on a forthcoming Arctic expedition. He would immediately write a letter for me requesting temporary membership in the British Medical Association.

Next evening he was back again, he was staying in Great Neck, to tell me he had spoken to his father by transatlantic phone and put him right to work on Sir Hubert. It was certain I could go north. Captain Romney was going to be in New York only a few more days, because he had an engagement to speak in Baltimore on psychiatry. Professor Adolph Meyer had invited him. Then he was to leave for England. He would like, though, to take me to dinner two days later. The following afternoon I was surprised to have him suddenly appear, breathless and agitated. He had been to the World's Fair and lost his wallet. He didn't know what he would do. He was too polite to ask for any money, but I urged him to take ten dollars, which he reluctantly accepted, and then I forced eight more on him when I found he was planning to stay at the Waldorf until he could get to his bank in the morning. He embarrassedly thanked me and left. The moment the door closed behind him, I felt something was wrong. I rushed to the phone, a long distance call to Baltimore revealed that Professor Adolph Meyer had never heard of Captain Romney. The police, on the other hand, knew him well. He had taken the librarian at Columbia for five dollars and had lectured on psychology at an assembly in a New York school and sold books to the teachers which, in spite of generous prepayment, had never been delivered. Worst of all, he had lectured to a Boy Scout troop and taken several scouts home in a taxi, ducking out at the last moment and leaving them to pay the bill. I sorted vainly through the photographs at the Rogue's Gallery, and philosophically concluded to myself that it was almost worth twenty dollars to learn such a lesson; and I stopped packing for the Arctic.

I'm almost as bad as my father. He was swindled four times by people who claimed respectively to be stranded college friends of my brother, of me, and of my sister. He grew philosophical about it, too. The second time it was worked in my sister's name, he didn't even wait for the end of the touch. He resignedly asked, "How much this time?" He was afraid to risk being thought hard-hearted by any of our friends.

Saddened by this revelation of falseness in my fellow man, but happy that my servitude had ended after 40 days and happier yet at the prospect of returning soon to Newfoundland, I paid my visit to California.

On my return East, I somehow found myself on a Colorado train between Pueblo and Denver. There were few passengers and no Pullman. In the friendly smoker, I fell in with a kindly, gray-haired, fattish man who wore a railroad uniform. In the breezy western fashion, we were soon intimates. He was telling me about his syphilis and showed me pictures of his grandchildren. He admired my generous head of hair and, with one thing and another, I was soon recounting for him my dolorous experience with Captain Romney, the confidence man. He was fascinated and shocked by this tale of eastern perfidy. "Tsk, tsk," he said, "I wish you would tell my friend, Blackie, about that," and he soon returned with a younger man, also in railroad uniform, who sold Indian jewelry for the benefit of tourists. Blackie was shocked by my now-embroidered story. "You know," he said, "I trust people and people trust me. Nothing like that ever happens. Everybody along this line knows me and, when the cowhands are broke, they come down to the station and ask me to buy a watch, or some silver spurs, or a ring. I give them what they think it's worth, and then I dispose of it in Chicago for about the same amount. I never have lost—but I don't plan to make any money at it, and it's a lifesaver for those boys. Now just this morning I gave a feller eight dollars for this." Out of his watch pocket came a beautiful, shiny gold nugget the size of a hazelnut. "A peach, ain't it?" he said, hefting it. "I'll get eight bucks for it, but it sure feels like more. Wouldn't want it, would you?" I hesitated, and he quickly stowed it out of sight and made as if to leave. "Let me see it again?" I asked. It was obviously worth about $40.00; in my haste to give him the eight bucks for it, I even dropped my thinning wallet on the floor. At Chicago, the three of us bid each other the fond farewells of lifelong friends. Need I record what a chemist friend told me of his test on this nugget? I forget just what the analysis showed, but the assay ran 18 cents to the ton, and I had something like an ounce and a half.

The Return

July, 1940—Twillingate

My homecoming to Twillingate was in rather a different style this time. I had expected the place to stand still during the year of my absence, but there were sea changes. Waddell and Tommy had taken up a practice in the settlement of Wesleyville at the northern mouth of Bonavista Bay. My place had been filled for the year by Chalian, a Hopkins classmate. The Olds had made themselves a new home, after the destruction of the Cottage by fire, on the top floor of the hospital where the water pressure is too low to allow its use as a ward. Edith was married, and had left to go live at Springvale, Green Bay with her Ranger husband. The Hardys were still at Twillingate, I am happy to say.

Since Waddell had wanted to get home to the States for a visit I covered for him at Wesleyville for about two weeks before settling in at Twillingate. It was a strain to work at a place where there was no hospital for emergency surgery. Waddell had established a firm place for himself in the local hearts. On his return I took the *S.S. Segona* as far as Carmanville.

Ted Drover met me at Carmanville, our plan being to finish the journey in his skiff. It has a small, two-bunk cuddy forward and a telephone booth of a wheelhouse, the stern half-open.

We picked a civil day for our trip. That was to prove fortunate. All was quiet until we had left the open shelter of Bacalhao Island and started

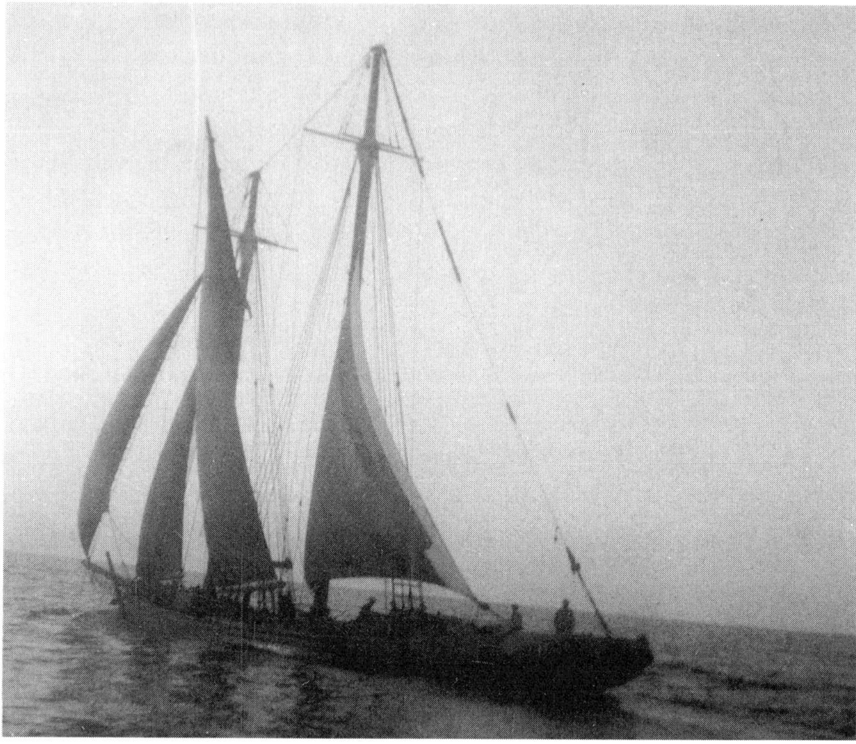

Wearing the mainsail, the *Dorothy and Ruth* heads north with a cargo of salt after dropping off Ted Drover and the Doctor in the dark somewhere north-east of Twillingate. Author's photograph.

through the open sea between there and Twillingate Long Point. It was getting dusk as we spied, against the setting sun, a big, heavily loaded schooner pointing north for the Labrador. "That looks like the *Dorothy and Ruth*," says Ted, "Let's go aboard and see the old skipper, Jim Wey." We put on steam and turned out to sea. They saw us and slowed until we got a line aboard. Jim was glad to see Ted, and invited us below right away. The *Dorothy and Ruth*, 200 tons, was once a smart craft. Zane Grey had used her for a long cruise. The saloon was mahogany paneled. Now she was awash at the waist, so heavily loaded with salt for the Labrador Fishery. Jim was sorry that he didn't have a proper drink to give us, but on the cold saloon stove was a big aluminum cooking pot of what looked like weak tea. "I'll tell you what this is," says our seagoing host. "I bought an empty rum keg from the commission and let some hot water stand in it all night.

This is what came out. It tastes like rum." We started quaffing from big earthenware mugs. It tasted mild, but the conversation grew animated and the hours vanished while the schooner beat her way northwards. It seemed such a short time before Jim jumped up and said, "Great Scot! You boys better get in your boat. It's a small one for this water and we're way outside now."

On deck the northern evening was peacock blue. We couldn't even see Twillingate Light, and that is 300 feet from the water. We got our course and climbed into the boat. I didn't like it too much—the idea of being out of sight of land on such a small boat. We pointed for Twillingate and watched the *Dorothy and Ruth* wallow away from us. The rum washings had not seemed much to me, but Ted was making heavy weather. In an hour we raised Twillingate Light, a seeming assurance that nothing could go wrong now. Suddenly, to our complete mystification, it vanished while we looked at it. We uneasily kept our course and in another two hours made landfall. It was at a completely unfamiliar place, a narrow indraft went between the cliffs. "Damn if I know where we are," says Ted, "but let's hurry!" We put on speed and cut a line down the middle. After half an hour we realized that the current had carried us south and the light had been blocked out by the high rocks of Burnt Island. We had been speeding through Burnt Island Tickle, a kind of side entrance to Twillingate. It is full of rocks and by the chart it is impossible to take the course we did.

At the wharf, I stood outside telling Ted where the rocks were. There didn't seem to be any response to my observations. I looked in the wheelhouse and Ted was, shall I say, asleep over the wheel. Others might say asprawl. I berthed the craft, roused Ted and got up the lane to the hospital. As luck would have it there were, even after midnight, a few loungers on the wharf. Next day the story of our unskillful landing was all over town. "Dr. Hackie had come back." There was also some comment as to the sobriety of the event, but it bore no relation to the imbibing. What convinced them was that I had "come ashore in underwear." Actually, I was wearing very smart white tennis shorts, but in this country no man in his right mind would appear so unclothed. The men are so modest that they lock the door to change a necktie. "Rum washings" is not that strong. Ted must have already had a load aboard.

My friends were glad to see me, though a little discouraged to note that I had brought another Irish setter—this time a little two-month female given me by Marianne to replace the still-mourned Dudley. I pushed my luck and called her Dudley II, though it's no name for a lady.

By the time I had settled down and helped a bit with the summer's rush of operating, it was time to take the *Bonnie Nell* to the people of Notre Dame Bay.

September 2, '40. Roused up at seven thinking I would be late for the start on the *Bonnie Nell.* I might have known better since it was almost eleven when we slipped our moorings. Meanwhile, good-bye was said several times, especially to the students who will be gone when I come back. Then I sped over to the boardinghouse of the bank manager, to get the bottle of rum he had borrowed but it hadn't come. Endless trips had to be made on the cycle to get all the stuff aboard. At the last minute Dudley II disappeared so the getting off was delayed. Betty and David came down to the wharf.

There was a nasty sea on and Spiller's Rock was white with breaking water, the foam and surf of it roaring as we passed. The sea gave us quite a roll and I did quite well not to get sick myself as I cleaned up after Dudley II. We made Change Island with no trouble but the *Mescol* was tied up at Billy's wharf and we had to wait out in midstream until she cleared. Bates came out to offer his wharf, but there was too much sea on. He's a young American who fell in love with this part of the world, after spending a summer on the Labrador—couldn't sleep when he went home for thinking about this place. Now he keeps a machine shop and has helped the people form a cooperative.

I examined a good many on Change Island and pulled lots of teeth. We sped through the beautiful tickle to tie up at Jack Roberts' wharf for the night. It was pitch black, with a little light rain falling as we drank cocoa for the first night on board.

September 3, '40. The United States declared war on Greater Germany today, to all intents and purposes. Fifty destroyers will be of great help to England. I don't see why Germany can't consider us an enemy now.

We had a busy morning at the wharf, where I made the acquaintance of the dynamic Jack Roberts. You can't say no to him. He is force and drive itself. I'm glad the hospital has made peace with a man so really interested in the general welfare. I made some shore calls and sent an 80-year old man to the hospital with appendicitis. I couldn't call it anything else. He had no fever but he did have a tender belly. Then a wire came from Horwood to see Joe West's daughter. We made sail and got there about seven. It was a lovely steam in a head wind, clear blue sky over a sea of azure. The dog enjoyed it. I had a nap then tea at sea. We passed several loaded schooners from Labrador.

The daughter had typhoid so I sent her to the hospital. We are now tied up against the *Grace Lorraine*, a beauty—seventy tons. I saw her at Fortune Harbor. The four schooners in here are loading Hodinotts' lumber for the new U.S.A. barracks at Quidi Vidi near St. John's. It's a black night and we have a snug berth.

September 4, '40. We are under sail now, after a quiet night in Horwood where we didn't see the skipper until noon when he came aboard to ask if we would honor the company scrip. He does seem interested in other things besides his own hemorrhoids. There is quite a bit of typhoid in this village but we have only two bottles of vaccine, so we can't do much about it. It will take a special mission "On His Majesty's Service." I told Hodinott to get his magistrate to communicate with the health commissioner. We heard Commissioner Puddister on the air last night, pointing with pride to the fact that not one of the recruits had been turned down for malnutrition. I'm at a loss to explain that. We have been examining recruits ever since the war started and we must not have thought of putting malnutrition down on the reports. Of course, in a sense, TB is a disease of malnutrition.

George Horwood is here again and had heard all about Ted's and my trip on the *Mary and Jane*. I saw him two years ago here during the Munich settlement.

After a modicum of examinations I made a shore call to the cleanest house I've ever been in. The front gate was a poem. The four corners were juniper knees and it was straight and true, homemade and new and clean and strong. I'd like to have one in my room, but I suspect that there it would look like a stuffed bird.

Now canvas is set and it adds a knot or so to our log. It looks nice and gives me a nautical feeling. I won't be happy until I've gone before the mast. Will Goodwin, a student here two summers ago, warned me about this "one more trip" philosophy as he had a ne'er-do-well friend who was going to make one more trip and was still doing it at sixty-two. I suppose I'll fall into that category. Now we are bound for Fogo, where I hope the mail has brought a dental syringe so I won't scram my hand trying to put novocaine into these jaws.

After Wester Tickle we shortened sail as we rounded into Fogo Harbor, though the wind was dead against us and very cold. Earl's wharf was a bust place. The cannery and the cod-liver oil plant were going full-blast.

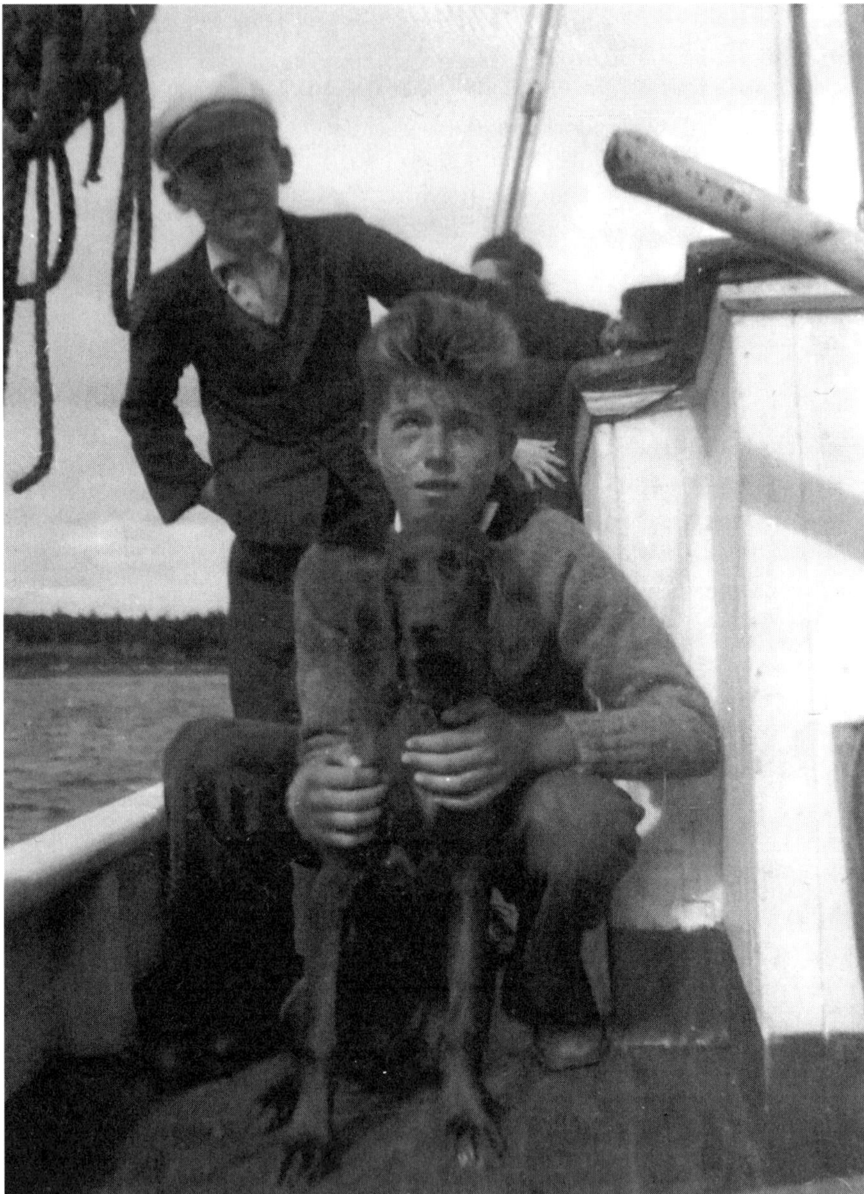

Dudley II had a fine time with the children. Author's photograph.

The men quit just after we arrived but I didn't seem to get a ride over to the other side so I washed up and hoofed it around the harbor. I met Mrs. Furz coming out of her shop. She was explosively glad to see me after I identified myself. Said I was fatter. Mr. Powell says I am thinner. Everyone else says I have altered. Meanwhile Dudley II chased some sheep and a goat. The sheep turned on her suddenly and while she was still skidding at the embattled ram with all her brakes set, she started to yip-yip frantically. At Change Island she had thirty chickens in the air all at once. We had to buy two dozen eggs to please the irate owner.

The hospital doctor here is new, Swanker. He and his wife have settled in here well but Johnson, the previous doctor did them a dirty trick—in selling every damn thing before he left. People are still coming in claiming they have paid for the hall stove, the treads on the stairs, the linoleum on the kitchen floor. Swanker is building a nice, big cruiser—forty feet and speaks of taking it around the world. Had a nice tea with them then he rowed me back to the *Bonnie Nell* in the pitch dark. The phosphorescence was lovely. You have to reach deep for it with the oar, but it lasts with the little vortex that swirls away from the boat. The bright northern lights were showing through the cloud rack after a cold blue and gold sunset. We had a drop of grog before Swanker started on his long trip home. My grog bottle fits beautifully into a locker made just for it in my stateroom.

September 5, '40. A little work today on Barr'd Island. We narrowly missed the rock coming in. I love those early morning sailings if I don't have to help get the anchor in. After breakfast at the wharf there were a few teeth to pull and some sick to be seen. Dudley II had a fine time with the children. We got four dollars for doctoring. At Joe Batt's Arm a few teeth came out and the day began to lower. Fog rolled in and the wind turned eastern. After winning back our anchor we sailed the hour or so down the coast to Tilting Harbor. It must have been two hours and it was rough because we were right out on the Atlantic. The bottom was smashed by lop and we did some fancy rolling and pitching. As usual, I took a nap.

In just a few minutes after we made the bottom of the long, narrow harbor a waiting list had developed. They seemed to have some money this year. All along this trip, I've been offering bargain prices for decrepit oldsters, only to have them drag out big bills. I did see one old epileptic from Barr'd Island who has begun to have a sensory type of fit. It comes all over him with bad tastes and a crawling sensation that goes down his arms and whatnot. It all started after he shored up his house, having been told not to work. He said his son was sick. Johnson had told him he had sprained the muscle of his leg. The nurse had told him he had a bad gland in his neck. I found him with a large TB abscess of the back with a contraction in his knee though there seemed to be no trouble in his hip. There was a draining sinus below the clavicle. He was pale and thin, and rotten in bone tuberculosis. I don't know how we will get him into the hospital.

At Tilting I went ashore to see a family and what with pulling a few teeth and taking off a big wart, we took in twelve dollars and fifty cents. Then came the long pull around stormy Cape Fogo for Seldom Come By, 14 miles with a strong easterly wind and fog. Cape Fogo is the worst point on North America, north of Cape Hatteras. The old schooner men all say, "If you round the Cape, you'll make it all right." It is a tough forbidding low shore.

Often the low-lying rocks are more uninviting than cliffs. It was fun sitting in the wheelhouse. At times, we would go over so far that the pipe would shift in my mouth (that's with my teeth on the stem). You could look to the east and south and west and you might as well have been in the middle of the Atlantic. It was so thick we couldn't even sight Cooper Island which is only a mile or two from Souther Bill. Lidge did a good job in bringing us right to the Union Wharf in Seldom. This place I remember well as our refuge from the storm which drove us off the Straight Shore two years ago. Here it was that the first Dudley refused to eat canned salmon.

It has rained all day but we are snug in the cabin where we were listening to the news when right in the middle of an interesting and successful bombing, the battery failed. While the radio was put on the charger I retired to my "stateroom" to type, while looking forward to the eleven o'clock news. The *S.S. Segona* will be along this shore next week to get our mail and bring me a drop of rum so that I will not get to Ted Drover's empty-handed, God forbid.

September 6. '40. Such a day, with a dirty wind from the northeast bringing rain and fog in it. Since work was light we turned to rearranging the saloon. It certainly needed it, an annoying mess for two years now. Helter-skelter piles of boxes and all kinds of junk. We had a good time condensing and hanging things up, nailed a box to the mast for bedpans and did all sorts of beautifying. Lidge Dalley made a rack for the dental tray under the companionway—it had always sat out on the locker before. It's almost a pleasure to contemplate the place.

We like-to-wrecked the skiff making a shore call on the other side to see a screwball who closed her eyes and trembled and cried out when I took her temperature.

Lidge made a backrest for the bunk near the radio with Dudley II helping. I bought the plank for it. With some pancakes and tea, somehow the evening flew by. Suddenly a lusty voice sounded from the wharf, singing some long ballad in the rain about how cold and hungry the singer was. I stood it as long as I could then looked out through the porthole. There was a ten-year old girl in a cotton dress, sneakers, cotton stockings and a little woolen hat. She certainly looked like the Little Match Girl, bedraggled and wet. Just then the men returned from getting a keg of water. She came aboard with them but immediately became very shy. She did show a little impetigo on her chin and confessed that she had missed several meals. We tried to get her to sing another ballad but all she would do was *Stand Up for Jesus* in a mild whisper. She wouldn't dance although she said she could. We gave her some food and sent her home in the rain, to her house with the blue door. Dalley remembers the house for it figured in a great drinking bout that the crew of the *S.S. Home* indulged in on their way to St. John's one year, to lay up for the winter. The men had gone ashore on the pretext of getting tobacco but went from house to house instead, intimidating the people to sell them moonshine. At this blue-doored house, pretty stewed by now, they tweaked an old man by his long, white beard, pulling him right off the couch. When they got back to the ship, a crewman was missing. Lidge was sent back and got his quarry, breaking up a cozy little affair to do it. In the morning, out of a crew of 32, there were three sailors, the captain, and one mate on their feet. Dalley took the wheel almost all the way to town. That one mate kept sending him back down from the bridge to get him a drop. Each time he would ask Dalley if he could smell it on him and of course, Lidge would say no (though you could smell it a ship's length in a gale). The mate eventually folded up and the captain sure was sore. When they reached town, they had about thirty liquor requests to claim at the government dispensary, forged in the names of people dead for years. There was a great party then, even the captain and his two sons joined in. The whole crew cleared out leaving the ship a mess.

September 7, '40. This is the day my family starts to California and I wish I were going with them. Instead, we left Seldom at daybreak to make some quick stops at Stag Harbor and Indian Isles. We ate my biscuits and gateau (the baking powder can was written in French) which I cooked in the hell-fire hot fo'c'sle while crossing the Sound of Sir Charles Hamilton. It was beginning to fog up and rain again. At Carmanville we tied up to a schooner and wasted no time in contacting the widow Hicks for a cake and some eggs. We saw one little girl, born about eight months after her father had drowned. He was drowned on the 14th of the month and ever since then the child on the 14th gets a sort of grieving spell—doesn't eat or sleep, but moans and groans and is sick. This has been very regular though at ten is beginning to wear off. She is a pretty, thin girl.

The nine o'clock news from England is not so good. There is a great raid in progress.

September 8, '40. Because it was Sunday, the day of rest, we could stay tied up to the wharf. Twenty-five patients came through the fine rain on what only began as a quiet day. I had very bad luck with the teeth. The first of these was Mrs. Something or Other from English Harbor, who wore a fur scarf and that's always a bad sign. As soon as a Newfoundlander puts on airs or gets a big white collar, they go kind of soft and funny. Everything about this woman was weak—her voice, her rare gestures, her complaints. But her scream when I nipped her tooth was something again. A little later I got the constable's wife. She had a large pearl earring in the way and before we were through, I had called her a hysterical female and charged her without getting the tooth out! I made an enemy there. The syringes keep breaking and that makes me furious. We still have no dental syringe and the bigger the barrel, the harder you have to push. My hand is scrammed and galled. I worked hard until six, when Mrs. Hicks sent her cake down. After tea we tried to pull a tooth on a boy but after three drops of novocaine he dissolved. He was out cold on the deck for an hour with the dog worrying him to get up.

That fine old bearded Sid Green came aboard to arrange about going to his wharf on the morrow. It was a lovely night, finally, with that clear light twilight that means fall. After our usual too-much-to-eat-with-cocoa, it's now to bed. Dudley II is quiet at night having finally learned that the foot of the bed is hers.

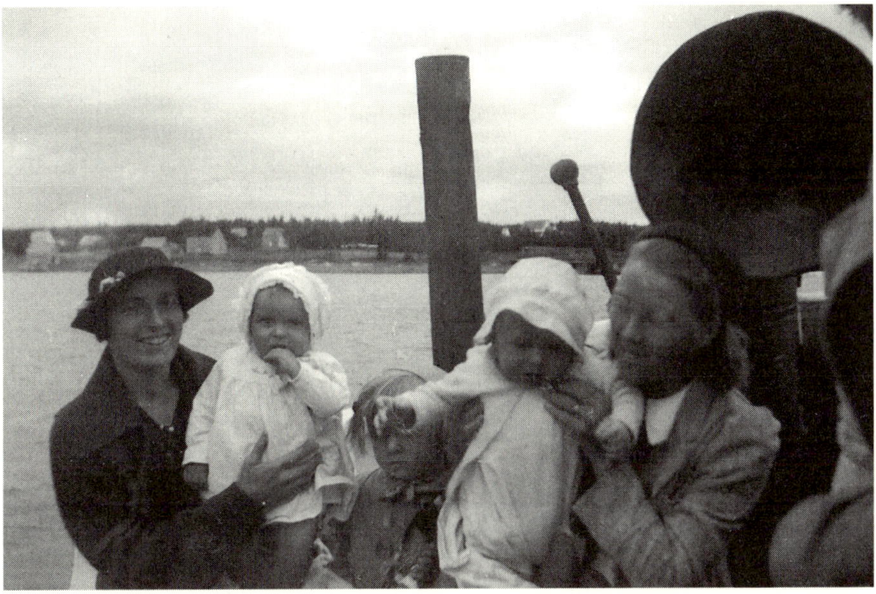

More patient patients waiting on deck. Author's photograph.

September 9, '40. I woke as we cast off, then fell off to a little snooze while we traveled. That's always the sweetest sleep—on a moving boat with a fine feeling of other people watching your interests. Since the only purpose of this boat is to carry me around, I feel very plutocratic. That fails me somewhat when I can't get into the bathroom to clean my teeth, which is the only thing I use it for, usually. It is the most awkward goddamn place in the world because you have to crawl on your hands and knees to get in and the light is bad because the lifeboat is berthed right over its porthole. When the boat rocks, which is all the time, it stirs up the rusty tank and makes the water brown.

I woke at Green's wharf to more rain. Sid was down already to be examined and to pass the time of day. I had a leisurely breakfast while we talked, then went up to pay my yearly call on Jim where I got my usual greeting. He put his fingers in his ears and curled up like a fetus. He's improving slightly. Downstairs they showed me some twine he was netting.

Then we moved to the unprotected government wharf where it was worse than ever. We banged and swung against it. This was too much to take so we swung off head-on and were more comfortable. Much to my

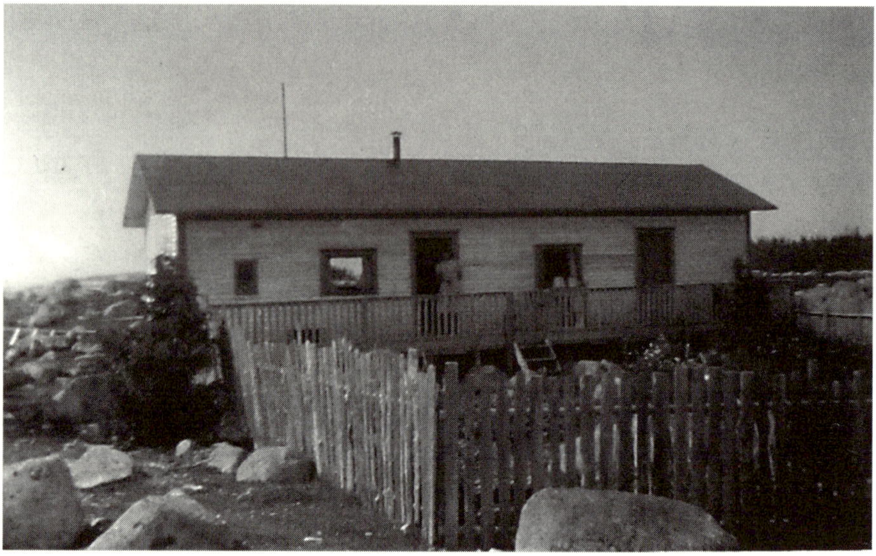

Ted Drover dwelling in Alder Harbor. Author's photograph.

annoyance, I had to start right off on a shore call, but not before Ted showed up and had a drink and apologized for finishing off my bottle of two-dollar rum which the bank manager had given him to bring me.

As I walked in the rain, Dudley II chased sheep and chickens. Along the way I saw Mr. Chalk who looked much better than I thought he would after reports of his death. Some emerging school children fell in with me, very talkative and friendly and crazy about Dudley II. One boy took care of her while I took care of the sick at Hicks'. They fed me and the dog some of their home-canned jam and salmon. I got back to the wharf soaking wet, laden with tobacco, bread, pickles, lobster and mackerel. The afternoon was busy. Toward the end of it the beneficent and kindly Willis Tulk came to ask me to make a charity call. As we talked, Ted came in for another drink and the wind changed suddenly, driving us against the wharf, breaking our rail. Dalley got kind of annoyed, started up the engine and coasted out to the middle of the harbor where we drifted. I got off on Ted's boat so that Tulk could take me to the patient—facial paralysis, deafness, trouble with her tear duct and a hole in the back of her head said to go up to the top of it all—the result of an overzealous mastoid operation.

As it got dark, Ted became worried and said we should hurry so I disposed of a few teeth and went below for tea while we steamed for Alder

Harbor with a pilot on board. We took the outside passage while Ted, with his smaller craft, went inside the island. Meanwhile we put on sail, scudding before the wind at eight knots before a fierce lop that couldn't catch us. It was clever and blustery and wonderful.

At Alder Harbor, I went ashore with Ted, taking one bottle of rum and leaving another for the crews' evening on board. Ted cooked some ham and eggs. The ham smelled like an abandoned sink trap, definitely bad but didn't taste as rich as it smelled. We survived it and talked until one.

September 10, '40. The ham smelled as bad at breakfast as it did last night. During our coffee, a wild-looking character broke through the door shouting something unintelligible, grabbed a shotgun and rushed out.

I heard a shot. It was a relief to find out he had killed only a chicken hawk.

We moved the boat into the wharf to see a few patients and to take on an old, White Co. marine motor. Even with its protruding pump removed, its weight caused much heaving and grunting until we had stowed it on our aft hatch. In taking the pump off, somehow Ted dropped it overboard. I dove for it. The water was so smooth that it looked to us as though we ought to make for the Straight Shore, rarely an approachable coast. I slept in the sun between stops at Apsey Cove and Ladle Cove. We did mostly teeth and I broke another syringe. Night found us in our dreaded Musgrave Harbor. There an old man came out whom I liked very much. He had his granddaughter, two-and-a-half years old, the size of a ten-months baby except for a big face. It must be pituitary. He was terribly concerned about her and said he liked her more than any of his thirteen children. It doesn't talk, it just sort of looks intelligent, had good teeth and no rickets.

We are riding at anchor in a lovely night, but in such a place that any trouble with the wind would wreck us. There is no safe berth in this place.

September 11, '40. Last night, except for a smattering of northern lights, we might have been on a tropical lagoon. I've seen Moose Pond, in Maine, rougher than this. We finished off the patients in Musgrave, in a manner of speaking. I recognized the voice of the Penguin Lighthouse keeper when he came on deck with his daughter who had a sprained wrist. Dalley told me he was tight but I didn't notice it and gave him a snort. I worked like mad until mid-afternoon. One deadbeat said he had only fifty cents, then pulled out a full purse.

We left for Noggin Cove with a fair wind and every stitch on. She clove through the roistering water, putting sea into the saloon. I foraged about for some beets with greens, some cabbage and two cakes.

After the British news in the evening, I examined a few patients, one with misgivings (remembering her spasms of two years ago). Lo and behold, without novocaine her six remaining teeth gave themselves up without a whimper. Doris, the nurse, went visiting the shore, and us with no cocoa!

September 12, '40. The engine woke me in the morning as we pulled out from Noggin Cove. My bunk being four feet from it could explain that. The approach to Gander Bay and the Island was serene but it is not always so, for here two years ago we dragged anchor and rolled out a storm that wrecked two schooners not ten miles away. At Mann Point we struck a run of uninteresting patients. Around the shore, giving the shoals a wide birth, we came to Main Point where it was calmer than ever. So on this nice afternoon I amused myself by climbing to the top of the mast where a patient found me. The first part of our interview took place from the masthead. Later I took a swim, so did Dudley II, so the next boatload of patients found me in the water.

September 13, '40. We are almost at the end of our southern trip and I don't mind, beginning to feel grimy in spite of the bathing yesterday in the bay. The morning found us in the channel at Clarke's Head. I talked with some Gander guides and would like to make a trip with them up the Gander River and down to the Bay d'Espoir. It would take a good two weeks. There were a lot of shore calls to make, then about twenty-five patients to see on the boat. I pulled innumerable teeth until my right hand is ruined by that damn syringe. Fine economy it is—not to have a dental syringe, since it takes me twice as long and I've broken six of them at two dollars apiece. There are a couple of things about this boat that are also insufferable. One of them is that seagoing toilet—every time you pump it you get a sprinkle of this and that.

Tonight it is blowing a gale so the skipper had to let out more chain. Tomorrow on to Victoria Cove, Gander Bay and home.

September 14, '40. I examined everybody and his grandmother. John Oake came aboard but was very quiet, contrary to what I had expected after hearing the way this benevolent despot runs Victoria Cove. We had well babies, sick babies, babies that weren't born yet, bed wetters and shore calls. Couldn't get away until almost three and we started to leave with patients still on board. They started to drop off one by one as we cleared Gander Bay. The wind was off the land then, dark and threatening. It started to get rough when we rounded the Head. I tried to make dinner but in the fo'c'sle the shocks, as she lifted her forward third out of the water and put it down on the seas, jolted the tea out of the cup. When we rounded Cape Farewell it was really something. I braced myself in the wheelhouse and, at times, it seemed that I could put my hand on the top of a wave before it touched the boat. She rolled, but we didn't put the rail under. The weather is off the port bow and we are not taking it well. I voted for putting into Herring Neck. We turned to the lee of Bacalhao Island where we put on a little sail to steady us. In the comparative calm of that tickle, a dirty darkness fell and through it I saw the *Kyle* bearing down on us. Lidge ordered the lights on, but that was a coincidence for he hadn't seen the steamer.

Behind the island, Lidge and the mate conferred, deciding to try for Twillingate. As we cleared the island, the full force of the wind took us. We started to put the lee rail under and once or twice we floated the punt, which is on top of the rail. I was almost getting used to it. I lighted my pipe and stood wedged in the engine hatch watching the water roll along the deck. We mounted a big lop and gave a sickening lurch to the port, sliding sideways into the trough with our whole lee deck under. With a crash, that White engine on the stern hatch gave way, broke its lashing and at the same time our lights went out. I was more than scared. I looked frantically for the steamer we had sighted for I knew we were lost. The next three lops we took the same way. Two oil drums came loose. That engine shifted with each crash until I thought the rail would go and with it part of the hull. I slid along the deck to the offending engine and tried to heave it overboard. Ted could have done it. I stood there with water breaking over me and could not budge the thing. There was no sign of anyone else on deck. We were listed way over to leeward. I was holding myself on by the thing I wanted to throw over. It didn't take a lot of brains to know that was a false position. I didn't see the drums, thought they'd gone overboard, and was glad of their absence. In fact, Martin, on the other side of the wheelhouse, had snared each of them with a line as they tumbled around on the deck. The skipper yelled to shorten sail and threw the helm over at the same time. I tried to get forward but the boom came at me. I ducked and it carried the chimney overboard, sending the deck plate scaling into the water as well.

Somehow we jumbled the mainsail down. We seemed to be riding easier. The geography was hard to make out but it became evident that we were running for Herring Neck, listed to port with our tail between our legs. The following seas hurled themselves on us and sucked us back, but we made it and a sorry sight we were when we got into the calm.

Below decks the stovepipe had come out in the saloon and lay against Doris' door. The front legs were off the stove and soot everywhere. Chairs were upside down, broken glass everywhere coated with soot. Medicine bottles all over the place, the microscope in the middle of the deck, bedpans, urinals, and pails. My clothes had come off the hooks, my trunk was across the floor. Doris couldn't get out of her room and when water had come through her funnel she had made herself busy with her prayers.

Our big White storage battery had come out of its braces, accounting for the light failure. We couldn't even get into the wharf because two schooners were there. It is too deep at Herring Neck so we said to hell with it as we let the chain out past the weak link.

We got the stovepipe from the galley so as to have a fire in the saloon for drying ourselves out and getting warm. I undertook to make an alcohol drink with seven cans of Malayan pineapple juice and we went on to have a gay evening to celebrate our deliverance. By a strange coincidence, when I made my way to the rail at 2 A.M. (there was something wrong with that pineapple) there I came upon the skipper and Doris with the same impulse. I got a terrible stomachache which lasted three days. The morn was blustery, beautiful, and rough.

CHAPTER VII

Ruminations

Why Live Here?

It is a good idea, I suppose, indulging in any form of living, to take a good stormy afternoon and do a bit of introspective stock-taking. As objectively as possible, one ought to list the benefits and disadvantages of the course one pursues or drifts on, as the case may be. The standard pattern doesn't call for this so much because no one criticizes you if you settle into the approved groove of home-office-home-movies-bed with a salting of club-night bridge and Sunday drives until that glorious two weeks in July rolls around so you can get a painful sunburn. The burden of proof lies on the (malcontent) (rebel) (idealist) (adventurer) (ne'er do well) (communist) (missionary) who crawls out of that quick-sand of respectability and chooses a regime which seems to weaken the ant-hill via vitae. Consider for a moment the lads and lassies who dwell in geometric apartment houses situated a hundred yards from the gaping maw of a subway station. Thither they plunge of mornings with no Virgil to guide them. The lucky ones work in a skyscraper boasting a subway station in its own bowels. Lunchrooms and bars and even cinema parlors lurk in the same building. One need never poke his nose out of doors except for that little dash from home to train. That, though, can be accomplished painlessly by holding the breath and running, say, as down a paddling line at a Beta Theta Pi initiation.

But I digress—I am not trying to point out the glamour of being employed at Radio City. I am trying to answer that puzzled shake of the head that my successful acquaintances make when they say "What—back to Newfoundland again? I thought you had gotten that out of your system."

I feel almost anyone who ever tasted Twillingate life would like it. It is not all beer and skittles, of course. It has such a consistent spirit—such an over-all purposeful flavor that every aspect of it has that same thing in common. Saying what is good and bad is like pointing to any one piece of a jigsaw puzzle and saying it is good or bad. The lines of demarcation are not coldly logical.

The pleasures will seem simple, the vices unsophisticated, the duties unadorned and sometimes arduous. The loves are deep and straight enough and the hates rather unprofound and difficult to maintain.

To mix things up I will start with the hates and they I am sure will have all the unconvincing qualities that ordinary social hates contain. I hated Arch Payton for quite a few years. In 1934 I had my heart set on working my way to Canada as part of the crew of the three-masted *Bessie Marie.* The owner said I could go. The captain philosophically and with the air of a martyr agreed also. The blue peter was flying and all was set when it occurred to someone that the permission of the Collector of the Port, His Majesty's local representative, had to be obtained. He was an old friend of the hospital. His d.t.'s had been fixed up by us. His broken leg had been repaired. John had even spent Easter Sunday trying to scratch Arch with a fly swatter where he itched under his cast. I buzzed happily over in the cycle. I was confronted by six feet three of Arch Peyton dignified and ministerial in his cutaway. The full significance of his position fell upon me. This was nonsense. Everyone knew I and my friend would be useless as crew (this really cut me). The ship's papers said ten shall be deemed a full complement. Besides that the *Morro Castle* had just burned. [Ed. I didn't know at the time that I had two cousins and their uncles on board it, only one lost]. Shipping rules were being tightened and of course we couldn't go. In a seething rage of frustration I told Arch I hoped he would break his other leg and I tore home on two wheels—the motorcycle was a three wheeler. When I returned three years later Arch and I maintained a polite professional relationship—for all I knew he had forgotten the incident.

I was sometimes Port Health Authority. No ship could operate until Arch and I had done our stuff. I lost my hate when we were making a boarding together in midstream on a stormy blowing night. We drifted down in an open boat to the accommodation ladder and missed it to come up under the six-inch stream of water from the ship's condensers. As the surprised Arch, somewhat hindered by his stiff leg, sat paralyzed under that flood, I forgave him.

Konopka, the dentist, I never forgave. Arch's frailties had a tendency to endear. The conflict with Konopka was more basic. He, for instance, probably could have licked me in a pitched battle. I have always been grateful I wasn't present the time he smacked Marianne. I never was certain whether he hated me or my Irish Setter or both. At any rate I am satisfied that he had the dog disposed of. There were other things though. He felt he, the first year out of professional school, should be paid more than the doctors because his department was the one that showed profit. I will never think better of him.

Waddell, I hated and loved by turns. We were in a sense competitors, I suppose. I didn't want to fight for my share and he was willing to wade in. Not only did I not want to fight, but surgery was so emotionally difficult for me that I needed it to be forced on me. John Olds understood that and made me do things (which I could do perfectly well, you understand) but it was too much to ask Waddell to force on me what he wanted himself. We wound up with a good understanding and mutual affection. He was a good man to drink with and play poker with or be with socially in any setting. Actually he was a good man to work with and my occasional flare ups were the thunder and lightning of my own storms. His wife Tommie I always was fond of.

Stan Hardy I was never really sore at. He was big, conventional and friendly. His involvement in what at times didn't seem too important could be irritating but his overall generosity and warmth made it always possible to think of him as a good friend. His wife Annette was of more keen material. There were flashes of sharpness between us but never real bitterness. We had a respect for each others' tongues and an occasional duel was good exercise of the wits and always drowned quickly in her ever forthcoming and welcome coffee. She often referred to me as Lord Hackie.

Business & Finance

There is nothing locally peculiar or mysterious about business and finance. I have never understood it anywhere. At home such and such a railroad has lost money every year. Yet you can't get a seat on it, they buy new equipment, people buy and sell its bonds and it doesn't seem to make any difference. At this hospital a modest deficit is announced every year. The Board of Directors shakes its collective head, makes a united tsk, tsk, everybody still gets salary and the work goes on. What do people do with deficits? Does one save them like stamps or bottle tops? It is common knowledge that the Fentons' business has been bankrupt for years. The Fentons are there only to sort the dead bones. They still live in a fine house, run up to St. John's, entertain and seem quite undisturbed. By the same token another business in another town is reputed to have made a million dollars. There is still linoleum on the floor and there is no, shall I say, indoor bathroom.

The shops and their methods are a constant source of interest. It is next to impossible to pay a bill. When you ask for an account it is with an air of offense that it is reluctantly rendered a week or two later. They sort of feel you don't trust them if you want to pay for anything. Some are a little more driving in their manner but on the whole a pleasant ease prevails in the marts. In one shop I was thrilled to see standing on a shelf, in a neat though dusty row, some Wellington boots. I have long craved a pair. They are water-proof and leather. They come to the top of the calf and a rounded little flap comes up in front to protect the knee. The price, as near as I could tell, was the wholesale cost plus the modest markup. Radio parts were for sale on the same principle on the next shelf. Newfoundland feet are small so no boot would fit me. They were returned after trial to the shelf to wait the next buyer. The interesting point is that these boots, the original fishing boot, have not been manufactured since the invention of the rubber boot and that wasn't yesterday.

At one shop I made a great find—Christmas Cards, British ones — printed at least 40 years ago. They were quaint and good. There were no envelopes. The picture was a hunting scene, a jumping horse, bearing the legend "Keep Your Pecker Up." This was a progressive shop so the price was somewhat reduced.

Dr. Olds wanted to make an apparatus for cyclic drainage of chest abscesses. He needed a small motor. At the largest shop in town he found the spring motor from a dictation-recording machine that one of the up-and-coming partners had affected some years before. He was dead this decade. There were no more wax cylinders, the machine was not usable and no one dreamed of ever using it. John asked the price of the motor. The merchant looked up the dusty record to see what he had paid for it and added ten percent to that. This was too much for John. There were no hard feelings. The machine was put back in the shed to await the next customer. There is not a doubt that if Froude's Hill should turn into an active volcano (not likely) in the next civilization archeologists will ponder this Pompeian Twillingate and try to figure out what this machine was for—still for sale at purchase price plus an increased mark-up (storage charge) and still just as useful to the average Twillingater. The ice creepers I bought were patented in 1902 and made the same year I would guess by the state of the elastic, and had a price marked on them only once. They lasted three steps.

It is pleasant when solvent to enjoy this credit and casual dealing. The situation of the impecunious fisherman is quite different. He is the helpless participant in this fanciful system. I never actually studied the setup but writers have described the fisherman as sharecropper of the sea. His whole financial life is lived on books of the merchant who so to speak backs him. The merchant advances fishing supplies, groceries, and the other necessities of life. To pay for these advances he buys the fish caught. The fish market has been notoriously capricious. The tendency in recent years (pre-1942) has been to lose in the fish-dealing as such. Many feel that the basic difficulty in the merchant system is the effort by the merchant to make enough profit over the counter—that is in the supplies he advances—to pay for the losses in the fish business. This puts fishermen in the middle of the fish business and the grocery and clothing business and I think it is a little bit like the red-hot approaching walls in Poe's story. One attempt at solution has been the establishment of cooperative fish handling with cash as a result. The cash is then the fisherman's and he can spend it at a cash store or a cooperative merchandising effort.

This movement has not prospered as one might think it should. The reasons are not too clear. There was some disenchantment with the cooperative movement when in one instance the elected management proved a little less than completely selfless in devotion to common good. The Newfoundlander has more than his share of the spirit of independence. The cooperative society more patently is communal. By some illusion the merchant system is a more individual concept. The fisherman feels that when he deals with the merchant directly the business between them is that of two independent people. This independence was brought out in the blanket system of insuring communities in our prepayment health plan. Although it is individually cheaper when a whole community signs the plan there are cases where the individuals take out individual contracts with the result that more money comes from the community to the hospital and fewer people receive the benefits. This same independence makes the Newfoundlander, in wartime, difficult to handle in groups but it also makes them the best snipers and foragers and small boat handlers in the Empire. Wherever individual, independent skill or bravery is at a premium, that is where the Newfoundlander shines. Wherever blind obedience or thoughtless following is required, don't look for Newfoundlanders. The Royal Navy puts at least one Newfoundlander on every vessel.

My *via vivendi* at the moment is not one calculated to bring me into competition with J.P. Morgan or any of those boys. I think I have a good time, however. I don't know what other business would have allowed me on one beautiful day we had, to go wandering over the marsh with my dog until, under our incredibly blue sky, I found a perfect mirror of a pond. We both dove in and had a grand time lolling about under our intense, precious sun with the only sign of human life a distant schooner we could see from the hill with her white wings spread, headed for the Labrador.

I wanted to write a lot more but the afternoon was suddenly taken up by a girl who had had an illegitimate baby about three weeks ago. She had decided that the shame was too much and refused to eat or drink and now she is in a deplorable state. I am certain that she will be all right. The local aids and maids will help her to see that her situation is far from unique.

With the drying of the wells, we get a lot of dysentery and some typhoid. When we go around the bay in the government boat giving typhoid shots we fly the hospital pennant from our forward masthead and from our mainmast the Union Jack. That makes us a belligerent vessel and I hope the Jack continues to fly with undiminished prestige from whatever masthead she chooses.

Thoughts

Eating in the homes of patients was always fun no matter what was served. The hospitable, hot black tea of the fisherman's cottage is among my happiest experiences. It's the proper drink for the long cold trail. The fruitcakes and the meat pasties and the good homemade bread and jams are good, too, but it's the tea that turns the trick. Just go up to any door, high carved and paneled or low broken and hingeless and you don't even have to ask for a drop of tea and a bit of loaf (bread). Clotted or Devonshire cream is too much of a luxury to be often available. When it is though,

Heaven kisses the earth. It's good on berries or jam. It's good on anything or alone. I never tried it on iron filings, but I'm sure that would be good.

We have a road on the hospital grounds that goes up to the pond, our source of water. It is called the brown flour road. For some years after the big collapse of the finances in Newfoundland, when the St. John's government failed and Britain took over, many Newfoundlanders had to rely on the dole to live. Among the staples distributed by the government were lard, tea, sugar, and flour. These items were, as you know, devoid of vitamins. Beriberi took a heavy toll. Dr. Parsons, the first hospital chief, persuaded the government to distribute brown flour, hoping its vitamin B content would lighten the beriberi. Instead of money, the Government once gave the hospital brown flour and Parsons used it as money to pay for the building of the road. This was an unwelcome form of cash because people do not like brown flour. By some strange perversion many attributed their ills to brown flour, when actually it was a cure for them.

Again and again I feel how good it is to face the basic problems—fuel supply—travel—food—shelter. These problems are only good, of course, when they are soluble. I don't suppose it is any fun at all to drown, starve or freeze. Last winter, for instance, we probably wouldn't have starved, but there would have been an awful lot of difficulty hauling food over the ice, if the last supply steamers of the navigation season hadn't been able to land the winter supply of flour and other staples for the island. Bad weather and other factors slowed the schedules of the *Clyde* and the *Segona*. When they approached, low in the water with food, they found our harbor choked with untimely ice. Captain Butcher and Captain Knee called respectively for full steam and rammed their prows as far as they could into the rough ice and leaned on their whistle halyards. Every dog and pony in Twillingate that could put one foot in front of the other and bear the weight of a harness was pressed into service. Anything that would slide on the ice was attached to the dray animals. It was an inspiring sight to see the diverging lines of teams making their ant-like ways between the ships and the store houses. Two bags of flour was a load for many. A tierce of molasses was a big load for a horse. Hundreds of tons of food came ashore that day and the ice was rough—ridged and hummocky. I fell into the water myself that day, but not from lugging flour, I was trying to get aboard the *Segona* for a bottle of beer.

The position of the doctor in Twillingate and of the hospital in the community is about what one would expect under the conditions. The people respond in the same way they would in any American rural area. It

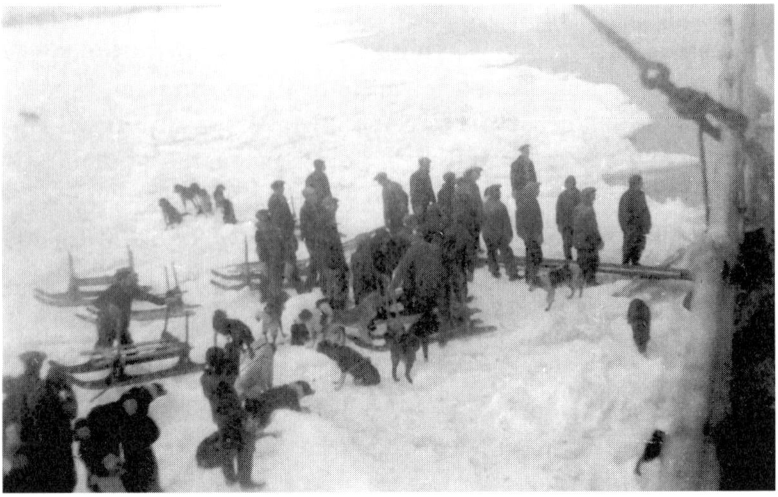

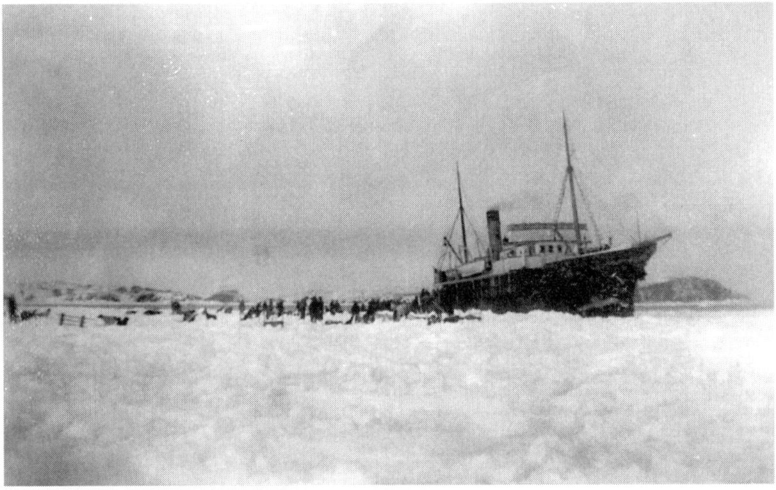

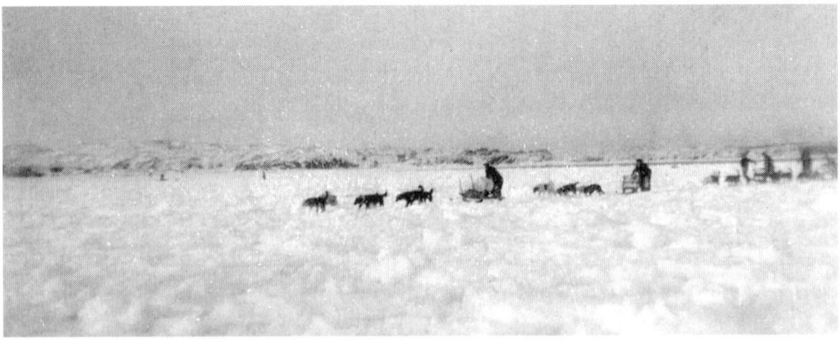

Unloading the *Clyde* on the ice. Author's photographs.

does happen that our standard of living at the hospital is rather higher than that of our neighbors. We have running water and steam heat. For most of the bay people we are the only hospital and the only doctors available. That in a way puts us in a spot. A bad act on our part means for them that doctors are bad. A good deed works the other way. The combination of our better living conditions and our indispensability gives our ensemble a slight "manor" quality. This probably exists in our own minds more than in the minds of our local people. The framework for social distinction exists. All the elements are present for prejudice or class feeling. There are rich people, poor people, teachers, clergymen, first families, merchants, people with learning and people who can't write. All this is there for the describing, but somehow it doesn't mean a thing. Unearned income or even large, earned income does not especially increase a man's stature. Anyone with a notion to put on airs soon learns he might as well conserve his energy. The man who is respected is the man who works hard, who fishes well, who can build a house or a boat. The true aristocrat is the man who has skippered a ship well or is a good pilot. I'm in complete sympathy there. I look with awe on a man who has taken a forty- or fifty-ton schooner down the Labrador summer after summer and brought her back safely through the buffeting capricious seas and dark threats of unfriendly shores. When he has done that he can stand on his two feet, supposing he hasn't shoes to put them in, and tell the world to go to hell.

Those older rugged characters tended rather to look on doctors and gentlemen of the cloth as people you had to call in once in a while, but on the whole were luxuries that the women folk seemed to demand. Their tolerant humor with regard to us was never irritating. I enjoyed their hospital joshing. If you traveled thirty or forty miles by dog team to visit their "weak nerved" granddaughter or their son, "spoiled by too much reading," they respected your having come much more than they did what you could do when you got there. Often enough, they themselves claimed our services in extremes. Nevertheless, they never gave up. One old skipper, just before he closed his eyes for good with Stan Hardy sitting by his bed, shouted to his woman, "Give the doctor a root" (drink of rum). Another old skipper groped in his terminal delirium and left the mortal scene with the shouted line, "That's a hell of a place to keep a bottle of rum." I tended one octogenarian in a bout of what looked like terminal arteriosclerosis of the brain. He reeled and rocked on his bed and clutched the head of it as if he held the wheel of a hurricane-harried schooner. With each surge of a dreamed-up sea he would yell orders to his imagined crew, to "Keep her off"—"hold her in." I was a little surprised to meet him at the post office a few days later quite in touch with reality.

Watched a patient die. Just made a few faces, reached for a breath or two, lifted his hand convulsively and joined his fathers. No matter how much of that you see you never fail to be impressed. There are many ways of dying. I've seen quite a few in departure. The line is not sensible in some but in others it is like jumping a fence.

These older fellows who didn't take the doctor too seriously are heavily outnumbered by the younger folk who have come to realize that medicine is here to stay. As in any rural practice we become involved in many aspects of the patients' lives. If a patient needs weekly treatments and lives at a distance it may be necessary to find a way for him to live in Twillingate—even to find a job for him at the hospital. It is not unheard of to lend a favorite patient a little money. The hospital is a sort of center in a practical way. Much food and other supplies are bought locally and considerable employment is offered. Then too, Twillingate is a shopping center for the bay and an arduous shopping trip is lightened by a visit to the sick.

I have pretty good luck with teeth. Some leave swearing I am the greatest dentist of all time and some steam off in high dudgeon making noises in their beards about "beating them all to pieces."

The ultimate in doctor relationship is manifested I should say in psychiatry. I took a flier at that as such. A young man of about twenty-three sat forlornly in an examining room. To my question, "What's the trouble?" he said, "Oh, not so much, only when I work I get weak and dizzy." Then he hesitated and in a lower voice, as though ashamed—"I even get weak and dizzy when I think of work." I thought here is a self-admitted neurotic case. I am very busy but I will give this lad some time, get right to the bottom of his trouble and fix him up in a jiffy. From my great wisdom I shot right at the heart of the matter, "What's your trouble at home?." He was amazed that I knew he had trouble. It quickly came out that he was the support of his parents—had to stay with them and yet couldn't earn enough to keep them if he did stay with them. He also wanted to get married. We soon reached the conclusion that he should go ahead and get married, leave his bride with his parents and go away to the woods to make enough money to keep them. (Dorothy Dix will sue me for malpractice). His face brightened with new resolution and he said he felt stronger and better. "While he's here", I thought," I might as well look him over." I put a thermometer routinely in his mouth. The temperature was

103. Startled, I examined him. He had classical rose spots on his abdomen, and the large spleen of a full-blown case of typhoid fever. He wouldn't stay in the hospital, but went walking off to do some shopping without even knowing how he would get across the bight to New World Island. Saddened and wiser I there and then abandoned that hair trigger, shooting-from-the-hip approach to Psychiatry.

When as a doctor I ponder my relationship with patients, with other doctors, with people in general, and with fellow non-doctor professional workers, I realize with a start that I am dwelling on "Ethics." I feel suddenly that strange, almost elated feeling, which possessed some oft-quoted old gent who suddenly found that he had been speaking "Prose" all his life.

Quick recourse to the big "Webster," gives me "A treatise on morals." Only way down in the third definition does he cite "medical ethics" but then only as an application of the general definition. I was pleased to find out there is nothing special about medical ethics—it is only decent behavior of a man when that man happens to be a medico. The lay have the notion that it is a kind of secret code among doctors to bolster each other in defense against the ailing, innocent, and defenseless public. What ARE the things peculiar to "Medical Ethics" and further, peculiar to our Twillingate medical ethics? This is not too easy for me to deal with because the school I attended laid no stress on the subject as such. They felt, quite rightly, that ordinary rules of human behavior would suffice for doctors too.

What do the lay think of when they think of "medical ethics"? Perhaps the first is "you mustn't advertise." That's all right with me. I don't think a doctor should. I think our civilization would be better off without most forms of advertising. It certainly renders a radio almost unusable. Of course it is useful to know what services are available or what products are available. Erich Fromm and Phillip Wylie are both articulate in their abhorrence of modern advertising. Doctors don't have to advertise. They have many ways of letting it be known that they are prepared to render such and such a service. This is the least cramping of the medical conventions. I know that we didn't have to advertise at our hospital. In moments of desperation we considered camouflaging the place so nobody would know it was there. We did look for business though. We examined schoolchildren routinely and free and urged many of them to seek our aid. We wrote articles for the paper and urged people to search out our services. I suppose we would have been open to criticism if such activity had increased our income. Doctor Woods, the local practitioner associated with us at the hospital, used to have a little notice in the local paper. In small print it said "If you can't see this"—then in larger print—"SEE ME." We all liked that little advertisement, if you wish, and it saved us endless trouble. He was the only man for the Lord knows how many miles who could fit glasses. Lots of people needed glasses and if that little notice made them know it, that was so much to their and Doccy Wood's good—and ours too.

"Doctors are not supposed to criticize each other—especially before the patient." Well, what doctors say about each other to each other, is nobody's business. That depends entirely on their standards of social behavior, their critical abilities, their cattiness or lack of it, their wit or any other personal attribute you can name. To coin a phrase—doctors are people. I have given critical accounts of other doctors' activities and I have heard my colleagues do the same. I know of no harm accomplished among intelligent people by it. On the other hand, I see no good accomplished by telling a patient that another doctor is no good. You can apply your own standards in treating a patient without pointing out the failure of the doctor who last treated your patient. It may even be honestly possible to condone and make excuses for some shortcoming. Before I left the States I knew of a ward patient who was scheduled to have her thyroid taken out by an eager house officer. I was convinced that she didn't need it, I crept to her bedside in the dead of night and urged her to scream for her clothes and get out before she got her throat cut. She didn't, but the resident changed his mind and left her neck intact. She didn't speak of my advice though or I would have had to pursue the rest of my medical life in Outer Mongolia.

In Twillingate our group of doctors is such a tight intimate one that patients are treated by all of us and suggestions and criticism are free and easy. There is never any need of criticizing a fellow doctor to a patient. Patients might report statements of other doctors that sounded like this breach of ethics but they could have been construed as unintentional. One of us had cause to do a delivery in the home. The baby and mother were fine except that the site of the hypodermic injection in the leg became infected and for a while troublesome. Another doctor treated her for this condition. In a later interview with the patient she reported that this doctor had said that the first doctor had used a poisoned needle on her. At first blush this sounded like a frontal attack and it may have been said in an effort to alienate the patient. I can however visualize the untutored woman asking simply why her leg was painful. The second doctor might have been put to it to explain how an infection starts. In any event, with our system, no harm was done. The thing to remember in this connection is that confidence in a doctor—even a bad one—and confidence in medicine in general play a large part in the recovery of many patients. One can also add this caveat: pick your doctor as carefully as you can.

A doctor is not supposed to take care of a patient being taken care of by another doctor without first having the permission of the original doctor. That seems fair enough. A doctor bows to a patient's will to change doctors. It is a good idea to know what the first doctor thought about a case. It is conceivable that double treatment on different principles would do more harm than good. I think that no one will argue with this medical conceit.

One also hears a doctor should not treat his own family or his friends. I don't think this is a law either written or unwritten. Most physicians will automatically shy from treating family or friends. It is part of the medical folklore that something always happens when you deal with someone in whom you have a special interest. There are countless creditable accounts of infections, embolism, obstruction, non-union in fractures, and many other unforeseeable outcomes of even the best surgery. My heart goes out to the prominent surgeon in a large New England city who took out his daughter's appendix and calmly explained, "I wanted her to have the best available attention." Sometimes circumstances force you to work on people who are important to you. Then your task is multiplied in difficulty and if anything your hand is less sure. Dr. Parsons, when he was alone at this hospital, had to do a caesarean section on his wife—herself a physician. She got into sudden difficulty with her pregnancy and the tale is told of his carrying her down from the cottage in his arms while a storm raged. Olds operated on his own son.

When I was alone at the hospital I had to operate on the brother of a nurse of whom I was fond. It was a simple operation but I hated it. It's even worse when you start taking care of yourself. Your judgment is very warped. I am haunted by the story of an old navy doctor friend of mine. A colleague of his in the early days was the only physician on one of our remote islands. He recognized in himself the signs and symptoms of a bad appendix. He begged his trained helpers to operate on him. They had helped him often and most likely could have done it. They wouldn't do it and with his trained eyes he watched himself die. On the other hand a nurse, posted by an organization to a far and isolated community, performed a successful caesarean section. She was censured and discharged because theoretically she did not have the ability to diagnose a condition as requiring such a radical treatment. It is completely possible that she saved her patient's life, but she may also have been guilty of exposing that patient to unnecessary danger. It's a nice academic question and I never could decide who was right. I didn't want to decide because if it turns out that the nurse was right it will disturb me for the rest of my days.

"What about fee splitting?" you ask with a sly indication that suggests that I was trying to avoid that subject. In a way, you are justified. I can't shed much light on it. In the first place you have to have a fee before you can split it. I don't seem ever to run into any fees. Trying to look at it coldly I would define fee splitting as the paying of a commission to someone who brings you remunerative business. I abhor the practice and at the same time ask if there is anyone in the business world in a position to attack it. Almost every non-professional person in these United States is tied up one way or another with business and finance. Of course it has no place in medicine. There is enough illness to keep every doctor who can flourish a stethoscope so busy that he has no need for agents. Most often they are actually such poor businessmen that they honestly do need assistants to collect even the unsplit fees. My friend, at the Twillingate branch of the Bank of Nova Scotia, told me that he hated to see a doctor coming to ask for a loan. They would lend to doctors, but it was under the heading of Social Service and they kept two fingers crossed until they got their money back. As a matter of fact the bank hated to lend money to anybody. I don't know what they did with their money. The only security they would accept was cash in the bank. In other words you borrowed at six percent instead of using your own money on which they paid you 1-1/2 %, but that's beside the point. I knew only one declared fee splitter in the states and he was such a generally reprehensible character that I wouldn't have been surprised to find him beating his grandmother. He didn't go to jail for fee splitting though. They sent him up for conniving with his patients at cheating the insurance companies. But there again playing games with the insurance companies is a pretty universal pastime too. To conclude: we have no fee splitting in Twillingate for various reasons but principally because there is nothing on which it can feed.

Nurses

Stella Manuel plays a large part in making life here a pleasure. She lives in the lower near corner of the nurses' home. Her fireplace is always going with peat, soft coal, birch junks or any combination thereof which will produce more than a smudge. Stella herself is slim smiling patient and witty. She was born in Twillingate and is the best interpreter of local character. Her supply of local anecdotes is delivered with gently incisive humor and an artistic control of the dialect. Everyone is always slipping over to her room at odd hours for a drop of tea. It is a social center. One long winter she taught me to tat. It was good exercise for a surgeon or would-be surgeon fingers. I was a little ashamed of such an accomplishment. The result was that I often needed to get out the knots incurred when I had hastily shoved the opus under a cushion lest I be surprised at such an unmasculine occupation. Stella's duties as head nurse often required her absence from her room. It was always a cooling disappointment not to find her there when between cases you felt like a cup of tea.

Joyce Scammel, bluff, big and easygoing, was a native of Change Islands. She was a head nurse but her heart was in anesthesia. Joyce's quiet ways could not obscure the fact that fires smoldered within. She seemed very tranquil as she mixed up some cheese biscuits to take to the Olds for dinner or as she went off down the lane in her Girl Guide Uniform to work with her troop. She has had moods though, which could result in joyful hilarity at a party or three days of complete non-speaking. I remember her best when I was a student. One of our student duties was to move patients who had died to the morgue which was at the end of the machine shop fifty yards from the hospital. Without going into indelicate detail I will say that experience had required the shed to be rat-proofed. To spare the feelings of other patients the removal would take place after midnight. I can see Joyce now in her white crackling uniform, her big blue cape flying, stalking down the hall ahead of us with a kerosene lantern in her hand. She would hold the door open for Dick Mirick and me to get the stretcher through and then lead us across the grounds. One black, blustery, moonless night in September stands out especially. The bleak dark shadow of her blowing cape flew out behind her and the purple and green northern lights draped a regal funeral curtain across the sky. We made a strange and noble procession of death. Then there was something strange and clandestine and Elizabethan about the silent transfer of the body to the orthodox coffin—larger at the shoulders—like a bichloride tablet. We had only one or two coffins which might or might not be the exact size—Joyce was up to all of this though and would even help on our rather makeshift autopsies. These were somehow more ghoulish than scientific. Her taste for the macabre was only thinly veiled by her round friendly smile. She was the one who pulled handfuls of my hair out by the roots in a moment of pique. I had careful respect for her.

Edith Simms Manuel made everything look easy. She was one of the best operating room nurses I ever saw. Trim and dark with a beautiful little figure. She was deft, skillful and brilliantly witty, dry and droll. In a snug group like this there are little by–words and common jokes that mean much to us. She was the master of these and the inventor of many of them. Her room was a center and there we hied at all times of the waking hours to find a cup of tea or coffee or to while away a spare moment. She was a good one to take on an outside call when there was work where a nurse could help. A nurse was never scheduled for outside trips but they were all willing to go and help on their off-duty hours. Many a hard baby case was made endurable by the company of one of these cheerful souls.

There is a special reservation set aside in my heart for nurses. I like to work with them and I like them when they are off duty. Once in a while they grow up and leave the bedside to become superintendents and night supervisors and they run into trouble. Authority of women over women is loaded with material suitable for atomic fission. That, of course, is another of those generalities. The superintendent of nurses at the Baltimore City Hospitals was to my mind a perfect woman and consummate nurse. On the other hand there was a floor supervisor at the Brady Clinic and, later in my career a superintendent at Brooklyn Hospital, both of whom I could use to frighten Genghis Khan. Night supervisors and superintendents are different. They become more like nurses. The long lonely watches of the night sweeten the spirit and strengthen human bonds. The night somehow belongs to the good of heart and the strong of heart—the heart that senses the yearning and the sorrow of the world. When the lingering blue sub-arctic twilight fades, our Twillingate Hospital drops into a different tempo. The busy office downstairs is closed and quiet. The diesel is shut off and the tired old waterwheel supplies only enough power to make the lights do a little more than glow. The kitchen is reduced to one or two maids who will serve the saved-over dinner for the night workers. The radiators stop their hissing and the patients who can sleep withdraw deeper into their beds and summon up their dreams. The doctors drop by for a final check-up on the sick and depart with hope that for once no call will come in the night. As the nurses and aids cluster around the ward desk making their reports and getting ready to leave, down the hall comes the night nurse. The tired rumpled day workers sense the aura about her. Her uniform is fresh and crisp. Her eyes have the bright shine of recent sleep. Her smile and manner have the relaxed quality that daytime sleep seems to give. Confidently she takes over the duties and responsibilities. Her colleagues leave her and she is Queen of the Night. She makes her comforting rounds with an ordinary railroad kerosene lantern. In her hands as she goes from bed to bed it becomes a tall sacramental candle in a gold holder.

When I come back from a call at two in the morning I wander through the wards looking for her and there she will be, leaning over a bed in a little island of friendly light. She has a cup of tea and some toast ready for me and we sit a few minutes in the ward kitchen and talk quietly. The atmosphere of a sleeping hospital is beautiful, hushed—almost religious. It can change quickly to busy noisy activity. It takes only an obstetrical case or two and a delirium or an emergency operation to introduce what can and sometimes does approach pandemonium.

The good assistance and companionship of nurses is what makes a doctor's work bearable. They lend courage to both the patient and the doctor. It is a very frustrating feeling to work without them. Their duties are especially hard here because we are lacking in any of the slick aids to housekeeping.

I would hate to contemplate living here without the nurses. There is something about their training and their experience with the less happy side of life that makes them know people—that makes them understanding and good companions. They don't mind doctors' shop talk. They like to go boating or on a little picnic or skiing. They like local square dances. They are always ready for a drop of tea. They will share a spot of rum. They approach life with ease and relaxation. It is not unusual for a doctor working here to find among them one whom he takes to be his wife.

Schooling

Examining the Twillingate schoolchildren is an interesting opportunity to get an overall picture of the people of our locale. The children naturally, in their manners, clothes, speech, nutrition and state of health give you a picture of the homes they come from. In addition, since they come in groups from a certain school and the school is always part of a certain religious group, one is able to draw rather general conclusions. In our school groups three general denominations are represented. The Church of England and the United Church are the two largest. The latter is a union of the less formal Protestant sects. The third group is smaller than the other two and is composed of the Salvation Army and the Pentecostals. The economic levels represented are pretty clear. The Church of England seems to be composed of the families with rather more money. More of the prominent names are on its rolls. The children are better fed and clothed. The United is only a little bit behind them. They are rather plainer people not quite up to the financial level of the Anglicans. The third group is distinctly less endowed with the world's goods and this clearly has its effect on the children. We have no Catholic community close to us, but I have had the opportunity to see two Catholic areas. The one at Fortune Harbor, where the admirable Father Casey is at the helm, is a model village—prosperous, industrious, and independent. The other Catholic community on Fogo Island is quite the opposite. I haven't observed it so closely, but from the patients I saw, I was convinced the economic and cultural standards are way below those promulgated by Father Casey.

There is obvious disadvantage in the local system of the church school. I know nothing of the intellectual aspect of this parochial teaching. I am here impressed and humbled by the tolerance and lack of hatred and bitterness. There is a tone of natural calm in the whole social set-up. This is helped by the comparative homogeneousness of the racial stock; I have never heard a clear denunciation of a member of a different economic or religious group. Bastardy I would not describe as accepted—better than that—it isn't even noticed. Nowhere in the world is it of less importance to be able to trace your ancestry. I don't mean by that that morals or whatever you want to call them are any different from those of an ordinary American community. I don't like the word tolerance. It means a conscious effort to "do the right thing." The tolerance of the Newfoundlander is completely unconscious. That island is separated from Nova Scotia by only a hundred miles. No one knows the meaning of the word "venom"—no one has had an angry cobra look him in the eye—until he has heard a Nova Scotian use the two letters "R. C." with reference to Roman Catholic. The very leaves on the nearby trees begin to drip with Prussic Acid. The Newfoundland tolerance is carried just a little too far. For one thing, they ought to scream at their government more than they do. All governments ought to be screamed at once in a while. They ought to scream about their roads and their economic level.

The lack of complaint doesn't mean they don't observe forces or events. They have developed a protective philosophy of humor. This humor is kind and quiet in spite of the fact that they always laugh when I bang my head in a low doorway. I stopped, uninvited, at a house in Virgin

Arm one day on my way back to the hospital. I was warmed and I tried to pay. This was as usual refused. I called a four year-old boy over to me and gave him a half-dollar which he immediately tried to bite. When I was leaving, the boy was playing on the floor but I didn't see the half-dollar. I said to the father, "I hope he hasn't swallowed it. I don't want to make the trip back here to fish for the coin." Without a change of expression, "Oh don't worry. I wouldn't send for you. I'd send for the minister. He's better at getting money out of people."

Frontier

It's a strange yearning I have for the remote and the wild and the lonely inaccessible. I have reservations and conditions though because I do enjoy people, and basic comforts. I enjoy contacts with my patients and my colleagues and I like my bathtub full of good hot water and I have nothing against a comfortable bed. I take a perverse delight in circumstances that make travel impossible and in the days when the ice is so bad the mailmen don't dare cross the tickle. The frontier keeps retreating though. When I first came here there wasn't an operating radio on this island. Gradually refinement has crept up on us. We used to have poor lights in the hospital, the diesel had to be conserved and was always being cut off in the middle of a poker game. I liked the flurry of getting out kerosene lamps to continue the game. The waterwheel made 112 volts and the diesel made 220 (beautiful planning). The 220 bulbs would make only a glimmer on the 112. For a while we used to shift bulbs but they would always be forgotten and in the morning would all blow out on the diesel power. This soon exhausted our supply. Now we have an efficient gasoline generator ready at all times. I feel threatened by "efficient" machinery and somehow it makes me feel inferior. We used to have to settle down to very plain food in the winter. Now Bert Pardy has destroyed that basic pleasure. He imports fancy canned goods and takes the risk of bringing in fresh tomatoes in the middle of winter. A big cold storage bait depot has been built. That means we can keep fancy meats and even have fish when nobody is fishing because the bait capelin is also good to eat.

The Tilt

The Tilt is a fine institution; it is a week-end log cabin on the far side of the island, perched among some trees on the shore of the Main Tickle between Twillingate and New World Island. There aren't any houses near it and it makes the perfect retreat. There's a good-sized living room with a fireplace, a bunkroom, and a little kitchen. It is called the "Tilt" because many Newfoundland families have a tilt, but not for purposes of pleasure. Though our Tilt was well-built, the usual tilt is very small and low and rough. They are just shacks thrown up on one of the inner islands so as to be near a fuel supply. People move into them in winter when the fishing season is over and camp there uncomfortably until the ice is gone. When the Olds or the Hardys get settled over there though, everybody who can goes over to visit them. The visitors are always welcome and everybody has a good time. I went to it once in the winter, determined to be alone for three days to search my soul and ponder the eternal verities. My only company on this sub-polar vigil was my team of four hungry dogs. Fortunately I found some good detective stories and a small cache of rum. With those and getting wood and melting ice and keeping warm and teasing the lighting system into action and taking care of the dogs, I never got around to plumbing the egotistical abyss. Only my psychiatrist would know what a quagmire I was saved from then.

Language

This isn't a dialect or an accent that is spoken here. It's a strong hearty vivid language. It doesn't dissipate itself with laziness, illiteracy, and intentional quaintness as our mother tongue does in some parts of this continent. Its starkness is eased by an Irish-like lilt. In its pure form it is hard to come on—like the mating of camels. You will find it in an older fisherman on any of the more isolated islands or you can surprise it on the party telephone while waiting for the line to be free. When it is used in the presence of strangers it is robbed of a little of its color. Much of the flavor comes from the use of ancient words which appear in Shakespeare or as the third or fourth definition in Webster. Sometimes they can't be found in any reference book but that is the fault of the lexicographer for they issue with the dignity and authority of centuries of accurate meaning. I have worked with many different groups of people who imparted a high seasoning to the English Language: Scotch, Cockney, French Canadian, Italian, Yiddish, Southern, Slavic, and Brooklyn. They all have their own charm and music. I like to hear them but I take care not to let them creep into my speaking. The Newfoundland speech I earnestly tried to learn and use. Something less than success was the result. The most elusive element was that rhythm and cadence which are the peculiar soul of any language. The best example is that short statement of a lad in answering a question. It was delivered with the mood of a slightly enlivened Gregorian chant. "I be ten sir, February gone." Giving up on that score, the next best thing was to adopt the phrases and figures of speech. The ultimate in polite agreement and/or disagreement in response to a statement is "I dare say I don't know I am sure." This is said in one quick breath with scarcely any pauses—there is no rejoinder to it.

Any male from ninety-three to a newborn (if he has been in the world long enough for a diagnostic glance) is addressed as "my son." The almost equally universal address "my dear" does away with gender difference. I was always pleased to be so spoken-to myself whether by our laundry women or a bearded old sea captain.

The word "boy" is used very often in direct conversation. It is softened and shortened to "b'y" and used without accentuation. One six-year-old patient in a body cast used to call me "Doctor B'y."

Certain phrases have special meanings:

To grease your rope = to have a successful seal fishery
Torn up in my mind = to be confused or undecided
To leg ("laig") one's self = to get up after a fall or collapse
To take your dodge = to take your time, proceed leisurely and with care
Go to the ice = to hunt seal
hood = an adult hooded seal
up along = Canada or the U.S.
leery = empty in the stomach
driving works = raising the devil—cutting up
strained in the head = demented
burning weather = cold enough to cause frostbite
on times—scatter times = occasionally
stellegan = crooked small evergreen stump—used for firewood, or evergreen sticks used for fence pickets.

bogey = a small wood stove
bogey warped = cramped from sitting in one position near a bogey.
swatch = a moderate expanse of ice-free water
swatching = hunting for seal at a swatch where the animals breath
lew warm = luke warm. This is Archaic, Scotch or English.
spall = splinter, especially used for pieces of wood knocked off a mast or keel in a storm.
stun = slow minded or dull of wit
gall = chafe
rames = skeleton or wreck of a vessel or for that matter a person
fitout = always used instead of outfit, and why not?
haul over = always used instead of over haul. This refers I think to the practice of hauling a vessel over onto its side for repair.
qualmish = on the verge of nausea
to urge = to try to vomit
glutch = swallow (as in eating—not the bird)
do it = any unidentified bird
bibber = shiver
dwy = an intense but passing flurry or squall of snow or rain.
skiver = skewer or wooden knitting needle
clever = handsome, amiable, blustery, strong and friendly, well nourished
neither = none. "I've neither copper in the house" means "I'm flat broke."
'ar = any or either.
n'ar = not any
wonderful = this word demands special treatment. It is used very often. It means a strong "very"—to be wondered at. It has no connotation of good. "Wonderful pain", "Wonderfully sick", "Wonderfully bad." As a matter of fact it tends to mean bad. If you simply say something is wonderful chances are it is horrible. It is a combination of Shakespearean accuracy and irony. This word can creep up on you, and before you know it, will appear three times in any paragraph you utter.
pitch = Settle, find, rest, go down. A nice word. I liked this one very much. When a gale dies, it pitches. When a hovering seagull settles on a grump or bollard, it pitches. When you fall off your roof you "pitch" on your wherever you make contact.

lun = in the lee of a protection from wind—a calm moment in a gale or a calm stretch of water (rare—the water is always rough)

yare = easy to handle, pleasingly responsive, when speaking of a ship; of a person, athletic, attractive, even handsome, always approving

Various sizes and forms of raw wood are called *splits, billets, junks, longers, stellegans, turns.* The most picturesque is a *cronic,* that's a standing dead tree.

There is a striking lack of vulgarity and profanity. This goes along with the British-inherited habit of understatement. When the steamer *Clyde* was prevented for three days from coming fifteen miles from Herring Neck to Twillingate, the *Twillingate Sun* reported her as being delayed by "Unfavorable breezes." As you hold on to a stanchion to keep yourself from being blown overboard, the polite comment to the captain is, "Blows a nice breeze eh?" The word "dirty" is reserved for weather that isn't fit for even a doctor to be out in. There is a term that is used to express the ultimate in repulsiveness and evil. I didn't hear it very often because few people or things short of Hitler and an occasional politician are heinous enough to merit this categoric denunciation. The phrase is, "It's not good enough." It sounds mild at first but after knowing people a while and understanding the circumstances that bring out this curse, you can actually feel its impact. In agreement with it you shake your head slowly and expel breath that expresses more sorrow than anger.

Only one local phrase really used to give me a start. I believe it is also in general British usage. Since I was continually being routed out for night calls I was frequently hearing the phrase. When a Newfoundlander goes to another person's house in the night with the purpose of making enough noise at the door to arouse him, that process is referred to as "Knocking up." I mention this only to point out that the fault here is clearly American.

The use of the word "Tickle" is an interesting one. It is used to designate any comparatively narrow stretch of water connecting two larger bodies of water. If it were larger it would be a strait; Webster does not give hydrographic definition of the word, but it appears on all the government charts. It is often part of a proper name, as "Whistle Tickle" or "Burnt Island Tickle"—it is however a definite aquatic entity. The word is used I would suppose because navigation in the tickles is unusually delicate and critical or, to use Webster's third definition of "ticklish," requiring careful handling.

The OPD (Outpatient department)

Probably some of the more recently recruited aids or maids would stand and stare at me if I asked one of them to rush down to the out-patient department on an errand. By the second day though, anybody would know where I meant if I said the "*OPD*." That's a standard term and every hospital in the U.S. uses it. One doesn't have time to use long words. When one thinks of a hospital, one draws on his personal or movie experience and a vista rises of long rows of immaculate beds with scores of crisp white sisters of mercy gliding noiselessly about in an atmosphere of rest and calm. Incidentally that's one of the troubles with frequent cinema attendance. Pretty soon you can't remember for sure if you have been captured by Arabs on the Nubian Desert or only saw it in a film palace. Well, we've got the nurses and beds and calm but we also have the OPD, and we wouldn't be much of a hospital without that never glamorized institution. I sometimes wonder what impression a more rural patient gets when he comes to the OPD for the first time. He climbs the ten concrete steps to the front door in the center of the face of the hospital. He hauls the door open, grunting against the force of the wind right off the harbor and it slams behind him with a crash that four or five times a year breaks the glass. Also as he opens the door, every other door inside the hospital swings in sympathy with the drafts. As he stands in the small square lobby, he is slightly dazed by the change in temperature and momentarily blinded by the impact of the comparative dimness after the keen glare of sky or snow. When his eyes settle down it will be clear that he is not the next patient to be seen. The lobby will have four or five people in it, the overflow from the bare-benched waiting room on the left. That space will be filled by a dozen patient citizens in their sea-going gear, with their bundles and coats and children all waiting for Bessie to invite them in through the other door to see the doctor. In an hour perhaps it will be his turn. Meanwhile he will have inspected the memorial plaque which describes the hospital as a memorial to the men of Notre Dame Bay who fought in World War I. Over the plaque is a small wreath, faded since its presentation last Armistice Day. Between the windows is a framed certificate wherein the College of Surgeons allows as how they consider this a reasonably good hospital. He may or may not be impressed thereby. Before he can rightly make up his mind he is whisked by Bessie into the inner sanctum. Here there may be something resembling confusion. The long narrow hall ends in a largish emergency room. Off the left of the hall are three examining cubicles. Doctors hustle about. Bessie is everywhere. A patient disconsolately waits in one corner for a laboratory or x-ray report. Through an inadequate screen a figure may be visible stretched on the operating table for the sewing of a laceration or the removal of a wen. From the other corner may come the vocal indications incident to the removal of a tooth. These sounds vary in sanguinity according to the skill of the operator and the emotional setup of the donor. The latter is by far the greater factor and the gamut is wide.

Bessie, an aide who has had all her training right here, is the breath of the OPD. She makes the wheels go round. The OPD without her is an unlighted lamp, an unmade bed, home without a mother. She is young, not very tall and just this side of plump. She is rosy of countenance and spirit. She is wise and full of local lore; her knowledge of the people and their stories is almost alarming. On a quiet day she will espy a patient coming up the hospital lane. Before the doorbell rings, Bessie will have given you a thumbnail sketch that would do credit to the dictionary of biography, with a diagnosis and outline of treatment thrown in for good measure. To do her justice, she does blush and sort of look at you over shyly raised shoulder as she makes the more delicate points. While Bessie is with us we don't actually have to have records. There was a slip-up in the OPD turmoil once. A rather inarticulate woman, of little will power, was already installed in bed upstairs before it was discovered that she had come only to sell eggs.

Maybe I'm wrong

In crepuscular moments, when a pause comes suddenly uninvited in the business of the day, I find myself leaning back in my chair by the study window. The same blue dimness—the pearly smokiness, that almost hides the anchored Labradorman in the harbor seems to dull the tooth as well of ordinary diurnal annoyances. "The world seems not so bad." The armor of my friends shines more whitely. Musing and introspection are inevitable in the gloaming—I wonder if I am right and almost cheerfully and happily I realize I may not necessarily be right. In the mind's eye, the days, the weeks, the months are reviewed and it is all too clear how ridiculous it was to be angry that I was not included in an operating schedule; how stupid it was to be annoyed when Waddell took a case that I didn't even want—in fact I was afraid of. When this imagined slight or that fancied insult fades then it becomes clear how dreamed-up and invented unhappiness can be. At the risk of plagiarizing, I conclude that unhappiness is within you just as much as happiness is. What a mistake it is and what a chore to go around behaving like something you think you ought to be. People are fond of you, for the most part, because of what they see in your unguarded moments. The studied manner butters very few parsnips I feel. A little reassured, I grope in the darkness for my stethoscope because I hear John yelling in the hall for Stella and that means it is time for rounds and after rounds we will have our cheering drink and then dinner upstairs in the Olds' apartment. My mouth waters as I remember that I overheard Betty tell Martin to bring back some caribou from the cold storage bait depot.

Hazel

It's hard to know what to say about Hazel. She is the gad fly in this medico-social unguent. She is one of the three or four best nurses I ever knew or heard of. She has an astounding, independent efficiency—like a perfectly tooled ball-bearing. She is most learned—she should have been a doctor. She knows the why and where for and how much of every drug. She is a good diagnostician. I felt it very high praise indeed when she told me she was perfectly glad to have me take the appendix out of her favorite brother. She knows as much about the laboratory as our good laboratory technician. She understands and can practice Pharmacy. When she watches an obstetrical case for you she knows exactly how the patient stands every minute. She has more than the average tenderness and solicitude in her nursing but in her thinking and acting professionally she is reasoning and objective. However on the social side we have a different persona: there is the female with all the guiles and wiles and charms of a Circe, Medea, a Josephine, a Lorelei. She is just the right height and slim and boyish and pink with pretty fair wavy hair, white teeth and regular features. There is a mocking in the smiling eye and a knowing what-are-you-thinking-about bow in the slightly parted lips. She is young and clean and fresh. Her air is one of innocence and good. Married women are well advised to take a defensive stance.

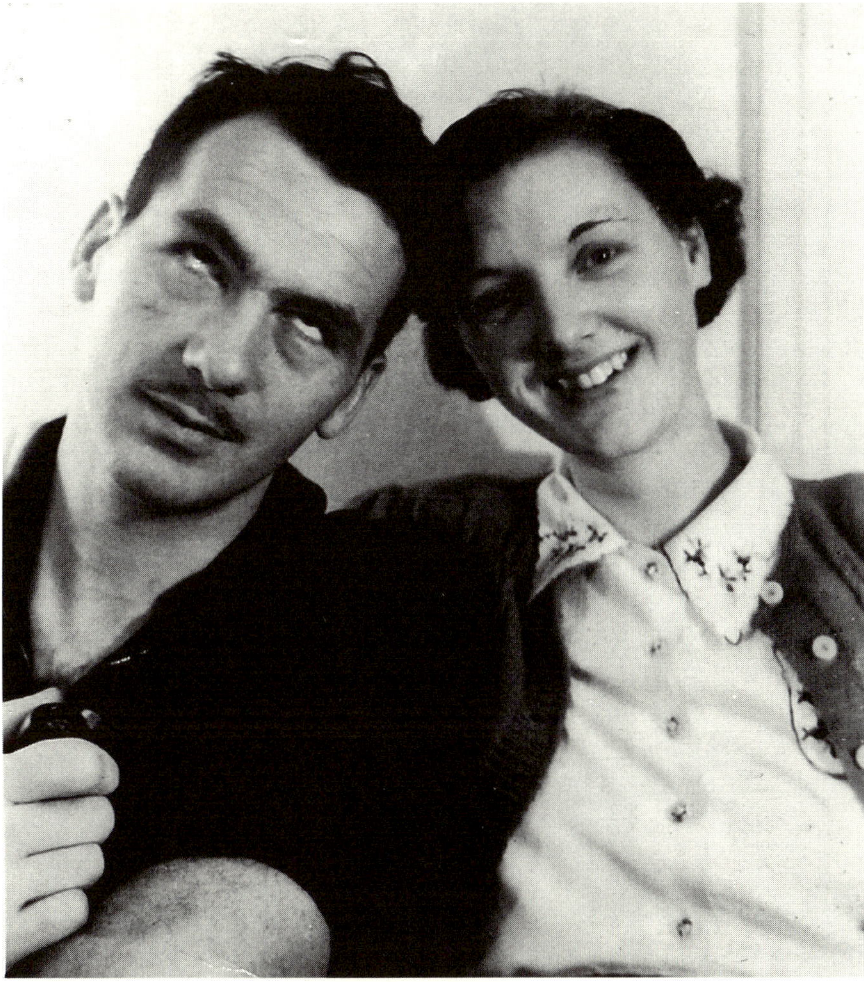

At a party—R.S.E. and Hazel.

Rita (nurse on last boat trip)

So Rita is my helper on this trip. Well, we'll see how that turns out. Rita has a faraway look. It comes from being in love with someone in the R.A.F. or else she chews betel nuts. A faraway look is not unattractive on Rita. She is an unstudied "Veronica Lake" type, only the sweep of her hair does not really obscure her vision. There are the same mouth and eyelashes. Sensuous nose and freckles heighten the exotic quality.

Ethics (again)

The great common interest in Medicine is not enough to make friends of all doctors. I speak somewhere else of the feud between the two local doctors. It waxed bitter before the hospital came and the hospital inherited it when one doctor joined and helped us and the other hated us. They both had their adherents among the people and the hospital inherited that difference. One day years ago, the cold radiators drove someone to the basement to investigate. There, almost dead from diphtheria, the furnace man lay in his little room. He had told none of the staff of his illness but had been going to the rival hospital-hating doctor to be treated for his "sore throat." This was years ago. He was too weak to resist hospital treatment and he was quickly injected with antitoxin. It was too late to help him. When he had died, his doctor loudly proclaimed to the public that the hospital had killed him. "Look," he said, "they stuck sixty thousand units in him. Nobody can stand that much of anything." This was strong propaganda. The fishing people shook their heads wonderingly. Sixty-thousand is a big number. What a unit was nobody had any idea, but they did know what sixty thousand fish or sixty thousand potatoes or sixty thousand turns of wood were and it was such a preposterous number that it would likely kill anybody.

Bone Grafts

Because of the prevalence of tuberculosis and especially of bone and joint tuberculosis, we do more than our share of bone grafts. When the spine begins to collapse from tuberculosis and pinches the spinal cord it becomes necessary to support it with a bone graft both to save the nervous tissue and to rest the spine. This is a fairly extensive and ponderous procedure but it is mostly one of engineering and things are pretty well under control. The spinal column is exposed and a bed is freshened either in it or beside it. The graft is taken from the tough thick bone of the shin and placed where it will support and stiffen the spine. The theory is simple and the act is simple but that does not take into consideration the vagaries of our homemade circular saw, a constant source of anxious uncertainty and even hazard to the operator. This makes an exciting event out of what might otherwise have been onerous. The patient for this occasion is well protected in a large cumbersome body cast of plaster and one feels as if he were working on a statue that bleeds a little and needs an anesthetic. Meanwhile on more than one occasion the housekeeper would be waiting at the door to retrieve the saw motor, since its original use is to power her sewing machine. The saw itself had been made by Olds—he cut it out of a Victrola spring.

Mastoid

The rarity of acute surgical mastoiditis used to bother me. Three times I saw youngsters who had had it and had not been brought to us. The condition had gone on to rupture of the mastoid region with formation of an abscess behind the ear and destruction of hearing but the sparing of life. As a student up here I saw only one acute mastoid in an adult. One summer though, we had the services of a well-trained ear-nose-and-throat man. He found a dozen acute mastoids that needed immediate operation. It was never clear to me.

One ten-year old boy was brought in to the OPD one day who had lain at home for two months during and after an attack of scarlet fever, complicated by mastoiditis on both sides. Both mastoid processes had ruptured into the area under his ears and he presented abscesses. He was emaciated to the point of dying. We tied a tube in a vein of his foot to feed him and filled him full of sulfa drugs. In three days he was strong enough to have the abscesses opened but not conscious enough to need an anesthetic. The complete mastoid bone was dead and loose on both sides and could be lifted out easily. We kind of adopted him and in three or four months he was a well-nourished little boy raising the devil in the children's ward but quite deaf. I am no psychiatrist but I think he was happy as well.

CHAPTER VIII

The Journal Continues

November 4, '40. This was a day. There were boats in from everywhere so I sent a note to persuade Stan to drop his tickle-side idyll and come home from the Tilt to work in the OPD, since the rest of us would be busy in the operating room. He returned somewhat annoyed and took over. I did a hernia using nylon sutures for the first time and liking them very much. The nylon has a good spring and is alive and handles well. Then I did three cystoscopies, including one in Pinsent. He had been condemned with a kidney tumor, but it suddenly disappeared and proved to have been only a blocked ureter.

Cystoscopy can be fun, for the surgeon that is. I don't suppose it could ever become a pastime for the patient. The procedure is a nice mechanical, practical one. As with many another medical maneuver it is exciting to see the mystery drop away from what seemed at first a secret, magic sort of operation. The first one you see is very impressive. It is usually done in the dark and that always adds to the effect. Naturally one doesn't expect to see into the inner cavities of the body—the bladder especially seems safe from the human eye except under very radical conditions. To take a tube then, fitted with mirrors and little levers and running water and a light, and insert it into the bladder appears at first to be formidable. To see the pink and red interior of the bladder you have to distend it with water. That is where the trouble lies. As the eye is applied rather intimately to the instrument in the search for those tiny openings of the ureters coming down to the bladder from the kidneys, the operator is usually encountered by leakage of the fluid used to fill the bladder. The size of this deluge varies but I never could get over the feeling of being like a salmon going upstream. It is not unusual to have to change even your socks after one or two cystoscopies.

The glass was falling all day, an opportunity to calibrate my homemade barometer against Stan's. During a meal of partridge Hazel came up to announce an OB call to Herring Neck which sort of automatically fell to me. I finished my tea and sat a minute. It was a cold crossing over the island on the cycle. The headlight was very poor; only by intuition could I stay on the road. When I got to the boat the waiting man said, "Quite a spell since we called—it's a matter of life and death." I detected annoyance in their tone and said very little, just huddled in the bottom of the fishy boat.

The engine quit off Gut Tickle but we got her going and cruised right through Salt Harbor Tickle. I had never been through there. The sea curled around the rocks only six feet from us and the only light was the angry gash of breaking surf. At the house I fell in with Mrs. Oxford, my favorite midwife, who always calls me sweetheart. The baby had been born even before the men had called from Little Harbor, so that exonerated me. The mother was fine, without even a tear, but the baby was moaning and all agreed that babies always died when they moaned. It looked all right to me. I fixed the eyes and the cord and foreskin. A jolly cup of tea was ready in the comfortable heavy gloom downstairs. The women joked about why we had babies and is it the men's fault entirely or not. One of the men spoke about cutting wood by moonlight and a woman said if he didn't spend so long in bed with his wife he would find time to do his work by daylight. The logic was obscure, the humor was clear and well received.

They brought me back in record time. The pleasure was taken off the trip though by meeting poor John, starting for Salten's on an OB call. I took his car back and left the cycle with him. I had only just crawled into the bedroom window, to Dudley II's delight, and taken up my ocarina practice when Stan interrupted to tell me he had a bad pain in his left chest and shoulder. He was worried about a coronary or pleurisy. His temperature was 101° so I gave him some morphine and he trundled off. I have forgotten which patient named Warren it was I went to see so I can't charge for the visit.

November 6, '40. The last two days have been really only one. Yesterday dawned bright and early with countless patients for the OPD but no one to work there. We started at eight with fluoroscopies and we had two tough operations planned after that—a difficult upper spinal graft which bent in two planes, and Clemmie's uterus. It was big and pregnant-looking and proved to be a tumor. It was dinnertime when I finished an appendix. I continued to work furiously in the OPD, slipping upstairs for scattered chores like tubing that prostate. Business roared right up until tea when we sent away five Gander Bay people. They had come so late. Tea looked like a great respite after long rounds, however we had an appendix to do after supper. During tea a man came in from Woolfry's Mill with three fingers made into hamburger. About eight I did the appendix through a small incision and had bad luck with the nylon sutures. Every one broke all over the place—even the purse string. Then we washed up the hand and took two fingers off and repaired the other. Feeling a little fuzzy, I went down to visit Stan and by his bed we had a drink. I got one of my speaking up spells (which are always at the wrong time) and sort of flared up at John because he didn't like my operating schedule. He was right, of course. I got to bed about midnight and goddamn if about three Hazel didn't have to shake me to get me up to go to Merritt's Harbor for a delivery.

Getting up was no fun, but I enjoyed it once I got started. The night was as dark as your hat, so naturally this was the time the cycle light failed completely. I groped my way across the island, standing up, with the engine in second, peering all the while ahead into the blackness. The irrevocable ditch lies on either side. It was nice snuggled coldly in the bottom of a big skiff. All three, even the helmsman, were lying down to get out of the wind. It was a picturesque sort of assembly, like that painting of Hendrik Hudson, *Cast Adrift in the Arctic.*

The delivery was an easy one – for me. The woman and Dr. LeDrew had had a bad time eight years ago with her first child. The midwife was a characterful old dame. She said to me as I was stooping to put on my hat in the five-foot-six kitchen: "Go up and see your patient again, you might as well do something for your money." I liked her and we had a nice time toasting a bit of bread and having some tea while we waited for it to be "a little handier to daylight." When we could see that Merritt's Harbor Rock wasn't breaking we started our bleak trip back in the rainy dawn.

After a tub, I dressed my appendix, which was bleeding from the incision—because I didn't order a binder. My side of the big hydrocele was bleeding too. After some breakfast I was ready for more fluoroscopy, then an appendix under local and next a graft job on an eyelid. Old Sid Green's hydrocele fell after that and we had to cancel another one to get down to the OPD because Stan is still laid up. There was more OPD after dinner. I got through in time to go see the infected finger at Ragged Point. Just as we started rounds, my OB went into the last stages of labor, making a great stink in a styled, grand sort of way and pushing not at all. I took her into the operating room where Betty put her to sleep, with the nerve-wracking help of an aide who had never heard about germs. It was an easy forceps, but she bled like the dickens. I threw the placenta on the floor in my hurry. She must have lost a thousand cc. Everything turned out all right. Tea was welcome and I played with David awhile until seeing him to bed. Now I'm going to turn in myself before I forget what my bed looks like.

November 8, '40. A lot of operating. Two bladder explorations and a hernia/appendectomy combined in a Salvation Army girl with a terrific aura of stale perfume. She complained that singing hurt her side. This operation then was to the Glory of God. There was another appendix and cystoscopy, at which I am getting red-hot.

This afternoon I walked along the shore to Black Duck Cove past Smooth Cove to Kettle Cove because I wanted to see a tendon suture I had done the other day. The path that way is beautiful. It meanders up along the cliff and at one point you can see down through the tickle into Friday Bay. The small Black Island just south of Twillingate Island looms up and you can make out the winter trail to Indian Cove. It is another world on that side of the island. The trees are large and it is very quiet.

This morning they put Jake in my apartment. He and Dudley II raised hell, tearing up the rugs and peeing on the floor. When the rain quit, I came down from the operating room, in desperation, to put them out in the garden, or tried to. Before I could shut the gate Jake had slid by me like a flash and followed by the puppy, was gone over the hill towards Little Harbor. He came back but not Dudley II. Now at midnight I have officially given up hope.

Stan is a little better but looks pale and says he feels stale. I think he ought to take the *Northern Ranger* and go to St. John's for a trip.

Last night I opened a bottle of rum by pounding on the bottom of it. I'm the only one on the staff who can do that.

November 9, '40. It was just as I thought. Wynn always has the local news; he came into work with it this morning saying that Dudley II had been shot, over at West's farm near Little Harbor. In the afternoon when I was free I cycled over, finding Mr. West mending his cod trap. He said, yes – a dog had been shot. Yesterday morning he had heard a rumpus down by the shore. He investigated and found two red dogs barking at sheep who had been driven into the ocean and were standing knee deep in the surf. I agreed that few things were as out of place as sheep in the ocean.

West had gone in for his shotgun. When he saw it, Jake had hightailed it over the hill, old hand at marauding that he is. Dudley II, though, was just a puppy and any man, gun or not, was another friend. He had run up to the man only to get a load of buckshot at point blank range. The man's version was that Dudley II had attacked him. West might really have thought so. In spite of the fact that these people depend on dogs, they do not understand them or have any real feeling for them. Every winter we see hands broken from striking dogs. Sport was considered a man-eater before he joined the hospital stables. Actually he is nothing more than an elephantine lap dog. I buried Dudley II at the top of the cliff at Codjack Cove and swore I would subject no more Irish Setters to this unfavorable clime.

Back at the hospital where the subject was, of course, the death of my puppy, I heard the tail ends of whispered rumors which I was never really able to piece together—having to do with the sudden disappearance of my first Dudley. The gist of them was that some person had hired someone I knew well to catch the dog and chloroform him and put him in the hospital furnace. The collar was thrown out on the Arm Trail so that it would be found; this was supposed to throw me off the track. I may be doing someone a terrific injustice, but I feel the culprit was Konopka, the dentist I feuded with. After I had left that spring, there was a party for some R.A.F. people at the hospital. In the course of it Marianne had accused Konopka of doing the dog in. He forthwith had slapped her hard enough to knock her down. He was planning to leave three days later but John made him take the boat that night. Konopka had also endeared himself to us when he claimed a percentage of his clinic take above his salary, which was already the same as mine. (They denied his claim.)

November 18, '40. We are becoming fairly international with a skipper and chief mate coming to tea from a Portuguese fishing vessel, a lovely four-masted diesel. The captain was Nordic in appearance but the mate was a standard Latin. They spoke the English rather "fewly" so we exchanged those little, red dictionaries. They spoke French, but no one of us was unselfconscious enough to try.

Our society is rather restraining. No one is willing to forget himself a little and if one does, the others sit around and comment.

The Portuguese profess great hatred for Franco, Mussolini, and Hitler and were shocked when I asked if they spoke German. I trust that their reaction was not studied. Anyway, I managed to get a good picture of their vessel.

This morning I did two appendectomies and a hernia and then helped on a uterus. The first appendix bled after we got the gut back in the belly and it was tough getting it back in because the anesthesia was poor and the peritoneal opening too small. We fished the gut out again and found a small bleeder in the mesentery that had been torn by manipulation. The second time the ether was better so we had no trouble.

Let me see what we have been doing these past two weeks besides lots of surgery. Stan had been feeling so rotten that after John got back from his hunting trip, he and Annette took two weeks off for a trip to St. John's. I've not been taking any time off because there's no place to go and no one to take my place. So I read about travel. Scott's diary of his trip to the Pole is a moving document. It is interesting to see how, on a project that was planned right down to the number of toothpicks, when they came to some really important steps they found themselves improvising. They changed the numbers in sledding parties. Some had skis and some didn't. They should have left men at the nearest depot, to help them back. It was a crime to be that near home base and die.

November 19, '40. There are two dying in the house now—Edwards with TB all over him, and Mr. Earl. He had been told it was hemorrhoids but we found him full of cancer.

In the evening John, Betty, Stan and Annette went to the Portuguese ship for dinner (I was invited but elected to mind the house). They dined by a printed menu—soup, cold meats and pickles, salad with LETTUCE no less, ripe olives, salmon, stewed beef, pudding with cheese, honeydew melon, port wine, *vin ordinaire*, coffee and cognac. They had a good time. Ate until midnight.

I couldn't sleep; too disturbed by too much coffee and by reading the last of Scott's journal. What a time they had lying in their tents, waiting to die. They could have been saved had they only relayed more food to One-Ton Camp. They could have kept a man on the lookout in that area. They weren't so far behind schedule. They should have planned to have relief parties much further out along the trail.

November 20, '40. The blusteriness and the snow of yesterday continued through this morning. A few operations, a terrible cancer of the lip in a 39-year-old man who couldn't tell us how long he'd been sick.

With a good stiff drink to bolster me I went off to the church supper with Betty and Stella. Stella is a lot of fun, a Twillingate girl trained in St. John's. She's the head nurse now and lives in Edith's old digs. Stella keeps the teakettle going in her fireplace and many of the happy moments of the day are spent having a drop of tea in her room.

I got nicked for the taxi fare and the tickets which got us a dinner that was all right at the fancy church (Church of England). We got a plate of turnip, peas and some kind of fresh meat, undiagnosed. All kinds of cakes, as usual, and tea. The Portuguese were there, having a little language difficulty—mixed up over Ashbourne, aspirin and ice cream. I walked home with Annette, had a nap and then had to go out in a roaring rain over Froude's Hill on a call. I was tired all day so talked John into delivering Mrs. Pollard if she comes off tonight.

November 21, '40. Here I sit in the last half hour of my 30th year and I somehow feel that it marks an important point in my life. I hesitate to take stock but, at the same time, there must be a few things on the credit side. At least I have a trade which can feed me now—one which has fared well in all the cataclysms of historic time. It has even thriven on the woes of the world. I wasted the day—read trash the whole morning and evening except for time out to do an appendix. I must organize my activities a little, at least write something each night and even carry a bit of paper with me on overnight or longer trips. If Captain Scott could write on his deathbed, I can do this. However, I suspect it is easier to write on your deathbed than on a casual evening.

I will soon receive my Ted-designed made-to-order wonderful overcoat. It would be just the thing for Southern California. It is calf length, black sheep leather, sheepskin lined, a high fur collar, generously double breasted, with a big protected pocket for pipe and tobacco. I can hear the frustrated whine of the parried wind. I have had great pleasure in the corduroy coat and short Austrian ski jacket brought home by my brother. It was just right for the fall and will be warm enough for most of the winter. The ski trousers I have not had use for yet. My fine frontier trousers you may remember suffered a serious tear on the anterior-lateral aspect of the left thigh in the course of my birthday celebration. Now I sport a fine big soft leather patch which adds to the decor tremendously.

With the coming of snow and cold weather, people are taking down their gates and removing strategic portions of their fences so that travel is more direct. That means that sheep are taken in and the dogs are unleashed and allowed out of their cages. If I could have held on to my fine beautiful Irish setter Dudley II just two weeks longer than I did, she would still be sharing my bed and board. It makes me furious. She was registered in the American Kennel Club on the very day she died. I almost think I will give up.

I was recently given the book *Kabloona*, which I've heard a lot about and am anxious to get at. Right now it is packed in my duffel for those few minutes at night when we have shooed the last patient off the boat and I am tucked into my narrow gasoline-smelling, damp bunk for a well-earned night's repose. I just got one letter from a professor at Dartmouth who says, "I have ceased to include myself among those who hope." My sister Kathryn is progressing, it seems, in her attempts to follow her career in special education. I will feel much more secure when there is someone more in the family from whom one can bum a dime for a cup of coffee. I feel more and more uncertain as my ne'er-do-well but pleasant course unrolls itself. I will leave here, to be sure, with a thousand dollars or so in cash, but my plans call for squandering it.

The Portuguese ship pulled out into the stream early this morning, making for Fogo. It was a lovely cold day and I didn't put a nose out of doors, but neither did I put it out of joint.

John has done a tremendous job here. Despite the great responsibility of this whole business he is still youthful and courteous. He is daring and skillful. He is here because he is a success. Stan is here because he loves it. Why am I here? I couldn't even tell the diary why. I'm not sure I know why I am here, but certain black shadows rise as possibilities.

November 24, '40. The events of Friday have left me sore all over with every new motion revealing undiscovered aches and bruises. Friday was my birthday, memorable for being unusual and uncommonly pleasant. It did dawn dark and threatening. After doing an appendix I helped take that cancer off the lower lip. It was plastic surgery—moving two big triangles from the cheek; to see the whole face laid open was a shock to me and made my stomach feel queer. After dictating notes and cracking some membranes I had two drinks before dinner since I was free by then to take the afternoon for my natal holiday. At that moment Dr. Wood called me frantically to his car just outside where he had a violently bleeding woman in her seventh month. It was an obvious placenta praevia. Stan offered to scrub since I was technically free that afternoon. Nevertheless I brought the woman in in my arms soaked with blood and I started an intravenous glucose while John did the section. Suddenly I was handed an unbreathing infant, and I rushed the baby out to the sterilizer to work on it. In a moment out came Dr. Wood with another. His breathed at once. Mine was slow and limp and white. They called me back to restart the glucose and then I got oxygen, after yelling for the wrench to turn it on. The child got red and breathed well.

Then I had a drink with George, the orderly, and finally took the cycle to Codjack Cove. There isn't a house to be seen there. It's a gloomy nightmare of rock and sea. Great, ugly buttresses and pillars jut up from the surf. It was also snowing and dark. I tried to climb a cliff but was frightened by falling rock. Then I sat there in a niche and smoked my pipe and thought of various things. I composed a letter to Sarah Maud, my high school drama coach, which I suppose I will never send. My spirits rose when I came back and had a drink with Bud and John and Lidge Dalley (in that order). Annette and Stan were giving the dinner. Annette has a genius for making any place beautiful. She had dressed the table up with her silver and her lace cloth. There was enough to drink and the night was exhilarating. We fought with one another, even dear Betty insulted me, but I was very flattered when they told me that though I had never acted very mad, my eyes had more anger in them than any they had ever seen.

They hinted around that I should go get the ice cream but I would be damned before letting any host make me work at my own party. The dinner was a success and John opened that bottle of fine old port that the steamer captain had given him. Somehow we waxed acrimonious. Raising my voice, I demanded not to be laughed at—if I wasn't to be considered a part of the organization, I would go away.

At the height of my ranting, John rose from his book to pay tribute, saying that his birthday present to me would be the pronouncement that in his eyes I became of age today instead of ten years ago. To my Peter Pan psyche, that was not unpleasant. He also said I took hell from him and stood it well. I denied that. A few drinks took us to midnight. John suddenly had the idea that I should spend the night at the Tilt and that he would take me in the panzer.

The panzer needs explaining. It is a weird, three-wheeled contraption made out of spare motorcycle parts and an outboard engine (from a boat). It steers by a stick like an old electric motor vehicle, or an airplane for that matter. It does seem able to cover ground but has two bad habits. When you throw it into gear it is a little inclined to rear like a horse and, once going, has a great reluctance to stop. Hazel said she would come for the ride.

It was cold, especially on the front where I was sitting with both legs hanging out. Not safe but there was no place else to put them. All went well as far as Edgar Warr's, this side of Purcell's Harbor Bridge. We careened off a rock on the starboard and the creature unpredictably leapt to the same side of the road, overturning with the motor still going. Hazel pitched out on her head and split her eyebrow. There was that wild unrecalled moment when you struggle to preserve your bones without emotion. We untangled and I was surprised to find myself functioning. We pushed on to the Tilt, where I discovered I had lost the food for breakfast at the accident. We built the fire and had a drink.

After spending the night freezing, I woke up early to suddenly wonder where my movie camera was, much pleased to find it on the kitchen table. Breakfast was not next to it. In pursuit of something to eat I walked up the road to the scene of the previous night's debacle to find my breakfast usable, but run over. My other find was a bloodstained Norwegian mitt. To augment these provisions I stole a piece of moose from a cache of Mr. Warr's. The rest of the day was comfortable and drowsy although I couldn't smoke much because my mouth was burnt from last night's bout.

Back to the hospital to be plagued all night by the night nurse who kept running in for this and that till I was crazy.

November 25, '40. In reading Shackleton's life I am impressed, as was Scott, by his colossal luck. I didn't get to bed until midnight and then couldn't go to sleep, but it didn't make any difference because I had to get up for a delivery in the small hours. I stepped on a rat in the downstairs kitchen. He 'laiged himself' and escaped into the utility room, much hurt. Today was busy in the morning. We opened a belly I never thought had an ulcer and he didn't; it was polycystic kidneys. The pond is frozen.

November 26, '40. This is a howler of a night. Sleet has been beating against the windows and the barometer has dropped to the lowest yet: 28.1. When it started up, the wind rose with it and now has a gale force right in from the northeast. The *Bessie Marie* is at the same anchorage she had when she blew ashore three years ago.

The morning was not heavy. Among other things Mrs. Price's leg was put in a jelly bandage and a cast. That will teach her to ride on handcars that go too fast. Speaking of travel, I finished the life of Sir Ernest Shackleton. It was a glorious story and I wept when he reached the Falkland Islands. That journey was better than the polar one. He died the only way he could, I think—on his way to Antarctica again. We had tea upstairs.

Betty is the hospital housekeeper now and it makes her a little irritable. I started to talk about the difficulty of getting marmalade for breakfast and she went right off the handle.

November 27, '40. After tea I sat in Mr. Earl's room. He is dying of cancer of the rectum but doesn't seem annoyed. He is only a year older than I am. He told me how lovely it was up around his home in New Bay, and how big the trees are.

November 28, '40. Thanksgiving. We decided this should be a holiday so I got up late, but first thing you know, I was doing a caesarian section on a baldheaded syphilitic. We got a boy out of it. Right after dinner I had to go to Squid Cove. There was talk in the air of someone going to Fortune Harbor; Stan glibly trying to talk me out of it. But John put in a shot and we decided to draw.

Meanwhile, this other call came in and I went off into the roaring snow on the cycle. It was slippery in spots and bad on the tickle. The boat was small and I took solid water in my lap several times. The child had diarrhea. It was dark as we left to beat our way back so they took me over to Stuckless' instead of Purcell's Harbor so I had a hot, wet walk over to the cycle.

There were twelve of us for a fancy duck dinner. We played cards and one thing and another until it was eleven before I knew it.

November 29, '40. A first class wind blowing tonight. Not so strong as the one that rolled up the linoleum in my bedroom, but pretty damn strong. Playing cards over at Annette's tonight we could feel the sun porch shake and that is made out of concrete blocks.

The evenings are short and the sullen sun sinks into the bight very early. I love it and we have a whole month before the days are really as short as they can get. I will have to spend a winter sometime in the land of no sun.

November 30, '40. This Saturday a dead day. I wasted it reading *Action at Acquile* and a detective story. No operating and no patients. I brought soup and canned strawberries for tea at Annette's where we sat around and played cards with Hazel and Stella until 1 A.M.

December 1, '40. My coat came yesterday. Ted designed it and had sent the drawing to St. John's for execution. It's fine horsehide leather, sheepskin lined, with a big fur collar. It also comes down to my ankles and has great big pockets and a belt. This morning I planned a hunting and exploring trip with Mr. Earl as my guide, for next February; he is to bring his dog teams—all he wants is his food and tobacco which I will supply. It would be fun. I like him. I only wish he was going to live more than a week.

I tried twice to get up Yates' Hill on the cycle, but it slid all the way down backwards, after almost making it each time, so I walked it, to find a sixteen-year-old girl all covered up and crying; afraid of the doctor. The mother thought the gas was getting up around her heart. She was afraid to let it go any longer though the child's face had been swollen over a week. The mother allowed as how it was the kidneys because of the way she puffed and all her children get kidney trouble sooner or later. She was right and the girl was swollen and had a temperature of 104; probably getting pneumonia in the bargain. I think the outlook is damn bad. I slid down the hill again and came home.

December 4, '40. We took out a kidney or most of it. A few naval recruits came in. There's a lot of snow down so the afternoon was quiet. I got the cycle out but couldn't get it back to the hospital. Snow is drifting around the garage. The *Clyde* is due any minute. God knows where she's been most of this time. I got off seventy Christmas cards. I sat with Mr. Earl while he died tonight. He just made a few faces, reached deeply for a breath or two, lifted his hand convulsively and joined his fathers. This passing never fails to be impressive. There are many manners of departure. In some the line is not sensible—in others it is like jumping a fence.

December 5, '40. I've been reading *Of Lena Geyer* all day. It was wonderful. Every time she sang, I wept. In the afternoon there were hundreds from the *Clyde.* Wood and Olds and Hardy worked in the OPD which was full to bursting. I couldn't somehow do anything in all that mess and I got the impression it annoyed them.

December 9, '40. I suspect there is much I don't remember about Friday, Saturday and Sunday past. Friday morning we operated and found things to do, though I was eager to start what I thought was to be a day off. I tried to take the prostatic pack out of Perry, but sensed that the string would break so I got John to pull it. He did and it broke. We had to give Perry chloroform to get the pack. I suspect it was taken out a little early, for in a moist area like that it should have been softer and less adherent. I finally was free—whereupon John and Stan went out leaving me to stay in. I suppose I had it coming to me for on Thursday I did think they got kind of short with me because I didn't pay any mind to the *Clyde* patients. But Doccy Wood was working out there and with the two of them there wasn't any room for me. They were definitely miffed. I didn't care, because I was reading *Of Lena Geyer*; read the whole thing thinking it was a biography, but I'm sure it's a novel, though I don't really know. I heard her every time she sang and wept every time she sang. It was like *Trelawney of the Wells* with Helen Gahagan and Pauline Lord. That was in my high school days. I wept every time she got up on the piano stool and sang *Ever of Thee I Am Fondly Dreaming.* Friday evening after tea we had a kind of party at Stan's and played cards until late. Saturday morning I made a call I should have made during the night, but it was blowing a gale and cold and the *Clyde* was due back. About 2 A.M. Austin Roberts had asked for me and told me his wife had a pain in her side. I told him I was busy but would come myself in the morning. I have delivered two of her babies and am going to explore her one of these days for that pain. He had been planning to leave on the *Clyde*, but didn't think he could get on her anyway, as there were so many dog teams and horses and men going back to the woods for the winter season. I saw his wife in the morning and found a bit of pleurisy and not much else. I wore my new leather coat. It certainly is warm. Betty and John spent the weekend at the Tilt. We spent a lazy Saturday and I read until 2 in the morning.

Sunday, I didn't get up till 10:30 and got a few chores done. Stan went off to Fridays Bay right after dinner while I was watching Mrs. Bascom for a transfusion. She had passed a lot of placenta, but looks like the dickens. In the evening we had tea in my room and it was fun. We heard the BBC news with a late cup of coffee in Stan's and I'd just gone to bed when Hazel dragged me out to go to Herring Neck to see Stella Bath, reported to have a temperature of 103. She had her appendix out here only two weeks ago. It took some finoogling to get me off, for there was no way to ride across the island. Stan got Mr. Stuckey and Mr. Stuckey got Claude Cooper who got Don Moores, who got his horse and slide. I suggested wheels, but no. So we went half a mile when the snow gave out and we unhitched the horse and walked. At Little Harbor, Mr. Pardy agreed to bring us back and Don left. We crossed the tickle to Merritt's Harbor and went over the Neck to another boat, then down the Arm to the Nook in Herring Neck to the very prosperous menage of Oliver Bath. The girl had a rotten pair of tonsils if I ever saw one. Though I wanted to come home, it was dark, dirty and rainy, with a big sea on. We chatted while I made toast and about three I was shown to a clean bed where I laughed to see the dozen blankets and the great bolster which holds you upright. They had put a hot water bottle in the bed. It was a luxurious night. In the morning we went back to Merritt's Harbor and got Mr. Card up to put us across. I can see him now, pulling on his pants and peering out of the window into the gloomy dawn to find out if the sea was breaking—it was. Little Harbor was full of whipped cream. I woke up Mr. Pardy and walked on ahead while they hitched up. We arrived at the hospital just as they finished the first operation. I had time to have a bit of breakfast before taking out Daphne's tonsils, the ones she had her syphilis in. They came out hard, she bled like hell and tonight she is a stricken woman. I worked the afternoon in the wards and the OPD. Stan gave 600 cc of blood for Mrs. Bascom, but it clotted before we could give it to her. That left him in a weakened condition for I was able to win a game of Ping-Pong from him. I finished *Fire in the Wood.* It speaks too mildly of the Nazis.

December 10, '40. Up early and feeling very low. My sleep deficit always catches up with me the day after, rather than on the first day. We had a long two-hour job in which we cut out the lower third of the radius for a giant-cell tumor and replaced it with the head of the fibula. The result was good and I have hopes. Then I took an appendix out through a hernial sac and we repaired the whole thing in one step. I know it is dangerous, but we never seem to get infections. Then I dictated for awhile and played the ocarina. Jake, John's Irish Setter, who stays around my room now, disappeared when I started my music. While I was having a nap Jake woke me up knocking on the window to be let in. Tea at Stan's and then over to Stella's for a lesson in tatting.

December 11, '40. Things started to freeze up after the nasty thaw. It snowed on and off all day. The glass is wavering up and down with quite a breeze of wind tonight. There was no operating and I wasted the whole damn day. The evening was bad too—I spent time showing David how to dive over the sofa on his face. Today Sidi Barrani, Egypt, fell to the Axis.

December 12, '40. Blowing a gale. No operating. Practically a holiday.

December 13, '40. Another lazy day.

December 14, '40. A call came in for a baby case in Herring Neck just as the day looked to be another easy one where I could get in a chapter of a detective story. It was six below and blowing a gale as I went to ask the captain of the *S.S. Glenco* if he was going to Herring Neck. He said no unless I telegraphed St. John's for permission and so forth. So I just got Clarence and put on everything I owned, setting off on the winter trail. It sure was cold but I was warm. The ponds were hard but the horse put a foot or two through the brooks. We stopped for a warm at Purcell's Harbor. The waiting boat was low in the water with ice. We faced the tickle. The lop behind us got larger as we neared the other shore. We rushed forward on the crests. It was "vapory"—the top of each lop blew off. I was awful glad to turn into Lobster Harbor. The walk across the Neck was not so bad. On the way we stole one of Mr. Smith's fence rails to hold the bag. He will never miss it on top of having his store burn down with all his gear and winter food and fish. With the bag swung between us, we made Goshen's Arm. With the wind behind us we were soon in Herring Neck, but the way that water boiled around those rocks was a caution as we turned into Too Good Arm. When we faced the wind it was cruel. A swipe with the spray was like a lash of a whip. The men's faces froze. We couldn't land near our destination because of the ice. Finally we crawled in paralyzed, to learn that the babe had been born. My lusty old friend, Mrs. Oxford, greeted me as "sweetheart" and cooked up some home-killed lamb. It was good. I saw the patient, had a smoke and set off around the bottom for a hard, cold walk. We started up the boat again and faced the wind of Herring Neck. Believe me it was bitter. The spray froze the faces again while we played fast and loose with the rocks. The steersman was blinded. Joe White was waiting for me at Carter's Wharf. He rushed me into his office, stoked the stove, plied me with rum, wrung out my coat and told my man that he would see I got to Twillingate. We sat in the office and time passed very quickly as we polished off the bottle. Joe's Hotel was none too warm at teatime. After the news, we went down to find Malcolm Simms singing Christmas carols to his daughter's organ playing. I smelled turr as soon as we got in the door. Simms said it was too bad we had no rum so it looked like a dull evening but Joe was not put out. After a minute or two Pauline pulled out a bottle of rum which we worked on and things looked brighter. After a few, Simms confided to me that he thought I didn't like him ever since I gave his daughter ointment for her chin that was too strong. This was the first I knew that it was too strong. Apparently Dr. Wood had said that and they thought, because I never got very chummy, that I was mad. I reassured him and we ate a couple of turrs and had another drink before going back to the hotel. I crawled into bed with most of my clothes on. In the morning I broke the ice in my pitcher and had a wash. Down in the kitchen I met Isaac. He wore one bifocal and one plain window. We made some toast, had a sardine and tea and a drink of moonshine. Isaac piloted us down the Arm after the breakfast. It was no warmer and the spray was just as nasty. I wish I had a picture of old Isaac standing in the stern by the tiller with a bottle straight up in the air like Triton's horn; or like my brother on the prow of the ship in *Marco's Millions.* This didn't help his steering, but we made the Neck where Joe, in his triumphant way, made everyone carry my bag. At Lobster Harbor I stopped to see a patient and there we found a boat to put us over to Purcell's Harbor. There we got someone to say he would bring the bag over later, thus we could make better time walking. We were pleased, halfway over, to have John meet us on the cycle and were quickly home. The rest of the day was easy except that at regular intervals, someone on the staff would come down with the flu. My face is swollen stiff from frostbite.

December 16, '40. After a couple of operations I set out for Purcell's Harbor on the cycle with Bud Young, our technician, and a couple of shovels. We had a good time— no trouble till we got to the long drift where the road rises and skirts the pond. We visited two flu cases who had come back from working at the airport with a whooping sort of spasmodic cough. We passed through Little Harbor with much pushing help by school children and flying of snow. Ten minutes after we made it back to the hospital a man called for a doctor to go to Herring Neck. It was too much. The woman had already been sick on Sunday when I'd been in Herring Neck and now they call at night just missing me in Little Harbor. I kept my heavy clothes on so I could go if I lost the toss. John went after we had a nice tea at Stan's. I was just getting ready to turn in when he got back so I sat up with him over a couple of drinks until one.

December 17, '40. At five, as usual these days, a call came from Herring Neck. I went off in a fury on the cycle which I was going to leave at Smith's, but the man who had come for me groused so that with his help we pushed it through the snow, got up the hill, only to stick where it had the other day. The second man who was supposed to be waiting for us with a boat wasn't there but we picked up another man and together set off in the small boat down the tickle in the very pitch dark. One man said something to me which I couldn't catch so I laughed in my flat way. He leaned over and shouted, "Don't set on them hors. You'll break them!" (oars) Unreasonably annoyed, I sat on the bow. It was warm, smooth and lovely through the dark. If I hadn't had the flashlight we never would have gotten under the low bridge which came as a surprise, though I know now that I have been in that part of Merritt's Harbor before. As soon as I got in the house they started in about not being able to take me home that night. The wind started to blow at once. The midwife was there, the crusty one who scolds me about making toast and smoking. The patient had just miscarried and lost a lot of blood. To get home we walked four miles down the island, in and out of the mountains, to Lobster Harbor, into a kitchen full of people. They said it was impossible to get across that night. I believed them as I listened to the wind shake that roof. Finally an aged gent, after walking down to the shore and coming back, said we might just be able to get across. After a little bustling about we were soon taking solid water over the bow. They thrust me off the end of the boat in Purcell's Harbor and turned around without stopping. I started the cycle, closed my eyes, and plunged into the drift. I got through. By now it was cold and blowing a gale out of the north northwest.

December 18, '40. Hazel called me at 3:30 A.M. because Clarence wanted the stretcher for a very sick woman on the *Clyde*. It had made a special trip for her. I got dressed while they telephoned again to ascertain – "a sick woman. Very, very serious." Wedged into the little saloon I found a woman in her fourth day of labor. A doctor had been trying all this time to deliver her with forceps. It took a lot of turning and twisting to get her around the companionway corners. My training as ambulance doctor in

Brooklyn tenements came in very handy. At one point in the procedure, with one end of the stretcher on the *Clyde* and the other on the wharf, the *Clyde* slacked away from the wharf. We got her to the hospital though and a low forceps lifted out a child long dead. She is o.k. Betty and John had a drop of tea in my room until seven in the morning and I went back to bed.

December 22, '40. Since Wednesday very little has happened except that the epidemic of flu has been raging—Stella, Mildred, David, Stan, Betty, Doris, Wyn, Minnie, eight or more maids and eight or more aides. The diet kitchen had to be given up. We stopped all treatments except the most essential; we stopped operating and admissions. We discharged all we could. People have thought we were overworked, so in spite of the fact that half the population is down we have not had many calls. I did go to Gilesport twice after dark and have been getting out most every day. Poor Stan has been in bed a lot in the past few months. John and I have been great pals. After we did an autopsy on Mr. Woodfords and found the shot adrenal and acres of bowel ulcer, we drank until one. My *Clyde* OB has done well. Since then I have had another difficult forceps case.

I don't expect to catch the grippe and would rather die than complain of anything that wasn't obvious to everybody. The *S.S. Northern Ranger* came from north and we heard the rumor that she was going back down north instead of to town. We got the patients over in below-zero weather, to find we were wrong. The *Clyde* came back with lots more mail and now is in Lewisporte. Botwood is frozen fast and Stan walked on the ice on Gut Arm. Our tickle is impassable; there is lots of slob ice which will catch if there is no wind. Stan is having trouble with his elbow; it makes it hard for him to use the cycle or drive the dogs.

January 4, '41. Only two days to Twelfth Night, and what a lot of water has gone up the chimney. An hour after getting to bed I had to rouse out to deliver a woman. Next, a cup of coffee or two in Annette's with Annette and Hazel accompanied by the unhappy groans of Stan. I hoped to God he was asleep, for if he was awake, we have a maniac on our hands. He is in his fourth day of pneumonia. He had come back from the Tilt with a temperature of 104.4 and spit blood so took sulfa for a day. That made him vomit, he had to quit and now his temperature is up again. John had a bad sinus and didn't want to go out, so I've been doing all the outside work.

Having had so much coffee, I took a Nembutal which gave me a late start into today. Soon after rising, I got a call to Merritt's Harbor and was glad of it. The sun was like February and the large snow crystals shimmered everywhere with refracted light. Travel was good and we had good horses. I stopped at Manuel's Cove to urge a woman again to send her boy to the hospital. I had seen him two days ago when he seemed to have a respiratory infection. The next day his neck was stiff—all the signs of a full-grown meningitis. Ordinarily that would have meant TB, but we had a spotted fever come in the same day, so it could be that. There at the Cove I did a lumbar puncture, verified the meningitis in the hospital and sent a horse down for the child but she wouldn't bring him in. He was a lovely, bright, handsome, little boy. This time she agreed to use my horse when it came back from Purcell's Harbor. I rowed myself and the two men over to Lobster Harbor Point and beached the boat on the ice, then continued by horse over the ridge up and down to get on to the ice, then continued by horse again over another ridge up and down to Merritt's Harbor. There I found Mrs. Card not very sick. Eighty-eight-year-old Mrs. Adams had a flu and Lucy Adam's baby had a temperature. A man walked down over the gulf with me. In the house he had been scared and dull; on the ice he blossomed out: "It's a cold day today with regards to the temperature"; "It's good walking with regards to the ice we'll say." Across the gulf I saw an old TB patient of ours. His young wife had a meningitis. I tapped her and I have about a drop of it left to be looked at in the morning. I started out with more but it was hard to carry what with the vicissitudes of travel. The ride back was fast in a pleasant evening and we launched the Rodney again, getting into ice for a regular standing-up George Washington on the Delaware act to Purcell's Harbor.

When they went to put the meningitis boy on the slide, they found he was dead.

We had quite a Christmas. I took a Benzedrine and scintillated with the same success as at Sarah's party in Baltimore; made up poems and gave Joe a bottle of rum and insulted the dentist, who stayed until two after the party to air his grievances to John. We had a good dinner and Hazel was a little tight, taking her turn at insulting everybody. Betty, just up from the flu, felt like the devil. I had been out the whole night before on a useless trip to Salton's. We had walked all the way around New World Island and pushed through the slob in the cozy cuddy of a skiff with a fire aboard, to see two children. I did hear that one of them died afterwards, but it wasn't sick when I saw it. I was tired and felt like the flu, but picked up quite a lot. Travel is awful. John has been out the same night and got home with Joe with great difficulty. Christmas day, Joe White was Santa Claus.

Stan had been hoarding eggs since Thanksgiving for the eggnog and he made one that packed a beautiful wallop. We stayed to dinner upstairs, though I was in a very disheveled state. In the afternoon Betty had an attack of hysterics and took to her bed where she'd been til yesterday with bad flu. John, much chastened, palmed David off on the Hardy's. Next morning the Olds left early for the Tilt and stayed until Sunday. Saturday night Hazel and Stella and I had tea with the Hardy's. Hazel made some crack about being unwilling to have a boyfriend who wasn't in the war and we sort of jumped on her. She went into a hysterical crying fit that lasted for two days. She worked one night and then came down with the flu and has been screwy ever since, finally taking to dark glasses. In distraction, John dragged her over to the private ward and put her to bed. She is almost irrational, lying in bed and griping and saying she vomits when she doesn't and keeps claiming that her temperature is up when it isn't. The Hardy's took their turn at the Tilt and came back New Year's Eve with Stan in the middle of pneumonia. He's been pretty low ever since. He lies flat in the middle of his bed with an ice cap balanced just on the top of his head and looks like the Pope lying in state.

My Virginia ham came and I had the New Year's Eve party—a calm one. We ate mostly and quietly retired. John read the whole evening and I had to put him out so I could go to sleep. I spent a whole day putting a barrel of apples in the base depot and getting two small packages through the customs. It is a sample of Newfoundland expediency. The Rangers spent a whole day posting the meningitis house.

On my last trip to Herring Neck, I went to the house where the typhoid was last year on Two Good Arm. While I was examining a child with pneumonia, a man burst into the room, very self-important, with a white crepe bow on his coat and saying the minister wanted to see me before he buried George Thompson. I went up and got into the middle of a funeral. The son was crying too much to pull the coffin the many cold miles to the cemetery. I took a look at the old gent, but couldn't give a certificate as I hadn't seen him alive. The wife was complaining to me about her troubles in a vacuous way, even as they carried her husband out. The men who brought me back were very amusing—they wanted me to lie down in the bottom of the boat and hide so no one would see me and flag us down. I couldn't ignore them in Lobster Harbor because I may well be stuck there some night, God forbid.

When I started out, the harbor was clear of ice. When I came back about a half past six to catch the boys polishing off a bottle of Main Brace in my room, the harbor and the ocean was bay ice as far as you could see. Today the bight is solid. Just before this the *Clyde* made a special trip with another of that same doctor's OB cases. I had to go round and haul her off the boat at one in the morning. She had been in labor for five days. I delivered her and she had a funny promontory, for the head came out easily but the shoulder resisted. Finally, after really sweating a bit, I got the child, macerated and smelling so bad that I actually experienced a few abortive urges to vomit into my mask. She is all right but I can't see why she won't pee. The flu is on the wane. Now we are scared of meningitis.

January 5, '41. No new cases of meningitis. I woke and got a call to Back Harbor. I couldn't get a horse until about eleven. When I finally got there I found a man who had a slight shock last Monday and this morning was unable to speak. This was all gone when I saw him; he belittled it, but in front of him the family insisted he didn't know how sick he was, and that he'd been unconscious and frothed and so forth. They made no effort to spare him any of the details or apprehensions. Yesterday it was the same way. The mother kept asking in front of the fully conscious patient if the patient had a chance to get well.

In Libya, Bardia fell, to our joy.

Stan is much better, though still wobbly. He tried to read a bit today. Hazel has lost all her insight. She lies there querulous and complaining.

The *Clyde* and the *Segona* came in tonight, the latter with three patients, two of them syphilitics that it took St. Anthony five months to diagnose. These are the last boats we can possibly have this winter.
Sir Wilfred Grenfell died this fall and yesterday Charles Parsons died. With those deaths, a link with the past is broken.

The *Northern Ranger* will stop here on her way south, then that will be the end of shipping till April. The harbor has broken up as far as the coastal wharf and the bight is clear of ice. Yesterday it looked as if you could walk across anywhere.

January 6, '41. I forget a good part of the day, but about eleven a call came in to see Nora Grimes in Herring Neck. We know Nora of old, almost every trip to her is useless. It looked like a quick over and back and so we started. Well, we got Mack out of the barn and went to Lowland Cove. There, in the face of a pretty ominous sea and a cold, gray day with no wind, we launched the Rodney and rowed to Merritt's Harbor. It was a long push and the men rowed right for the rocks, then detoured way around to keep the sea from breaking on us. It was obvious that they were wrong; one of the men was even facing forward. More and more often I see that my own judgment is as good as theirs in the things in which we trust our lives to their hands. It is very disconcerting. We made in at Merritt's Harbor where I went at once to warm myself at Steve Langdon's. The open-spoken midwife, who lives there, invited me in for a cup of tea. It was a chance too, to check up on a miscarriage they had had there. Then Steve took me up those cliffs and down the Gut to Nora's. It was as I suspected. From the front door I had a glimpse of Nora disappearing upstairs to get into bed. Her illness may have been real enough to her, but I couldn't find anything. By this time it was blowing a gale, snowing and getting colder. It was already apparent that we could not re-cross at the same place. The men had assured me I would be back at Lowland Cove by 2:30. The horse was to meet me then. There were a few other sick to see. The dame next door was peculiar. She ran down the hill with slippery abandon and beckoned me mysteriously away from my cup of tea to give me a drink of rum. She made me pay for it by launching into a recital of her woes. I finished my tea, got another drink and then saw a collection of various wrecks, one with cold, hot, crawling pain and numbness in one leg since Herman died.

Suddenly there was a hail and a breathless man rushed in to ask me to see Redick. He and another eighteen-year-old, Parsons, had been out by Calahan's rock in a Rodney. They were after turrs. One of them shot his big muzzle-loader across the Rodney and the recoil upset the craft. Parsons was lost. Redick cut the lines holding the guns to the tiny boat and sat in the water-filled boat. By a miracle, a power schooner, the *Young Hood*, happened to be going by. With extreme daring and foolhardy courage the skipper took the *Young Hood* in behind the rocks and picked up Redick. The engine stalled and it looked for a moment as if all hands would be lost. They dropped the anchor and there was only just room to swing about and come out forwards. Redick was taken to Malcolm Simms' house, given warm clothes and was lying on the couch by the kitchen stove. I gave him some Luminal and he'll be all right after a little sleep.

It was time I was getting back so I couldn't stop for tea. Pauline slipped some dark fruitcake into my pocket and I set out to cross the tickle, I knew not where or how. Before reaching the bottom of Gut Arm I decided it wasn't possible to get home so returned to Simms' just in time to have a cup of tea and eat my own cake. It was a good chance to know Mrs. Simms better. She is a stout, quiet-eyed, wise woman. She takes Malcolm's enthusiasms calmly and the three of them make a happy home. They fed me to bursting with roast beef and the fixings. In the evening I made four or five calls around the Neck and Simms went along. It was a bitter, bad night, and our path around the swatches was not clear in the low drift. Herring Neck is so broken up by water that they say of it, "You can't go to bed without using a rowboat." We wound up at the vicar's and sat with them in the kitchen with his wife as she cooked his supper. We left at 10 for Simms' and bed, a good one, pajamas out and everything. At half past four I heard a clatter on the porch and stuck my head out the window to be told that the vicar's wife was sick. I took my clothes down to the dark kitchen where there was still a little heat in the stove. I couldn't figure out how the woman we had seen laughing at ten o'clock could be this sick so soon.

It was awful out. I fought my way behind my guide to the patient, going in to my knees at the wharf. Mrs. Diamond had a full blown pneumonia. I took care of her and sat with the Reverend until daylight, drinking coffee and talking. I enjoyed the vigil. The Simms made me breakfast, after which I climbed around Herring Neck making all kinds of calls, the day being too bad even to look at the tickle for a crossing. I visited the Parsons, that fine household of many young men, all busy at nets and boats. I couldn't help but worry about the buxom, pleasant gal, Powell's daughter, who is their servant. I dropped back to the telegraph office to pick up Simms and while I was standing there, a man from Cobbs Arm came in, nodded to me and dictated a telegram to Malcolm. I couldn't help but hear. It was to Father Jones in Tilting. It said that the sender's little boy was so sick that he thought he was going to die. Would Father Jones say the necessary prayers to save him? Then he said good day to me again and left.

After tea Simms went off to an emergency meeting of the Fisherman's Brotherhood, to make arrangements for getting Stan Parsons' body. I wasn't called that night and the next morning it looked as if I could get back to Twillingate. Two men walked with me along Long Ridge to Lobster Harbor. From the top of the hill we could see, stretched below us, the tickle full of broken ice. No boat could make it. "Ah," said the men, "we'll skip and copy." I had long felt that sooner or later I'd have to do some of this jumping from ice-cake to ice-cake. Now that the moment was here, I was not enthusiastic. My reluctance was apparent to the boys. One of them got out on a piece of ice and danced around to show me how safe it was. I screwed up my courage and followed. It was about a mile from Lobster Harbor to Vincent's Point and I had to keep going like hopscotch, because most of the pieces were not big enough to hold me up. The idea is to get off before it sinks. I don't know where the term comes from— the skip part is obvious enough; copy, I think, means to balance.

January 15, '41. What a night! The midnight sky is dark and the wind screams without pause—from some frozen hell. It is well below zero and I thank my God that I am warm and indoors. This morning I woke sore and tired from my trip to Newstead only to find that those indefatigable Herring Neckers were here again for the doctor. That's four days they've spent trying to get me. They waited two days in Seal Cove hoping to waylay me as I came back from Newstead, but they missed me. I spent three days on a hard trip to Newstead—had to wait over a whole day because of rain. Here I would have to start out again.

All that rain has frozen and we are in the clutches of a "glitter." The whole world is one big sliding pond. There isn't anything in sight that offers enough friction for you to stand on. I sent down to Ashbourne for some ice creepers which had 'patent pending 1905' on the bottom and fell off after three steps. I threw them away. The horse was shod sharp for the ice so we didn't have too much trouble getting to the tickle. Two men took me with three dogs across the tickle to Indian Cove. I couldn't walk a step but held on to the sled which bumped like hell over the slick, rough ice. We were blown rather near the swatch. The men said that if I slipped in they planned to save my fine sealskin gauntlets. The men had chains wrapped around their boots and could just manage to stand up. After a warm at Indian Cove, a six-dog team took me over the delirious ridge. We scratched our way up the hill to the Merritt's Harbor road and blew down the Gut Arm to find the woman well! Maybe she had had a pneumonia, but she didn't have any today. Then to the minister's after a bit of fresh pork stew. His lady was pretty well over the pneumonia, but I examined his heart for the scattered flutter.

I went back to Indian Cove on a slide pulled by a skittish horse. It was so slippery on Gut Arm that the slide would start swinging, pendulum-like, behind the horse. After the fourth or fifth swing we would go far enough to turn the horse completely around and we'd have to stop, then start all over again. While warming at Indian Cove, I examined a poor old lady who had had a weak turn.

On the dog sled again for a dark cold bump over the tickle. That crossing was endless. Being unable to walk for the slipperiness, I froze stiff, but it was nothing compared to the cold of the ride behind the horse across the island. We got lost on Rocky Pond. Honest to God, I was so unhappy and in such pain that I wanted to vomit. I sat on the slide while the driver looked for the trail, and wondered what it would feel like to have hysterics. I planned, if I fell through the ice, to breathe the water and die as quickly as possible. I thought never to be at peace again. There were tears of pain in my eyes when I rushed into the hospital to give the driver a drink and to tear off my cold boots. Tea was one of the happiest ones of my whole life—Annette made it for me in my apartment and Betty ate with us. It was a great joy to be warm and in the company of these two people of whom I am so fond. I had to lie against the radiator to stop my chill; I hope never to have those sensations again.

John had to go to Summerford this morning. I hope he doesn't try to come back until travel is better; besides that he has Jake with him and Jake's not in very good shape. He seems to be sort of my dog now— sleeps in my room—even on my bed.

January 16, '41. Cold as hell and blowing fifty guns. I did the cystoscopy and pyelogram that John had tried twice.

Stan's apartment was full of coal gas coming from a crack in the laundry's chimney, which seems to be a three-walled affair like the one that set the Cottage on fire. They had to leave the place and since it was so cold upstairs, they all spent the afternoon in here, including tea. I found Jake in my room this afternoon hungry, lame and tired, so deduced John was back.

January 17, '41. This was a pretty nice day. John sprung a spinal graft on us late last night and we did it first thing. They're fun. We cut off a strip of shinbone and sewed it into a groove made in the spine. What makes it interesting is the little power saw that we use on the shin. The saw itself was filed by Skipper Dalley out of an old Victrola spring. The motor is borrowed for the occasion from the housekeeper's sewing machine and she's usually waiting at the operating door to get it back. The saw has a habit of coming off the shaft and whizzing past the assistant's ear. While scrubbing, John suggested I take the day off. I didn't know what the game was, but I took it. He's going to Herring Neck tomorrow to attend a meeting held to make arrangements to put a nurse or doctor over there. We have to do something to channel these Herring Neck calls.

I spent the morning hanging pictures for Stella and broke only one. Then I tried to go ice skating because my room was full of maids scrubbing it. When I got up to the pond I found myself trying to put on two left skates.

Ern French was here for tea and we had moose hamburger. We finally stirred up a poker game where I lost three dollars, but had a couple of drinks. Ern drank some of Burt Pardy's rum and promised him a drink in return. Ern came in again later with two bottles showing in his pocket but never delivered.

January 18, '41. Wracked today by a sinus and a stiff neck, controlled with codeine and aspirin. Finally I roused out to take some pictures to the carpenter for framing. He said, "It waits a dirty day to do them." John and Wyn had started for the Herring Neck meeting on this year's "Snow-Go."

Every year John invents a new vehicle for traveling in the snow, an endeavor related to but on a larger scale than the surgical power saw. This year it is a low slung model with a sled on the rear. The front is a frame holding the marine engine from the panzer, driving a great, big roller-wheel like a barrel. It has had some success. I saw two figures coming back over the glassy hill, walking dejectedly towards the barn. It looked like John and Wyn and that meant that the machine had failed. I then espied said machine in the middle of Mrs. Olds' garden. Inspection revealed shearing-off of the pin holding the axle to the wheel.

January 19, '41. A quiet Sunday. I did a few chores and about 12:30 John came back from Herring Neck with Wyn and Joe White. I was feeling a little low, but enjoyed dinner. John had not bathed or dressed by rounds, so Stan and I did them. I was suddenly invited to tea at Burt Pardy's where we had a nice assortment of their canned vegetables and some ham from Chaulkers that Mrs. Pardy announced was bad and then gave me some more. Burt came back to the hospital with me and brought my new radio (for getting BBC and WRUL). I listened a while, did some quiet vomiting and went to bed.

January 20, '41. I did the hernia and hydrocele of the cord on Eddie Gross and after that I got a haircut from the orderly, and took a diathermy and bath for my stiff neck. About noon a wire came asking for a doctor at Cobbs Arm and somehow or other it was at once my affair. I announced I wouldn't go today but about three, while we were listening to the thrilling inaugural (F.D.R.), Joe White offered to take me as far as Herring Neck with his dog-sized pony, Dolt. Soon we were off over the back trail to the Arm Trail and took the tickle at Brass's Harbor.

It was still so slick we hit only the high spots on the rough ice. At Indian Cove Joe said he was afraid to go into the Gauss' because he once made Mrs. Gauss cry by saying Sid was going to sleep with an Eskimo that winter on the Labrador, while the *Bessie Marie* was tied up in the ice at Mutton Bay. In the middle of Goshen's Arm Joe decided that a drink was in order and broached a bottle that had come on the *Clyde* as a gift. It looked official and the seal was intact, but somebody had watered it—Joe sure was sore. We had tea at Joe's hotel and then of course went to the Simms'—finding them getting ready to entertain the local capitalists, the Howells. There followed a pleasant evening of progressive auction, at which I was pretty poor. Joe kept the party going even in the face of Lester Howell getting a little tight. Lester sang and talked a lot for a completely unwilling audience. I went to bed with an even stiffer neck and a terrible headache.

I was surprised this morning to be able to move at all. Joe called for me right after breakfast and in the face of a little snow we crossed Redick's Neck and the Arm, up over the hill to the Wallet, across Two Good Arm and up over the cliff out over the country to see some flu at Cobbs Arm. The patient's brother said he would bring me back to Herring Neck, so Joe returned to send a wire to the hospital instructing them to send transportation for me. I stayed to have dinner with George Chaulker. The goodness of just a pick-up meal explained why George and his wife look so well nourished. They have built an attractive Cape Cod house about fifteen feet from the rock crusher at the quarry. It will be dusty and noisy. I don't understand them.

Two dog teams came for me and we walked, ran, and rode towards home, making good time. It snowed a bit and grew colder. We crossed the tickle to Granvil's where I dismissed the Cobbs Armers. The hospital horse hadn't come, of course, so I sweated it to Purcell's Harbor and had a cup of tea with Mrs. Jim Anstey while Jim got his horse ready to put me across our island. Just as we were starting, Doccy Wood hailed us and asked us to guide him across the mish. We went ahead until we hit Rocky Brook. There I changed to Doccy Wood's slide and came on home. The hospital had sent dogs for me, but the wire was slow and made it too late. I was in for rounds and a good tea. Now I am listening to the radio for news. Walter the dentist has been boring me with a dissertation on musical instruments and has just gone off to find a saw to try playing. As soon as the English news is over I'm going to bed—tired of looking at the rear ends of horses and dogs from 9:00 to 5:00.

January 22, '41. Tobruk fell today. (W.W. II, Libya, North Africa)

January 23, '41. Delivered a baby between midnight and dawn after a small episiotomy—the longest-haired infant I ever saw. The stomach operation of yesterday was fine. I tried to go to the Arm but was stopped by a cut tendon. Doccy Wood helped me sew it up. Finally I got off, wearing my new forty-dollar leather pants and ski boots. At tea Stan looked better than he has for some time. He saw the woman I thought was getting pneumonia and now she definitely has it; he left her some more sulfa.

January 24, '41. A great day. Dawned stormy. A low drift, snow and a high wind, with the glass wavering around the lowest point. Rather strangely, it seems to be coming from the northwest which is usually a clear quarter. John asked me to ski part of the way with him to the Tilt. It was easy on the way out but bucking the breeze coming back I was glad to have the fast-disappearing trail to follow. Another ten minutes and it would have been obliterated. I was feeling kind of lousy before tea, but a few drinks and a meal of the pork that Stan brought back put me right. Now to bed after scraping a good foot of snow from the window ledge.

January 25, '41. The fine sleet didn't stop Bud and me from having a ski. The snow was very soft. Jake came along making like a kangaroo, but after a while quieted down and followed our beaten track. Mrs. Penny has a pain like appendicitis in her side and so has Budgel, but the latter is moribund with tuberculosis.

January 26, '41. A howler all day with deep snow and lots of wind. We finished up the Christmas ham in Annette's. The story of the day is Mrs.

Chaulker and her baby getting lost. George sent them on ahead with the furniture, two horses and a dog team. He came on himself a couple of hours later. When he arrived there was no sign of them and those Cobbs Armers know nothing of this island. Search parties were organized. They were discovered about midnight at Gillard's Cove—no place to spend the night. Well, there was another event for the annals of medicine. Harvey Sharp wanted a doctor because his son had "swallowed a machine." He went on to describe it "as a part of a pleasure thing, a contrivance for making a noise, a part of a horn the size of a dime." Since he didn't have any symptoms I said I wouldn't do anything without taking an x-ray, and he said it would be too bad if the boy died with the hospital and all the doctors in town. Then I said it would be too bad if he died without being brought to a hospital that was as near as this one. He called again at midnight to say the boy had a pain in the arm. I surrendered and went to see him. Of course there was nothing for me to do. Nobody was even sure he had swallowed anything.

January 27, '41. Still storming like hell. I was giving a transfusion when a call came for Ragged Point. I sent the man on with the bag and went on over the hill on skis. Still storming like hell. You could not see ten yards. From the pond I took a compass course and started on the trail, head down and foundering. I found myself on the Little Harbor road but I didn't know where. Finally I bumped into that little house that was almost caught in a brush fire this fall. A man there gave me a new course and I found my house. The woman wasn't in labor so they put her in a box on a sled like a load of cabbage and started back with eight dogs. They stuck to the road while I cut directly across the island, really going blind and got back fifteen minutes before they did. You couldn't hold your face to it; I could have been lost between the barn and the hospital—as it was I found myself on the vegetable-cellar roof.

The woman is in labor now and I don't think I will get undressed but will lie on the bed in readiness. I had to chop the window open to let Jake out for a pee.

February 3, '41. The whole week has transpired and I hardly know what has happened. The woman failed to push and I had to put the hooks on, but I forget just when it was. The storm finally abated, followed by a day or two of wretched skiing. Then there was a pretty good day when I went to Herring Neck. Joe White went with me and I kept ahead of the dogs all the way to the tickle. The skis proved very good, even in a slob, better than Joe's snowshoes. We stopped at Sid Gauss' for a drink. On the Arm the slob was deep, but I could keep out of it well. I found pneumonia in a child and they sure balked at paying the driver. Charles Hussey wanted to be examined and we got two dollars out of him. John Farthing is helpless with arthritis; I wish I could help him. Bucked up by a little tea I was ready to mush home when Joe told us there was a call to Pike's Arm. I agreed to go now rather than do the whole trip the next day. That meant spending the night. Mr. Dalley was to be my guide. Back in December I had been unable to go to Pike's Arm once when he had asked me; Doccy Wood had gone. He allowed as how his sister would have died without a doctor because she had the bronchitis.

Well it was hard going. My feet were hurting by this time and I was glad to shed the skis when a horse came for me a few hundred yards from the house.

An old woman had a little diarrhea and I examined her husband, who had been caught between a couple of skiffs. I then mentioned I had stayed over at extra expense and had saved them two trips to Twillingate, would a dollar be too much? The patient from the next room shouted, "Don't give it to him." They didn't. They brought me back behind the horse through slob belly deep. We left the horse on Hundry's Island because the Arm is swatchy, and plunged over the Herring Neck Hills in the pitch dark. Joe revived me with a drink and we had tea at the hotel. Both my heels were raw. After tea I went down and had another tea with Simms. Joe came in after I'd beaten them all at Chinese checkers. Simms' mother-in-law, on a visit to them, allowed that Pauline had baked the beautiful chocolate cake for me, though it was supposed to be in her honor. I awoke stiff and sore the next morning, struggled into my gear and had a late breakfast with Joe, then had to make calls at the cove where I had passed the day before. I saw a leg much less painful than my own. On my way back the Gut Arm was a mire. We took the ridge in preference, but it was unbroken and sticky and I was discouraged. The forward lug of the sodden ski was crucifying. My heels were getting worse so I tried riding on sled, but with both of us aboard, the horse could hardly move it and the driver was damned if he was going to walk. At Mose's Marsh I took to the skis again in desperation, dying at every step toward the hospital trail. I got lost a little but finally arrived swearing I was going to take the rest of the week off. Stan and Annette were headed for the Tilt as I hobbled to the door. I took some blood for a transfusion almost before taking my coat off and had to get right to work. Rarely had a trip taken so much out of me. Since then I've crippled about in my slippers. Mrs. Samson passed a missed abortion this morning, thereby circumventing by a very few hours having her uterus removed. She had a peculiar history and we were justified in thinking it was a kind of tumor.

February 4, '41. Still in the house with raw heels. We operated on Mrs. March this morning. She sags at corners that other people don't even have. The uterus was all tied up and we would have liked to take it out but she was in mild shock.

The rest of the day I worked on my barometer that is almost finished. Sure looks professional (if it works). At tea I told David to stop kicking the dog. John said it is too bad when you can't even kick your own dog in your own house. We kind of flared a little bit and didn't get along any better when we took opposite sides on the British Colonial question. He was for our never having left British rule.

David and I have a good time. He asks me a thousand questions, demanding that the answers be as fantastic as possible, much to his mother's despair. She is all for the truth. I've taught him to slide on a hooked rug clear across the living room floor. He also can dive over the sofa onto cushions. He calls me 'Mr. Binx the Barber'.

February 5, '41. The day looked rough and the glass has been going down, according to my homemade barometer. We had a belly to open and I said quite plainly we would find cancer. John was intrigued but not convinced. Stan hadn't thought about it. We did find cancer and those two had to be impressed. It was very good for them and me too. I have an intuitive way of diagnosing bellies and my success is reasonably constant. The cancer was in the gall bladder, which was small and very hard to get at. After the school clinic I lay on the floor by the radiator and listened to an hour of symphony. It was good—Beethoven's Fifth but I fell asleep because I had gotten up at 4:00 to deliver Mrs. Mudford. The afternoon was quiet too, but, of course, I didn't accomplish anything. The mail hasn't come because travel is so bad, but if we get the storm that my new barometer promises, it may freeze enough to open the trails. In a few days my heels should be well enough for me to hit the road. We listened to the various editions of the English news until bedtime.

February 9, '41. Today I got to know how much fun it is to work in the machine shop. It gives a you great feeling of power to shape hard metal.

February 19, '41. A lot of time has gone but not a great deal has happened. The school clinic is busy and we've been doing some surgery. Yesterday I did a total hysterectomy, a fairly easy one but it took me an hour and a half. She took it rather well. I was beginning to get a little bit discouraged in my surgical progress and I think that John sensed it. He has great concern for others. I have spurts of doing all right and spurts of thinking I should be in some other business. I perspired over the operation but it went smoothly enough. I've been helping John in quite a few things that I should be doing myself.

Though I don't ask for anything, it does happen that John is good enough to almost force me to do things.

I've been enjoying *The Flowering of New England.* I sometimes think that was the time for me. The past week I've been doing a lot of skiing with the dogs; Spot, Watch, and Jake work well for me and we've been zooming over the hard crust faster than I want to go. I visit my patients this way, cutting way over the inside of the island, three times as far as we have to go.

Had to go to the post office to get a license for my radio; the department has been threatening me.

We had another go at the snow machine. It began with tea at Stella's following a drink in my apartment, for I was feeling rather festive having had the afternoon off. Stella provided a dead chicken, which I carved, and things progressed with more rum. About ten, John said with one of his usual inspirations for a late hour that he would take the Hardys to the Tilt. He told me to drive them over and we went out to try the snow machine. It got as far as Carter's pond with my pulling my guts loose several times trying to get the monstrosity out of snow holes. We turned back with me at the throttle. Some derelict who had helped us joined us, so I relinquished the tiller and ran a bit while he had a ride. He left us when we abandoned the thing at Stevie's garage and we decided we'd have to go to the Tilt some other way. The rest of our party had swiped what was left of my rum and were playing cards. By now it was midnight and John was willing to give up his inspiration. Annette, however, was not, so John hitched up the dogs and carted off the two Hardys to the Tilt.

On the way to French Beach yesterday to see a bad side, I risked my own side and a good deal more, hitched to the dogs while I skied. It had rained over the weekend and the snow was soggy soft. The three dogs and I went up Yate's Hill and started down the first Arm road with no track. I gained speed and guided the dogs to my right behind me. When I slowed, they caught up with me, then passed me on both sides. This wound the chain around my ankle. I kept going fast but I knew there would have to be a denouement. One ski dug in and I fell. There was a sprawling heap of dogs, me, snow, chain, and ski pole. I was sort of staked out with all the leverages and centers of gravity against me. I didn't know how to get up. One ski was pointed in such a bizarre direction that I hoped to God my foot wasn't still attached to it. It was. With superhuman effort, I freed my left foot and got the skis straightened out and was amazed to find that I could walk.

It's interesting to me that our American dog, which has had no training but is of a good breed and has been treated well, is the best dog. The others are so scared as to be stupid.

Father Hinchley fell through the ice in Southwest Tickle. It is calmly reported that they watched him for two and half-hours before they got to him. All they did was try to throw a rope to him. No one thought of boards or a ladder. No one went out to him with a line around his waist so he could be hauled back—that would have been without too much risk. It's a grim story. Why the inaction? They tell me that once the ice caught a schooner in Twillingate Harbor and kept her there until a robin had built her nest and reared her young in the jib gear.

My ankle tonight is painful and swollen, but ought to be all right soon.

February 20, '41. We had about forty in the OPD. Quartan, our consul in St. John's, seems to ignore my presence here, but the others got a note saying they had to go to St. John's to get new passports. I wouldn't mind going, but I'd hate to spend the money. My ankle is swollen still but with almost no pain. I was in kind of a paranoic depression today. John was kind of short, and the hell with the whole business. Lidge Dalley is making some progress on the ship's bed for my living room and that's a little cheering. [Ed: That bed, made out of juniper, is in the upstairs study now.] Every bit of ice is gone from the harbor. The glass is still down and we need a storm.

February 23, '41. After skiing on Friday, a day off for me, we had a few

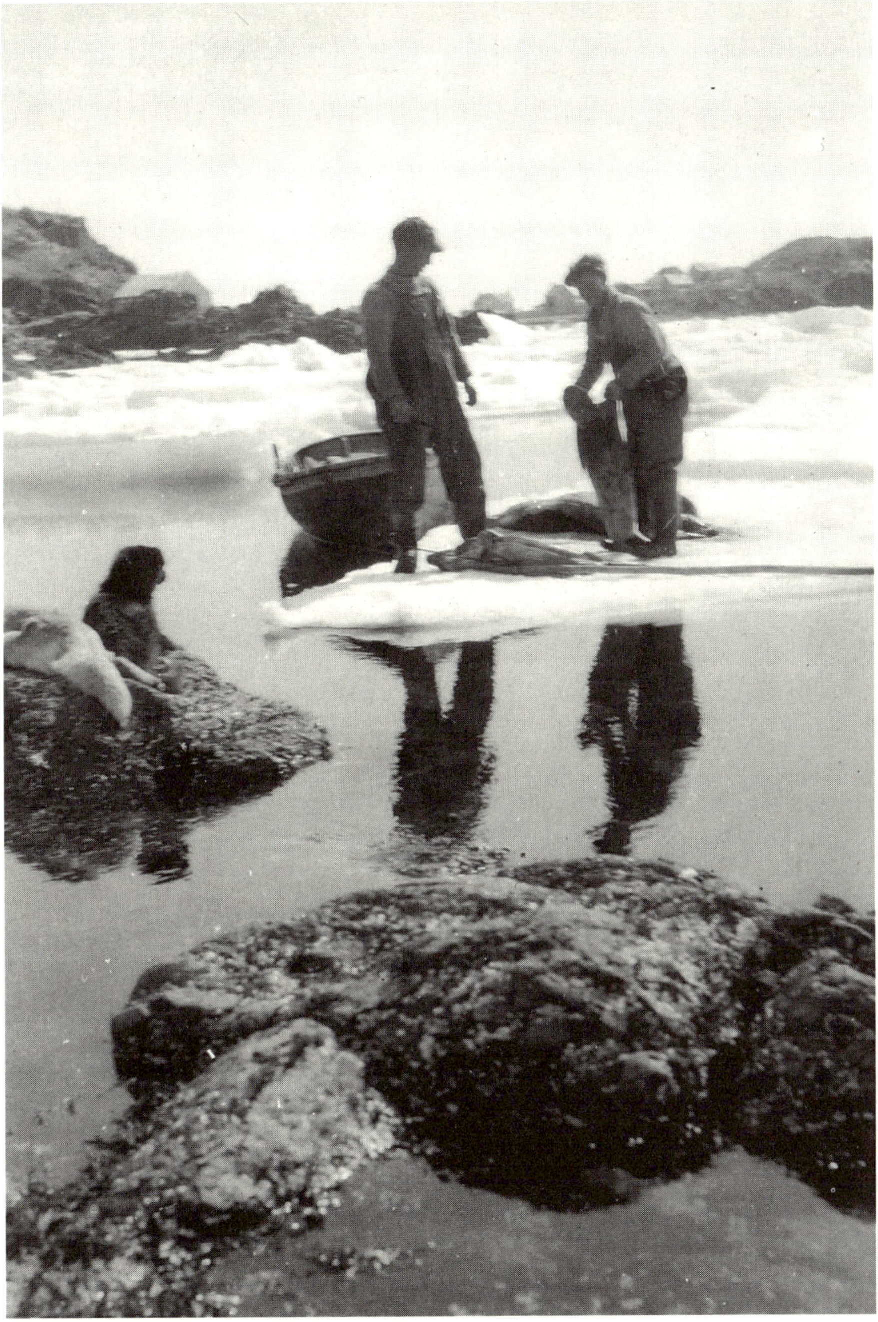

Local seal fishery. Author's photograph.

drinks during which Betty said I never liked her and never will. That was a shock, because I adore her and think she's beautiful. I thought our rapport was swell. Apparently she had taken this housekeeping job to heart with the result that all my smart-alec comments are construed as direct criticism.

I spent Saturday and Sunday making a table lamp for the Hardy apartment out of the brass boiler tubes salvaged from Saul White's tugboat.

March 27, '41. I think it's safe to record this day as a great one. I was thrilled to hear that Yugoslavia has revolted and forced out the pro-nazi government. It is a turning point of the war. I wept over the Canadian Jervis Bay broadcast from WRUL of the Friendship Bridge program. There's no question but what that is the best radio station in the United States.

Today was John's birthday. We had a mild party of caribou upstairs, but nothing came of it. Not much is going on. We had bits of winter. All last weekend we had a bad snowstorm, but the warm sun has made little of it.

I've hardly been out of doors since returning from that hard long trip to Carmanville when I covered 75 miles without stopping. It was a frantic call. By ski, dog, pony, and foot, I mushed to Carmanville to see Edison Green, a man about my age and size who had taken to his bed because his heart fluttered. There was nothing wrong at all. He was in better shape than I was. I only stayed about twenty minutes and came back by pony and cart to Horwood. That pull across the mouth of the Gander River at night is something I don't want to do again. Peter Hodinott and his wife took me in and were wonderful to me. She is chairman of the local Women War Workers who have made a beautiful bedspread out of embroidered squares of bleached flour bags. It was being raffled for the Spitfire Fund; I took 30 chances and won it!

The ice has been in and out and in and out. The men got a lot of seals for food but we couldn't lay our hands on a flipper. There was a report of six men from Western Head out on the ice when it was running and ground to slob near the shore. The Twillingate men had to come ashore on a rope and we never did hear how the Western Headers fared, but I suppose there was nothing in it. Stan went to the States with Annette two weeks ago, for a couple of months, which leaves a big hole in our society. Another appeal came to me to go to Alaska. The Episcopal Church offered

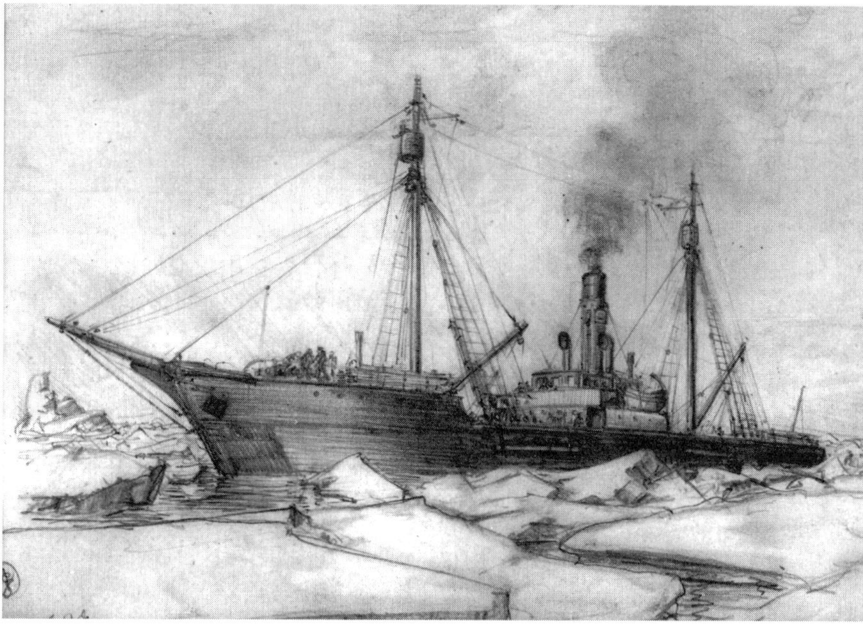

Seal fishery steamer *Neptune* in the ice, drawing by Ted Drover.

me a hospital just above the Arctic Circle at Fort Yukon. It sounds very attractive, but I can't leave here just now. John got his motion through the board of directors to allow him to go to Canada shopping for an aeroplane. He feels that a small plane would be the answer to these two- and three-day calls. I am against it because everything we have is improvised. I can't believe that we could alter our psychology so that there would be one perfect thing—the aeroplane. I'm sure it would have baling wire in it somewhere within a week. I predict here and now this will be his death, but not mine.

March 28, '41. I'm all beat out. My appearance at breakfast, late and in pajamas, was taken by others as a too casual approach to the day so John, a little piqued, announced the arrival of a couple of recruits for examination. I made ready and was about to start when a call came to go to Cobbs Arm. It was old one-eyed Pete whose former wife, Daisy, was one of the Saunders of Cobbs Arm. The third generation of that family has Olds' disease, that familial disease that John is studying—the one where the small bones of the feet come out. Daisy, however, is dead and the current wife had a pain. I knew without going that it would do as well if I gave him some aspirin and codeine. His dog team is measly, though they all are now this late in the winter, what with one herring a week and hauling wood all the time.

I took Jake and Spot, (Watch hid), and they certainly put the others to shame. They dragged every inch of the way and the snow was soft and deep, though slippery. I came behind with my mentor who, though thin and ragged, wanted me to ride. The way he ran along, I was surprised to hear later that last summer he was laid up with rheumatic fever.

The tickle wasn't so good, though it held us up. We could cut pretty well to Indian Cove Head, but we had to keep inside a bit where the ice was gone. In a few places there was a foot of water on it, but we got down Goshen's Arm to Eliot's Neck and on to the Wallet, through Two Good Arm and over the hills, through that vast shaved hinterland to Cobbs Arm where I saw everyone and his grandmother for real and fancied ills. The people there live in poorer houses than almost anywhere else. I was tired by the time we started back, but it was a lovely evening. I was waylaid just as we came down out of the hills. Mrs. Levi Cutler smelled me out. Then I went in to see a week-old babe who was doing something peculiar—never did find out what but it seemed all right to me. I visited another house there for a pain in a non-Center man, whose courage I so admired that I didn't charge him. I leapt a few rents and led the dogs around the hill to our other waiting sled, took the new sled on ahead and put my dogs on the second team to bolster them. I drove the dogs pretty hard and had good luck. At Indian Cove, the men were afraid of the ice but I stayed on ahead, retracing the morning steps and soon we were on our own island.

March 29, '41. Another project afoot; the weathervane I am working on will be attached to the chimney and have a dial with little lights on it in my apartment so I'll be able to tell what the weather is without getting out of bed. Otherwise I did a conservative mastoid and read *Benjamin Blake*, a good book. A smoked turkey came from father. John went to the Tilt in a roaring rainstorm. Of the outer world I couldn't get the news, though I understand it is very good.

April 3, '41. After snowing in the morning, Sunday afternoon was warm and with the window open, you could hear that sure sign of spring—the rushing torrent of water past the corner of my apartment. The first part of week was marked by the eating of the smoked turkey. It was on the road a long time, but was the best meat I ever ate. It was wonderful, reminding you of all the things you like, caribou, partridge, smoked eel, sturgeon, the smell of pine needles. It lasted until tonight, when we polished it off as soup and even that was good.

I am now as tired as one can be and still be navigating, having started for Virgin Arm at ten after doing a quick half of a double hernia. John meddled so much with my half that I was sore. Add to that that the weather was bad and travel a travesty. I took three dogs including Irene. She is half Jake (Irish Setter) and half Sport's wife (just dog). She ran just ahead, stopping every six feet. The others would come up short and lose their momentum. I was ready to give her a taste of euthanasia. I went ahead and found the trail myself—over Black Island to Seal Cove and through Tilt Cove to Fairbank, then out on the ice to the Bottom. The snow was like cotton. It dragged you and stopped you; torturous, but I made good time. My patient had either meningitis (TB) or a cerebral hemorrhage. It was a doleful place and I was afraid to take anything but a cup of hot tea so I've had no nourishment at all today.

Tea is wonderful stuff, the only beverage for winter travel. Often when I get to Herring Neck it seems as if I just couldn't start for home. After two or three cups of hot, black tea I'm a new man and ready for the trail. I confess it drops out from under you in about half an hour, but by that time you just have to go on.

The road back was inside Trump Island to Manuel's Cove, with the slob ten inches thick and Irene sort of pulling until we got past Trump Island. Then she sat down and we dragged her backwards a long distance while five or six sleds watched. I begged, pleaded, swore, and cajoled and finally broke my ski stick. I had to slip her and think she'll never be any good. She was tired and figured quite coldly that whatever I did, it was little enough to pay for getting out of harness. I got home ready to die. Three books came in the mail: *The March of the Barbarians*, the *Life of Finney* from Marianne, and a book on the Russian cinema from my brother.

April 4, '41. Roused out at 2:30 A.M. by a gent who wanted me to attend his wife who was in labor though only eight months gravid. He had tried Dr. Wood, but Doccy has the diarrhea from eating too much seal. John was committed to go to Herring Neck at 5:30 A.M. for a shoulder out of cup, so I informed him there was no doctor free as I had to stay at the hospital. He would have to try Wood again. He was loath to do so and couldn't understand why John wouldn't go to his house instead of to the other person's. Waiting for Wood to call I had a cup of tea on the ward, but he didn't call so I went back to bed about 3:15 only to be awakened at 5:30 by the curses of John looking for Jake. At 9:00, I was awakened again for a catheterization—at which point I decided it was time that George, the orderly, learn to catheterize. I let George do it. Apparently Dr. Wood had gone on the OB case because he didn't turn up for his day in the OPD; so I took on his chores: fingers, eyes, sores, prescriptions. Dinner upstairs with the Olds', the first seal flippers of the season and they were good.

In the afternoon I took the poor tired dogs and Irene behaved beautifully. We went way around the North Island to see a baby in the care of its grandmother; the worst grandmother yet. She was afraid I would scare the baby into fits and she leaned over it, talking to it so that I couldn't get near the thing, so bundled up to give it more fever than it had.

We all had a drink in my room before tea. David was in funny mood and he put on a show with his father. David went through his routine of throwing things on the floor. The trouble is that he is brilliant and knows just when to press his advantage. He is a good child though and I enjoy very much his liking me.

Here's a story about the aunt of the wife of the new Ranger sergeant. I heard it today. She was frightened in the minor earthquake of 1929 (twelve years ago) and has been hiccuping ever since. She had both the nerves to her diaphragm cut and has lived on morphine pills ever since. I suppose she wouldn't give up her hiccups for anything. I spent the evening with Stella and am beginning to be much better at tatting.

Travel is lousy. You wouldn't believe that anything having to do with water could be so sticky and nonskid as this ice is on both land and sea.

April 6, '41. Palm Sunday. On my way down the lane to Burt Pardy's for tea I could see two sealing steamers on the horizon. They are frozen in tight and drifting with the Arctic ice back towards Fogo where it is probably breaking up. From our line of sight the ice extends as far as you can see. This has been a great week for the landsman sealers as the main pack of seals come to our shores only once in thirty years. John went out on the ice four miles to bring one in and we've had three meals of it. Most of the people save the pelts and throw the carcasses away. The men kill more than they can get aboard. It seems a crime in a land that needs both fertilizer and meat that the carcasses are discarded. A Norwegian sealing steamer takes a whole seal aboard and not a hair is wasted. For them a successful voyage means only a quarter of the seals required for a successful Newfoundland steamer. The Norwegians can the meat and make fertilizer as well as using the fat and the leather. The Newfoundlanders consider this unfair competition. For the most part they use just the fat and the hide leaving the carcasses on the ice. Stella's grandfather once fitted out a schooner in Twillingate to go for seals and he filled it without leaving the wharf.

The war swept into the Balkans today and I wept as I heard the Yugoslav anthem over BBC. I prayed for the Greeks, the Slovenes, the Croatians, and the Serbs, and it must be that they will win.

There are tales of a seven hundred-bed army hospital in Botwood. That would be the end of us. A seventy-bed one would be the end of us because the government would take it over in peacetime and cut off our grant. I believe all St. John's is only too willing to cut our throats.

April 7, '41. Newfoundlanders have retained what seem to be archaic past participles. The name for what I woke up with today is a bit of 'hagrod'. I suppose hagride is the correct word. You hear 'sove' for 'saved', and 'scrope' for 'scraped'. Reminds me of a hysterical girl I was called in to see. She had been to a Pentecostal church meeting. In a burst of religious enthusiasm she had fallen to the floor. When a gentleman in the congregation hastened to assist her to arise, the mother intervened, "Don't tetch her, don't tetch her, leave her lay where Jesus flang her!"

With a jelly bandage on my poor ankle I headed down to Gillard's Cove with the dogs. Jake did not take the lead because he doesn't feel well. Spot stepped right into the lead and behaved nobly. Irene pulled like a little tractor except that on some of the fast hills we took her backwards on her behind. Gillard's Cove is nice. There I saw all the old crocks and received a dollar's worth of what Old John owed me, in seal flippers. The war is going slowly after yesterday.

April 8 and April 9, '41. These days have been like summer as far as work goes. On Tuesday we did four operations in the morning along with x-ray and lots of people in the OPD. The next day I was left alone in the OPD with eighteen patients, the baby clinic, and syphilis treatments, after two operations in the morning until I was so tired I fell to bed.

My ski ankle has been doing not very well. I keep putting jelly bandages on and taking them off. We have been having lot of seal to eat but I don't think that is what is wrong with my ankle.

More stories from Dr. Wood who came in ostensibly to tell me why Paul Moore had had a gall bladder attack. Maybe that is related to eating seal? Anyway before he was done I learned what every single one of the Osmonds in Moreton's Harbor had died of and how much each of them had left. The connection to Moore's gall bladder was that his mother's second husband had had something to do with the settlement of the estates. I kept wanting to read my mail which I managed only much later and was gladdened to find the announcement from father that he was sending me another ham.

April 10, '41. Since no operation had been scheduled for early in the morning, I slept on through to hear John with his arms akimbo asking what the hell. There WAS an operation, an anterior-posterior perineal repair and I had to do it with no breakfast. Doccy Wood had been scheduled in the OPD or I would have been up anyway. Now it's teatime already and I think John is going to the Tilt though I haven't been informed. It would be all right to tell me because I have to do the work when he's gone. An x-ray of my ankle showed nothing, though the ankle makes peculiar noises, feels funny, and is swollen. After reading *White Oaks* my interest rekindled in *Finch's Fortune* so I swept right through it.

April 22, '41. *The Twillingate Sun* published three health articles I wrote for them. I wish now that the first article hadn't told them to put a hot water bottle on the side if they had appendicitis. Apparently someone had sold them on an ice bag for that condition. I don't think it makes any difference which is used.

The sun was so hot I took off my shirts on a pleasant walk to Little Harbor; partly walk, partly lunge—in some places the snow was waist high. It made as much sense to go over the hills direct, for the winter trail and the summer road are no better than the moors. Jake started out with me, the other two caught up as we hit Minty's barn. On the way back I fell through the ice on one of the ponds and got quite wet. While we were planning a poker game yesterday, Swanker came in with the body of a fourteen-year old boy who had been struck in the forehead by the fist of a teacher and knocked over a couple of benches. That was in February. He had seemed to be rather ailing and had headaches, but was able to go out on the ice after seals a few weeks ago. Four days before death he had been seen by Dr. Swanker with signs of cerebral difficulty and pulmonary edema. He died and the feeling all over his town was that he had had a head injury. Our x-ray seemed to show one. Swanker was convinced that the blow had done it all. Doccy Wood wandered in during the autopsy and grunted his disbelief in that theory. He knew the whole family. He said we'd find tuberculosis. Autopsy showed no fracture of the skull, but did show lungs full of tuberculosis. It showed me the value of the family doctor, the one who knows your family and your town and everything about you. There's a wisdom that comes to the doctor with long association.

Rose Black is in a restraining sheet and we are feeding her through a tube. She won't speak, eat, or move. My emotions are a little Middle Ages when I see such people in this land where the work of everyone is needed. Her mother is almost as bad. Rose was here years ago when only ten and even then she was talking about dying; we thought she was screwy at the time.

On the subject of dying, John is carrying on again about an aeroplane, but I'm talking as much against it as I can. We would have to have a full-time mechanic pilot to run the thing. I don't think our methods are good enough to fly through the air on.

We are well through the ham, which is not so good as the others, but beats the one Mrs. Pardy forced me to eat. Ham is still a luxury here so we will eat anything that resembles it.

I was talked into doing a caesarian section; I still think she might have made it by herself, though her measurements were small and the risk is always great when the first baby is a breech. She hasn't voided since. When I pulled the baby out I think the womb was infected from below by the suction. We gave her sulfa at once and there has been no rise in temperature. There are three fathers, but it can't be pinned on any one of them.

April 23, '41. By noontime I had dictated about thirty charts and a call came to Kettle Cove; it had warmed so that after much debate about what method to use, I got Clarence and his horse and uncomfortable wagon. It is just a light flat surface on four wheels and like all means of conveyance in this country, grueling. The horse plunged, ran, trotted, and fell down, but we got through the deep snow to Manuel's Cove. There we left the horse and walked the mile or so to Kettle Cove. Mrs. Chappell, the object of our visit, was in bed, "that weak," her tongue clove to the roof of her mouth. She trembled and shivered and didn't know what she would do in the world at all whatsoever. Her 'laig' is all drawed up and whatnot. My legs feel "drawed up" too after plunging through nine-foot drifts.

Back by six to find young Lemuel Smart waiting with a ruptured appendix. Betty and Stella had gone to the church supper and promised to be back by 7:00. They arrived six minutes after 7:00 but John was already furious. Later on the girls and I played rummy while John sulked. We three had hangovers the next day but John had been smart about it.

I must find out which hymn it was that Mr. Smart sang to his son, Lemuel, who was at the tiller coming to the hospital with his ruptured appendix. The father sang the whole way to cheer his son, interspersing song with, "Keep her off, Lemuel! Do you think we'll make Twillingate by dark—hold in, Lemuel!"

April 24, '41. A beautiful day but I didn't get out in it. Word of a big steamer going into Botwood this morning—one of Northcliff's paper boats. Things must be tight in England to have it running so early. I think Botwood is still full of ice.

April 25, '41. We had a terrible time this morning. John took a tumor out of a thyroid and it was a tough job, soft and bled like the dickens. I've rarely been so glad to see the skin sutures go into a live patient. The boats started to pour in with patients and we were busy the rest of the day. In the late afternoon I rowed Wyn's boat across the harbor to pay some bills and to visit a sick hospital aide.

April 28, '41. We were busy as hell in the operating room. I did a tubal pregnancy that was not diagnosed beforehand. It had felt to me like a cyst. There were lots of casts to be put on people.

In the evening a call came for Back Harbor to see Robert Simms with a stroke. I took the cycle and Stella but the former got only as far as over Church Hill. We walked the rest of the way in very poor going. The old man was in bad pain, a sort of angina. He was spitting a little blood. I gave him morphia and wrote out his will: the house and land to his wife, to go on her death to the daughter; the fishing room and land and gear to the son, from which he was to give a bit to his mother on times; the gun to grandson, Robbie.

April 29, '41. The ice was twelve miles off by last report, but you could see it creeping in all day and by noon it was touching Cuckold's Point, advancing well into the harbor by teatime. It is rough and is packing up the bight too—the wind still blowing by evening after raising hell from the northeast.

I had a quick baby tonight. The whole day went quickly after an abdominal operation in the morning. I fixed a hernia on the woman to whom Jack Spence promised the price of a set of false teeth by way of recompense for favors received. He came to see her and brought her two chocolate bars. Then I took out an eye in a man and another in a little fellow with cancer. He was four years old. It had gone through the sclera and invaded the optic nerve. I hated to do it.

April 30, '41. A lovely day for the last of April, snowing and blowing like hell and it never was clear enough to see if the harbor was full of ice or not. The mail due two days ago hasn't even reached Comfort Cove. We fished a loop of gut out of Mr. Chaulk this morning and put a tube in. He has cancer of the stomach but wants to live long enough to go on one voyage with his twenty-five-year old son to see how he does as master. That son and another were in here with multiple TB foci. The former will have to make a living for the family and there are ten children.

The spinster postmistress astounded the village last night by having a baby. She must have been frightened at the amateur concert when Dr. Olds warned the people that they would be expected to take patients in with them in the case of air raids. I sometimes think I've taken all the gaff I can. I get bits of depression nowadays. It's been a long winter. I think I'm homesick. The old man whose will I made the other evening died the next morning at 4:00. I am reading Van Wyck Brooks' *New England: Indian Summer*. My friend Charles Burnett is a product of that golden New England—an Emersonian.

May 1, '41. We managed to get Billy LeDrue's terribly angulated thigh into some kind of alignment, though I fear the hip is somewhat rotated. He is a fine kid, in spite of the effect this deformity must have on him. He even fished with his father last summer and caught four quintals, for which he got eleven something. I skied to a patient in the afternoon, but the snow was not in number one condition. The ice is still in tight with a wind out of the northeast.

Mrs. Boone, with her fits and spells, sent a wire to her husband saying, "Feeling terrible, having a heart attack every day. Come at once." John edited it as it went through the office to read, "Feeling much better." She was annoyed to get the answer, "Glad you are feeling well."

May 2, '41. The ice still tight. No mail. In the snowy wet morning we did an elaborate operation on a cancer of the intestines.

We celebrated Betty's birthday last night with alcohol and lime juice; in spite of all the lime juice my blood vitamin C is only half of a milligram per hundred cc.

John is writing a paper on vitamin C, towards which the laboratory tests show that we are all on the edge of scurvy. We have not found a patient or staff member with a normal vitamin C blood level, yet—interesting—we see almost nothing that could be called clinical scurvy.

May 5, '41. Still no mail, for more than two weeks. I went to Bluff Head on the cycle in a cold rain, taking Bud along in case we got stuck in the snow. I saw Claude Brown, whose TB is not much better. Our bowel operation (Miculikz) is doing well, it is retracting into the belly though only four days old. Mr. Chaulk, with his stomach cancer, is vomiting from a high obstruction. I'm afraid he'll never see how well his son can captain a schooner. A patient fooled me and had her baby on the ward before we could get her into the operating room. I've been reading a disturbing book, *Fame is the Spur,* and can't decide whether it laughs at labor or not.

May 7, '41. The ice is still tight but the mail finally got here and a poor one it was for the waiting. Only a letter from Grace Patten Sparkes apologizing for what she said about my name and I don't remember what she said. John did better; a thousand-dollar donation for the hospital from Betty Washbourne. She worked here as a nurse when I was a student.

Yesterday I did a difficult spinal fusion of the Hibbs, Albee, Olds, Ecke variety for a lower back difficulty undiagnosed until explored. That circular saw still amuses me. The operator has the greatest confidence but the assistant is always apprehensive. Then I did a fifteen-minute appendectomy on a red hot one about to burst.

May 8, '41. I can hardly remember the day. Mr. Chaulk is worse and my graft has a high temperature. I woke at 4 A.M. not knowing what woke me. I heard later that it was an aeroplane.

May 9, '41. Our water main is plugged and John was scheduled to cystoscope the pond so I went out groaning to respond to a request for a doctor at Cobbs Arm. By 9:00 I had hitched Dolt to the sulky and was off to Little Harbor on a springy ride but having to lean back so far I had the feeling it would lift the horse off the ground; a characteristic of sulky riding, at least of this one. After I got the horse into a barn and gave it some hay, I walked with the men way out to Jones Cove and climbed over the cliffs to the Point. The tickle was full of loose ice, some of the pans were big and thick, jammed against the near shore. The punt was forty yards from the water and with some difficulty we launched it over the ice, stern foremost.

Finally aboard, our troubles had just begun. We pushed and shoved while the bottom ground on the ice. With three men standing, we were often on our beam. The men would jump out and walk it along a pan. The precariousness of our situation caused me to feel frankly rather sick at the stomach. Bear in mind the tickle here is a mile across and after half an hour we were fifty yards from shore over cold water. The young fellow with them knew I was worried and he purposely pushed it into the ice to see me wince. Even in the comparative clear the lookout let us bang into pans. Once out of that it was a hot rough walk three miles along the Bottom to Redick's Neck.

There I was amazed to find the same punt, this time stranded by low water fifty feet up the shore. It was on the wrong side of the Neck so it meant a long row before we could get into the bight. It could have been shortened but the ice had shifted and cut us off. We had some more poling to do. After all of us had to get out on the ice and drag the boat for twenty yards; we ran aground and finally abandoned it. Then we were in for a long hot walk again to Cobbs Arm. I cooled off on the porch and then saw three children, vomiting with red throats. The boy had it, the mother has it, and the three young children have it. This did not prevent my being asked, "Is it catching, doctor?" Then I saw the teacher and a girl with a boil on her bottom.

Back at Green Cove, John Blandford had been waiting for me, but had gotten tired. He tired awfully easily. It hadn't been two hours. His wife had erysipelas and the hired girl no periods, so I prescribed for both and Blandford put me over to Carter's room where I found Joe White. We stopped at Malcolm Simms for a hospitable drink and went on to Redick's Neck where I saw a girl with the white mouth and another who kept butting in to have her chest examined.

We were soon poling again in the leaking skiff. At open water we changed to a fast motorboat and banged around with Joe signaling from the bow like Eric the Red. The ice was strong, blue, and threatening.

We skinned one berg 40 feet high. That's a bad practice. These bergs have a habit of foundering when you disturb the air or the water near them. They tell a story of a fairly large steamship, I think it was the *Segona.* To please a passenger the Captain blew his whistle near a big iceberg. The berg broke in half and rolled over. One minute later a half came up under the ship and for a sickening moment lifted it clear of the water, then rolled slowly and launched it again without harm.

At Little Harbor we hitched up Dolt again, but Joe and I were a big load for that outfit. The whiffletree came off at the top of a big hill. It would have been bad in the middle of the hill. Since I'm no hostler I had to take the harness all apart to get it off. Joe sent me a bottle of rum for bringing him home. It embarrassed me. There was no need for it after all he's done for me. I do like rum. There may be an OB call tonight at Crow Head but I think John will go. I hope. It's Doccy Wood's case but he has gone to see his son at Sydney.

May 11, '41. Sunday and a bad day. I watched the fort. Lots of patients came to the OPD. Mr. Chaulk went home refusing to take any food. He says he is not going to eat or drink until he dies. A little boy came in, eleven years old, with a story of eating a half-pound of prunes two days ago. Last night and this morning he had two loose stools, not surprising, and a pain in the belly. He had no pain or temperature when I saw him—the abdomen was soft and he denied any tenderness. I sent him home. We were busy then for a while, admitting seven patients. The boy's mother came again in the afternoon and asked if I couldn't send some medicine—the stomachache had come back. I went down to see him instead—good thing too—I was really shocked to find a board-like belly. The boy still denied pain and had no temperature. We opened him up and found that his appendix had been ruptured for at least two days. We gave him sulfa and cut down on a vein for a continuous drip and he may pull through.

May 14, '41. These two past afternoons at 5:00 we have had to do emergency appendectomies. I have a feeling now that every child with a pain in the belly, proved or not, should have the appendix out. I'm not sure I am completely innocent in the matter of Ernest Bulgin. If ever I wanted a patient to get well, he is it, but he doesn't look too good—sort of tense and a little distended although his chart is all right. Tonight I put a tube in his stomach.

All day I was on the road, starting with Herring Neck this morning for a bunch of liars who said the call was Herring Neck when it was Pike's Arm. Said the patient was terrible sick when it was an old gent of seventy-nine in his third or fourth year of mild bronchitis; said they were up on the books when they were two years behind.

I stopped at John Blandford's to lance an elbow; there I got a wire to go back to Two Good Arm to William Young. I don't get along with him but his babies are always really sick and worth the trip. I got home by 2:00 in Carter's roomy skiff, steering by compass because it was so foggy. The Merritt's Harbor rocks look very unfamiliar when they are all the land you can see. Saw patients until about 8:00 and listened to news about Rudolf Hess parachuting into England. At 10 PM it's not really dark.

May 15, '41. We rose early and were soon off on a dirty misty day into three operations. I did all three; partial resection of both ovaries for cysts, appendectomy with removal of an ovary for a funny hard little tumor, and another appendix. In between we did fluoroscopies. Late in the afternoon I went over to Dun Ansteys' and found that his little girl had appendicitis. They got her ready while we were on rounds and we did that only to find that the OB was about to pop. In the small hours I was called to see Ernest Bulgin who was beginning to look as if he would make it. At 6 A.M., I had to go to Crow Head.

We were glad to see Stan and Annette get back. Stan's elbow was in a cast. He brought me a nice pipe and new hardware for my stethoscope. I am getting right to work with the new typewriter ribbon he brought me that mother sent unasked—very thoughtful. Of course, it will make my letters more readable.

Arriving in Crow Head at dawn I was greeted with "I didn't know if you could get all the way over, doctor, so I gave you plenty of time." What I found was a woman eventually going to have a baby but not right then, her cervix admitted only one finger. She may be a couple of hours and she may be a couple of days as it is her first, so I've come back to help take out a uterus and do a caesarean section meantime. Then I'll call up and find out how she's doing.

May 18, '41. Well, that Crow Head OB business turned out to be something again. I did a nice section and a few chores and then, looking for trouble, called up to see how she was getting on. They said she wasn't very good and wanted a doctor. I hurried over and found her very little advanced. I sat around, I had tea, I read a mystery sitting in the open door over the sea. It was a lovely afternoon and you could see over the beautiful Crow Head all the way to Cape St. John. I watched a little stream of snow water running under the house. I gave a little pituitrin. I had more tea. She was terrible. She screamed and crawled and howled and rolled and inched and yelped and refused to cooperate in any way. I got desperate. The father cried and her mother cried, though she had had eleven children herself. The grandmother cried and she, as a midwife, had 'barned' seventy-five. I had the four of them bawling at once. I offered to take her to the hospital, phrasing it in such a way that it would look like their idea but the patient balked. At 6:00 that evening old granny Elliot came in to say that the hospital called to see if I needed help. I was touched by their concern, at the time, and said yes, I could use a nurse. The family called for another doctor but I told them they couldn't get one. In a little while Stella came, right from the still-busy operating room. My patient had been in the second stage for three hours and made no progress in her labor, though she moved a great deal about the room. Stella put her to sleep and I put on the hooks. The head was high. I would have done a version if there had been fewer germs around, but with the mother and grandmother at either leg, fiddling with the drapes, I didn't dare.

The baby came with only moderate traction and a deep episiotomy that went right through the midwife's heart, from the shudder she gave. I sewed and though there was no hemorrhage, the bed and room were blood to the ceiling. The patient was soon happy and we got home by 10:30 that night, for a game of rummy and dinner in Stella's room. I decided I was sore as hell at that offer of help from the hospital—which had been done as a joke. It's a nice commentary that a joke is what would ordinarily be a Christian deed.

Saturday I didn't get up too early and when I did the OPD was soon in full blast. Stan had to write letters at crucial moments and John came in for an hour in the afternoon just ducking Mrs. Reverend Gill. She plans to have her baby in the hospital in about two weeks. I saw her and in a few days her blood pressure had jumped from 130/35 to 162/100. This looked bad to me so I told her to come up Sunday morning. I finally got through the cases and was just about to go to Crow Head when Stan got a rush OB call. In a few minutes he brought Mrs. Lewis Blake back, bleeding badly with a placenta praevia. I did a caesarean section as fast as I could.

Since Mrs. Gill's blood pressure was 140/105 this morning I told her to come back in the afternoon to be admitted.

A sick baby came in from Bridgeport and I thought it had infantile paralysis. That was bad news for John, meaning he had to assemble the iron lung which Lord Nufield had given the hospital. At one clip he had donated 500 iron lungs to hospitals throughout the Empire. We have used ours a lot, but never for a case of paralysis. It was a gold mine of useful things: the machine was put on the tonsil suction in the operating room; the rubber mattress is used on the delivery table; the rubber hose is on a blower in the x-ray room, and we use the top of the lung as an extra bed when we're crowded.

We've had eight emergency operations this week, counting Mrs. Gill's. When we took her blood pressure this evening after the news, it was 165/122 so we did a section at once and got a nice babe and I think just prevented really serious trouble for Mrs. Gill.

The *Clyde* came in this evening, docking first at Ashbourne's to take on fish.

May 19, '41. That baby did not have infantile paralysis, but we did get the iron lung together.

May 25, '41. Well, we've recovered from a week's visitation from Ted Drover. Although I know he is fond of me, he is so dynamic that I wear out. A case of rum did too. I don't like it in that quantity.

The week saw thousands and thousands in the OPD; forty in one day. Lots of operating. On one I cut the nerve to a diaphragm right after John did a quick one. He was helping me. He said there is the place to go in, I took his word for it and we searched and searched only to find we were not in the right place. When we got oriented, we had no trouble and although I looked bad it wasn't all my fault.

By the grapevine I heard that the Green's had not been satisfied with my call on Edison. That was the one where I covered seventy-five miles on a winter day to tell him there was nothing wrong with him. There wasn't anything wrong with him. What did they expect me to do? He has been working ever since.

The week dragged on. We opened an intact hymen to let out a great collection of old blood and removed some ribs to collapse a chest. On Saturday morning things got quiet and John suggested that I take a weekend

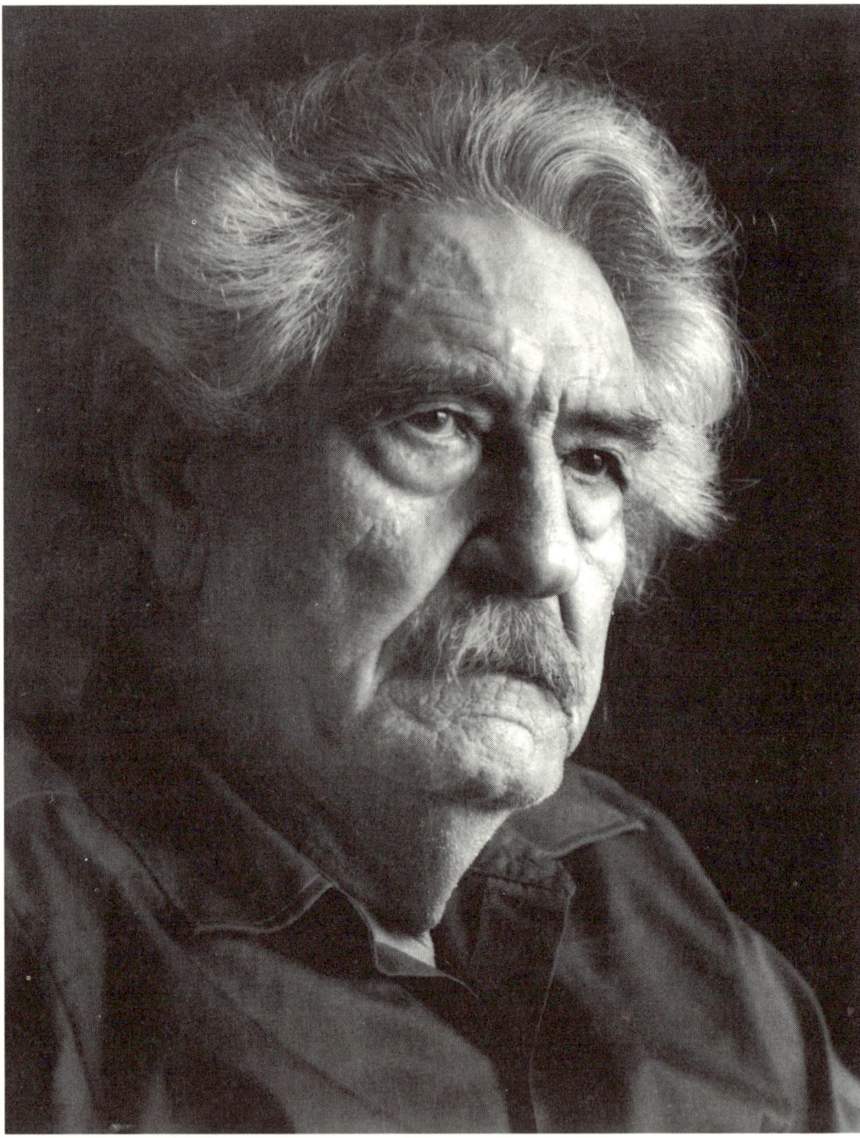

Ted Drover: fine artist, genius, seaman, and great friend, 1976

off and persuade Ted to go with me. That we did although I wasn't feeling very well. I had been slightly nauseated for three days.

I allowed myself to be governed, and we started out of the harbor on Ted's boat. The *S.S. Glenco* was just coming in. While she was still moving we tied up to her and climbed aboard. When she docked, the wharf idlers were mystified to see Ted and me at the rail, when they had just seen us leaving. I was introduced to Captain Snow, a fine appearing, stern-visaged, blue-eyed man who didn't seem even civil. He ordered me to hurry up and find out about his fireman, who was in the hospital with TB, a bad heart, and syphilis. His force was such that I hastened to comply although the ship's nurse was just about to offer me a drink. I walked up to Hodge's to telephone but couldn't raise the hospital. So as not to disappoint the captain, I made up a message and he didn't even say thanks. Ted and I lost interest in the *Glenco* and started off again.

Our boat was yawing a bit to windward, I think as a result of the rock we hit off the breakwater. Ted would set the wheel and we would both go below for a drink. We did that with no one at the wheel most of the time. Just inside Cobbs Arm we happened to be on deck when we passed Paddy Miller in his limestone-laden schooner. We went aboard, but unlike the *Dorothy and Ruth*, we had to bring the skipper back to our boat for a drink. We made for Roper's Harbor, our favorite picnic spot. I stood on the peak and signaled away from the rocks. It's a completely wind-free, land-locked harbor with a natural rocky wharf. When we tie up beside it, juniper branches brush against the porthole. We pulled some herring nets hoping to steal a few herring but they were empty. The owner came along while we were doing it and gave us some herring. We paid with rum. We scoured the bottom for lobsters, but couldn't find anything but flounders. We ate and talked until midnight and then I had a very uncomfortable sleep. I was awakened early to a dull day by an aeroplane overhead. I took the wheel part way home and was feeling worse. I had a deep, nasty-looking ulcer on the inside of my cheek. I took a long nap and mourned the loss of *H.M.S. Hood.*

May 26, '41. The day was so clear you could see Cape St. John Gull Island. The inevitable little island off most of the points and capes is often referred to as Gull Island tacked on to the name of the point. I took out a uterus and went to take the stitches out of that OB case at Crow Head. I sure am happy to call that case almost closed. We heard today that one of our nurses aides is unconscious. She had a peculiar spell when the dentist had his and we thought it was a paratyphoid, but she didn't seem to get well. She came back to work but didn't feel right and has been home ever since. Doccy Wood saw her and thought she had meningitis. I did a spinal tap for him and he was right. She's gotten rather worse since. I stopped at

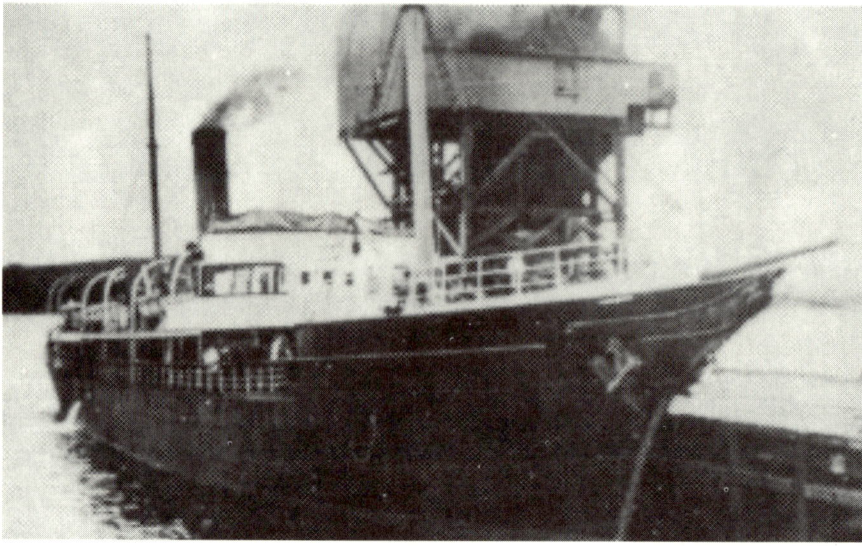

S.S. *Glenco.*

the lighthouse and lay down on the edge of the high cliff. The sun was bright and there were gleaming white icebergs in the distance. The surf was too far below to be noisy. It is hard to realize that with no land between us, there is a great sea battle going on—the Royal Navy after the *Bismarck.* If only I could see far enough. All day we heard aeroplanes. One went over this morning towards Greenland and came back tonight. They all seem to use the hospital as a landmark and it makes us uneasy. The feeling of war seems to come closer. A heavy cruiser dropped into the harbor. Mackay and Banting, discoverer of insulin, crashed near Musgrave Harbor. We see soldiers in Lewisporte and Botwood. There is talk of aeroplanes at the airport and of flights to Greenland. I donated twenty-five dollars to the Spitfire fund.

May 27, '41. Now it seems that the very aeroplane that we saw Sunday was in search of the *Bismarck.* It was fine to hear that they got her, though the cost was terrific. Tonight I listened to President Roosevelt issue his proclamation of unlimited national emergency and the hair stood up on the back of my neck. I was almost in tears and in a way, scared. It sounds final and I am sure that no such state of national emergency can disappear by lysis, it will have to come by crisis.

Today was pretty good one. I did one belly. It had sounded and felt like a tubal pregnancy but turned out to be just a large leathery ovary. I had to leave the next operation because of my cough and my voice today has been below low G. My throat is getting sorer and sorer, but in spite of that John sent over at 11:30 as we were waiting for the Fireside Chat to tell me there was a call waiting in Purcell's Harbor. I was griped as hell but Stella offered to go with me. I sat till the broadcast ended and then found John in my room not having listened. He was angry and rushed off to Purcell's Harbor himself. I don't give a damn. He had no right to push it off on me anyway and he had all evening to go if he was in such a hurry. I can leave here anytime. We examined sixteen recruits today.

May 29, '41. I sort of forgot yesterday. We did some operating. John was kind of surly all day, so I just let him go hang. I have taken a course of only speaking when spoken to; I'm tired of making conversation when I'm not sure it's welcome. Let him go on reading and keeping quiet. The hell with it.

This morning I was awakened by the passage of two big planes going north and tonight about 6:00 they came back. The poor things have been in the air all day—looking for the *Prinz Eugen* I suppose.

This morning I took out the tonsils and adenoids of a thirty-five-year old woman. It was her own idea. I hate to do surgery on order by the patient. It's like tailoring. Then a gal came in and we couldn't push the baby's head into the pelvis, although she was at term. I did a quick section, and couldn't see any obvious cause of her difficulty.

The afternoon was quiet. We had lobster for the third time this week. I've agreed to take the students into my apartment this summer. We will be kind of crowded.

An airman told Wyn that planes have been going to Greenland from here and the Americans are pretty well set up in Greenland. The *Esmond*, a German ship captured at Botwood, was torpedoed with two men from Twillingate on board. One, Jim Gillette, was saved. The other, Arthur Gillette, is missing. The *Portia* has been sunk and so has the *Humber Arm* and one other paper boat.

May 30, '41. A fine Decoration Day. It snowed and blew like the dickens and is getting worse tonight. It really was a bad winter's day. The ice is so close though that the harbor didn't get rough enough to catch the *Bessie Marie*, who, as in most storms, was at her fatal mooring.

I got a start tonight. During our poker game, Burt Pardy told us that they were planning, mind you only planning, a road to Philips Head in Botwood and Goering said over the radio that there was no sense in building the road because the airport would be gone in a week, and the same day that the Black Watch left for overseas and were replaced by the Queen's Own Rifles, Germany announced the fact.

I took off a male breast this morning and we used sodium pentothal. It worked pretty well but cost $2.50 and requires the services of a third doctor. Stan had quit the poker game because of the reaction from his typhoid inoculation.

June 2, '41. Oh dear, I am beginning to get that waiting feeling again. I have the same sensations one has during the too-long intermission of an amateur show that has started late. I've had it before and it usually leads up to a resignation. I had a moment of panic today when I watched John palpating a belly and making up his mind to do a gall bladder. I had examined the patient and it hadn't occurred to me to take out the gall bladder. I felt very inferior. I don't have any trouble deciding to do caesarean sections, but after all it's not too hard to be sure, at least, that there's a baby under the knife.

I had a feeling on Sunday that I was going to die in this war—this is to be noted especially by my biographer. [Ed. Early in the war, my body was rumored locally to have been found on the shore of the Strait of Belle Isle. In fact, in 1942 I had sailed through the Strait in convoy.] The planes continue to fly over us—two yesterday, one went for Cape St. John and one for Ireland. Only one came back. The nurse's aide died today and there is gloom over the hospital. I know of course that TB meningitis can't be cured, but people always have a hope that a miracle will happen. The combined staff announced last night that it needed sleep, would I take the calls? The night nurse was even instructed to call me. That handed me a laugh. She knows perfectly well whom to call nights. Let them go, I say.

June 3, '41 This gets worse. Instead of taking all the cutting I can get, I am happy when John decides to do the operating.

I am working against myself. I wake with a nausea at the pit of my stomach and approach the incisions with dread. As soon as I get warmed up, all is well. I'll be a good subject for psychoanalysis if I don't watch out. We heard today that the *Terra Nova* was sunk between St. John's and Halifax. I don't believe the location but it probably is gone. Our acquaintance with ships is not great but a tremendous percentage of those we do know have been sunk. The U. S. is too slow at getting into this war.

Today I helped on a stomach then did a skin graft and snapped off a breast in no time at all. I am getting pretty good at that. It's not so long since I laboriously snipped away a little at a time, but now I get right down to the muscle. We are beginning that dreadful expedient of putting the small patients two in a bed— "that way madness lies." Stella got the most pitiful paper-flower wreath for the aide's funeral. It is a sad business— those paper flowers for funerals. They certainly emphasize all that is remote and drab about this place. It looks like a cheap spring hat for a flighty dame. Then there is that custom of typing messages of condolence on the white ribbon tied to the wreath.

June 5, '41. The war closes in. The *Northern Ranger* and the *John Cabot* have been sunk. The *Bessie Marie* was called to St. John's by the Custom Department last evening, probably to be commandeered by the government.

Yesterday was a heavy day. I took out a uterus, an appendix, ruptured some membranes and removed some tonsils. Today I took out an ovary, an appendix, and helped John with a normal gall bladder. That last helped my state of mind. It was the case that depressed me so when I couldn't diagnose it. The trouble proved to be her appendix. Today, closing the skin, I kept catching the thread double. I did it once and blamed the length of the thread. The second time John said, "Isn't the thread just the right length? I've drawn this to your attention twice." Doctors are too much wanted in England and the States and too hard to get here to put up with this kind of talk.

Tonight we had enough lobster to send some back to the kitchen and then a couple of drinks with Stan and Stella. It's blowing a gale. The dormers are shaking. The glass is steady withal and the rain is coming down. Last night at 5:00, I woke to find myself sitting up in bed fishing around under the covers. Suddenly a furry object leapt against my chest. I batted it around until it disappeared. It must have been a rat under the cover of my bed. I got out and looked around, but it took me a long time to get back to sleep.

• • •

The Burnetts, Brunswick, Maine
August 25, 1941

Dear Sue and Charles and David,

News from you was very welcome and I would have told you so long ago but for the great turmoil we are all in. What with the students camped in my room and all over my desk with their clinical clerkship, the usual summer rush, and the presence of my sister and a friend, I haven't even been writing in my diary and there has been lots to put in it. We run about 107 patients in bed, and twenty or thirty in the outpatient department, and three or four operations daily, and too many outside calls. I just had a weekend at the Tilt and came back early this morning (Monday) and I didn't get a chance to clean my teeth until 6:00 this evening. We operate to the left and to the right. Babies appear from everywhere. Sick people come by the boatload and we chase the treated ones away before they should leave. Our annual report shows an increase in every department but staff and that is smaller. Each year we have reached our limit but the next year is always higher and now it looks as if we will have no dentist next year. The army has them all. I will hate to go back to pulling teeth.

Olds and I had a bit of a spree. We went to St. John's to the medical convention. Olds had a paper to read on vitamin C and I went along to support him. You would have loved the trip, Sue, we went in the *Bonnie Nell*—very much the private yacht. We took a crew of three—master, mate, and cook. Dr. Olds, his wife, and I were the passengers. If you look at the map you will see that it is an outside trip. We leave our bay and go right down along the shore through the blooming Atlantic Ocean. It was quite a venture for a not too well powered fifty-foot ketch. We had what they call a clever time of it—that is, lots of wind and waves but very little real storm. I must confess I am not as doughty as I might be. I do not like to be out of sight of land in a thing that can roll the way that boat does. All went well until we got outside of Wesleyville where we wanted to stop to see Waddell and pick him up to go on with us. It was just dark and the skipper called Olds and said, "Now this is the Stinking Island. You plot a course for the harbor." Well, the harbor is nestled in among bristling rocks. I had spent two weeks there and knew it was a graveyard. I remembered the man who wrecked his schooner in fair weather fifty feet from his kitchen door. We plotted and drew all kinds of lines on the chart and the

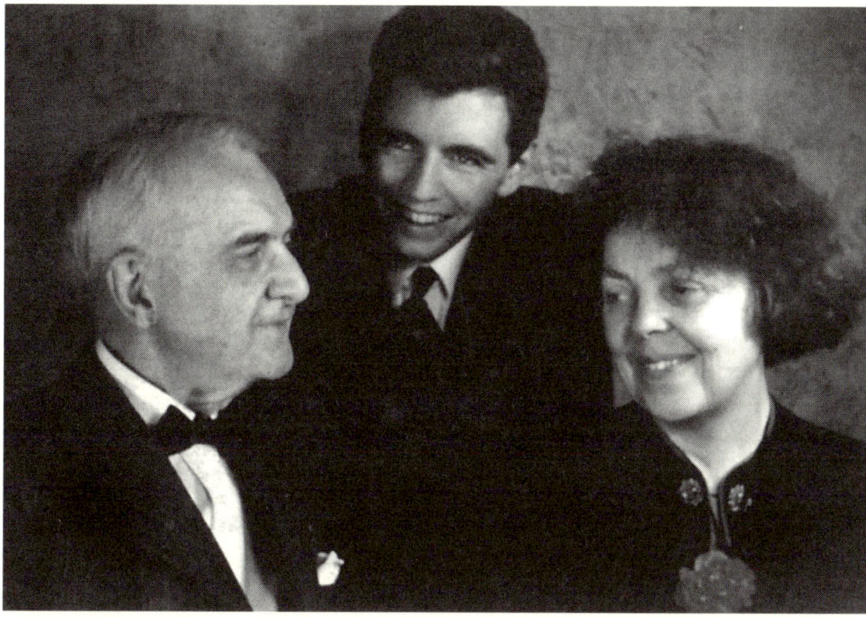

Dr. Charles T. Burnett, Sue Winchell Burnett, and son David. Author's photograph.

wrong islands turned up on the wrong side of us. Then we found the principal guiding light was out and what with one thing and another the skipper got so near the bottom of his bag of tricks that he even appealed to me for information. I said, "Do you see that light? Well, you keep it close on the starboard and bear right around it for that black spot on the shore and I think that is the wharf." Then I ran below, took six fingers of rum neat and put my head under the pillow. Our lights were finally seen and a sealing captain came out to pilot us the last few rods. The next day the natives told us they were sure we were rumrunners, for no honest vessel had ever been able to get around through the rocks on the course we had taken.

That next day was a daisy so we were off in the afternoon so as to arrive at St. John's early Sunday morning. It was glorious. Mountainous lops on the quarter and a stiff fair breeze. All went well until Olds shot a black balk. It is bad luck to shoot a bird (they were rising round us in literal clouds) and not pick it up so we broached to the sea and went around in dizzy circles missing the elusive feathered creature at each crazy dive at it. It was finally salvaged and with it my life expectancy, for as each sidelop sent us for the bottom, I uttered up an abbreviated but fervent prayer and at the same time a petition that the cause of this excursion would be visited with his just deserts. As we passed Cape Bonavista at dark I retired to my swaying bunk and we went on all night. I will never forget the sight that presented itself as I came on deck about 2:00 A.M. to find us in Baccalieu Tickle. Baccalieu is a very high island off the point of one of the capes. As you steam through it you are flanked on each side by great cliffs, and their sheer black mass against a brilliant night sky and reflecting water with a spanking breeze and a pleasant vigorous motion of our stout craft as she bolted along under full sail, presented a combination of sights, sounds, and sensations to live a long time. (I am not certain about the construction of that sentence. I was stopped three times in the course of it.) What I didn't find out till next morning was that the engine room had caught fire about midnight and the blaze had been extinguished without casualties.

Our entrance to St. John's, one of the most spectacular harbors in the world, was interesting on a clear lazy Sunday morning but censorship forbids detail. [Ed. There were nets and chains across the harbor mouth to thwart U-boats.] St. John's itself and the medical meeting were low-grade though we had a pleasant stay. We left on Wednesday afternoon to find fog closing in on us and our course back to Baccalieu was different. We steered by compass and knew we had made the tickle only when the foghorn suddenly blasted in our ear though we could see nothing.

After Cape St. Francis, Conception Bay had given us no trouble, but crossing Trinity Bay with the wind right on us was not amusing and again the saloon was filled with my false assurance and silent prayers. We gave up and scurried for shelter in Catalina but just as we made the Green Island with a delicate course to follow through the rocks, and quite committed, the light was closed in by fog. We had neglected to take a compass bearing! The rest was sheer luck and we anchored.

Dawn found me asleep in my bunk but the boat on its way to Wesleyville again to drop off Waddell. We made our landfall with no trouble and to our great joy, a gale breezed off the land so we couldn't try Cape Freels. We had a picnic all day in the sun. That night our crew rushed up to tell us that the *Lone Flier*, a schooner that had left St. John's with us and was well known to us, had kept on and been wrecked on such and such an island (censored). We were off early the next morning and went right up to the wreck to see if we could help. There she lay, poor thing, with the waves breaking over her and the disconsolate crew sitting in the rigging helping with the salvage. They refused our aid and we were home in half

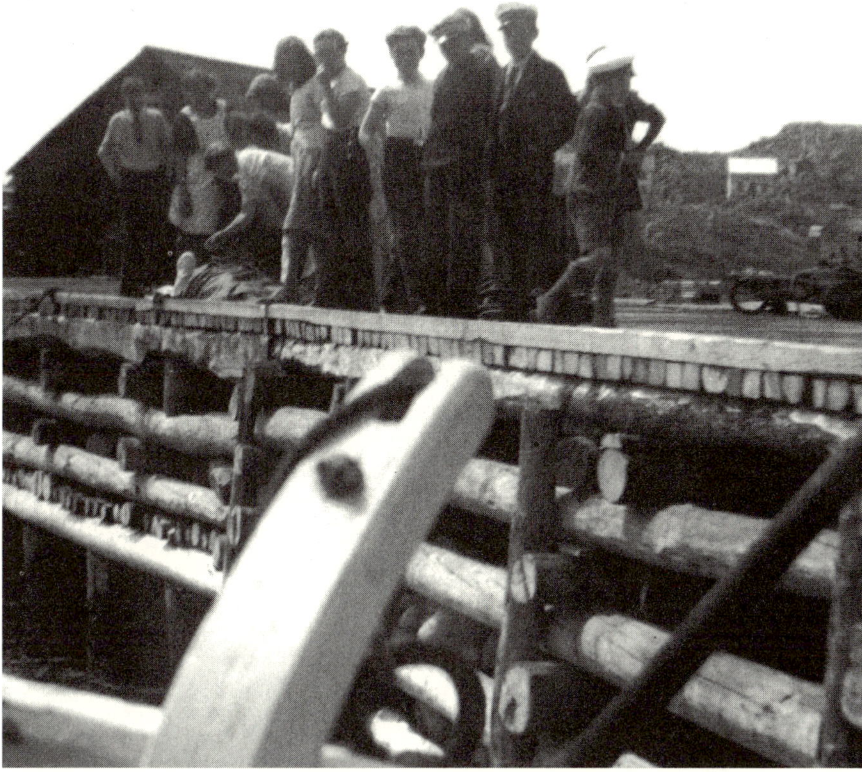

Wharf loungers in Wesleyville soberly appraise *Bonnie Nell*, identifiable by the cat's head (anchor davit) in the foreground. Author's photograph.

a day. There I found word of my sister and in two days she arrived with Dorothy Houghton of Kew Gardens. They have been here ever since and love it and I am delighted to have them. They are full of reports (second hand) of the Bowdoin commencement and when I hear of people having supper on your porch my heart fills and I get homesick. I am determined to make me a visit to the States around the close of the year. You don't know how often my thoughts go out to you and I wonder why I spend so many of my days here. I think I know why I do but I am sure none of the others give up so much as I. They can't possibly have such people as you to look forward to seeing. Now yesterday for instance . . .

I don't know what it could have been that I was going to tell you, for yesterday was three weeks ago and this letter has been in the machine ever since. It is not totally my poor character that intervened. This place is a merry-go-round. That yesterday must have been the day I delivered a baby down on the Arm before 6:00 in the morning, came back for breakfast, did three operations, two intubations of a ureter, saw two or three patients in the OPD, then was called for another baby down the Arm again. I cut across the island dressed lightly for a sunny day, walked two miles to see six patients in on a road by the sea where the cycle can't go. Just as we started home, I was hailed by a man who had been waiting an hour or so and with no warm garments or even tobacco with me and all my tools used and dirty, we were taken ten miles in an open boat to a forsaken part of the coast to deliver another baby. That proved to be a difficult and complicated job. We were there from 5:00 in the afternoon till 8:00 the next morning. We had missed our dinner the day before (one of the students was with me) and all we got to eat was a bit of bread and butter and some tea. It was a night in the ashes. I thought the dawn would never come but when it finally was bright enough to see the bedbugs on the pillow, we put her to sleep and did a fairly strenuous bit of home operating—a version and extraction against a rare condition of the uterus called a Bandl's contraction. It tightens down the middle and holds on to the baby instead of expelling it. Now that is not exactly a typical day but it is not far from it. We had babies at three in the morning three nights running. Relief of a sort is in sight. Tomorrow I start out on the lopsided *Bonnie Nell* again to go down north. It will be a month's trip starting at Cape St. John and coming south calling at all the little ports along the way.

Last Sunday I tearfully put Kathryn and Dot on the boat for Lewisporte and points south after a delightful five weeks. I had a wonderful time with them here and I hope you were home when they passed through Brunswick. I received Charles' letter last week and was glad to have the visit with you. You do seem to have a picture of my environs but you will have a better one when I show you my movies, which have been pretty successful. My lack of talk about war effort is mostly due to my deference for (or is it to?) censors. We have not been idle. Recruiting is active; we have a part in that. There is construction going on but the newspapers must be full of that. There are bereaved families and we talk to men home on leave. There is knitting. I suspect though that war activity is probably more feverish in your part of the world than ours though we may have more actual contact. I leave you now with my fondest as always and will not be so churlish the next time. Life will soon settle into a bit more of a groove and I will have my desk back and a chance to concentrate.

• • •

August 26, '41. La Scie, here we are—it's a long time since I wrote anything and a lot of smoke has gone over the bridge. Stan got back from his trip to Lockport on Friday. He had been called for On His Majesty's Service to investigate an epidemic of sore throats. By the time the appeal had gone through St. John's and he had gotten there, the throats were all well. One man had died. The man's father had planned to bring him to the hospital. The patient was well enough to walk down to the boat. On the beach he had dropped dead. It was hard to tell just from the histories whether it was diphtheria or streptococcus. Stan voted for strep.

John went off to the Tilt Friday night. Saturday was a busy day complicated at 8:00 P.M. by an appendectomy, not an easy one. I used eight clamps on the mesentery. I didn't want to operate with Jim, the student, because he has a hex on me and everything we do together turns out hard. Stan went to the Tilt when John got back and this was a bad morning to be short-handed in the OPD. There was lots of operating and I was anxious to get off on the *Bonnie Nell.* As it turned out, if I had been delayed another hour, we might have been lost. I helped John on a gallbladder whose blood pressure went down to 60 and told him to do the appendix while I took the OPD. He did a nine-minute job. He did the tonsil too, but it was a tough one and he was impatient and it took a long time. I was pleased with his discomfort.

We finally cast our lines at 1:00 and had a smooth trip across the bay. It was oily and calm but dark and I took the wheel almost the whole way. It closed in on us and we had to steer by compass. As we neared the cape, it rained and a minute after we rounded it and were in its shelter, it suddenly started to blow like hell from the southeast. The wind was terrific and if we had been caught out in the open it would have been serious. The skipper says we would have had to run before it. As it is now we are slamming the wharf and thumping and pitching. The wind in the rigging is making movie noises and the rain is smashing on the deck over my head. Every once in a while I stick my head through the hatch to enjoy how bad it is.

Cape St. John is a bitter ragged cruel jumble of rock. The worst hungry tooth at the point of it is called Mother Burke. We are snug in this berth under the bow of the *Young Harp*. We have berthed with her before. We had one incident today just as we got out of sight of land. Lidge Dalley, who wasn't feeling well, sat dozing beside me in the wheelhouse. I had my nose glued to the binnacle. I noticed smoke. I was vaguely conscious of it for ten minutes before it occurred to me to investigate. I looked at my pipe and it was cold. Lidge's pipe was out. I leaned out around the wheel house door and smoke was billowing out of the engine room hatch. "Don't look now," I said, nudging the skipper, "but I think the engine room is on fire again." It was a wild dash he made for the extinguisher. The fire was out in a second. The solid white fumes from the chemical rolled forward on the following wind right into the fo'c'sle, where Martin the mate was taking a nap. He appeared in the hatchway like a Jack-in-the-box. I've left the cash box at home. I will wire the hospital to send it with some money by the *Clyde.*

August 27, '41. Nothing to report. We lay all day in La Scie in the rain squalls, and business was way under last year.

August 28, '41. I woke as the engine started, a little worried because the wind was still up. I planned to take movies of Mother Burke. I knew I could tell when we rounded the Cape by the increase in roughness but when I finally got on deck we were past her and almost to Shoe Cove. It turned out to be mild in the bay. Shoe Cove is an amazing little scrap of beach nestled among 600-foot cliffs. It's no fit place for habitation—just a shallow scallop in the shore and the back of the town goes straight up. We lopped and rolled dreadfully and after killing myself on the anchor windlass, we faced a nasty bit of stuff. A storm broke while we were outside and she bucked to please anyone. It was a race as we rounded the point and got into the lee of a 700-foot clear drop of rock and there we were in Tilt Cove with more cliffs and the most utter desolation—millions of dollars in abandoned mining equipment. The wharf was double-decked and the whole shore had been formed in a pseudo-natural way by dumping hot molten slag that had hardened into a sort of conglomerate rock that may well mystify future geologists. There was hardly anybody here to do business with and we left just in time to catch another squall. A hell of a blow was coming out Round Harbor. That was a nice, well-protected place and we did a bit of work only to leave after tea, and face this keen north wind to get into Snooks Arm. It was punch and toss the whole way, but in the bottom of this great cleft in the sheer rock we found a quiet nest and here I did a bit of carpentry with stolen lumber and we had a few drinks, two patients, and a nice night of it. These villages are amazingly isolated, unlivable places, clustered around a waterfall coming off the tableland—just holes in the palisades. Snooks Arm is nearly a ghost town.

August 29, '41. Before breakfast I worked hard retrieving our heavy anchor. I had fair fainted when the skipper had said he was going to give her the big one. I worked so hard I was sick to my stomach and couldn't eat my breakfast. It wasn't long before we were busting around at anchor pulling teeth at the Indian Burying Ground. That was a clean place on stilts with no land at all but a nice waterfall. I saw eighteen patients and was quite busy until 1:30. I didn't have dinner until it was spoiled and ate it while the bottom crashed under the head-on lop as we fought our way to Nipper's Harbor. This is a good harbor. We had a job warping and the scion of the Noble family was yelling to have his teeth out before we docked. I started but he quit and has given us a bad name. We worked until 10:20 and the wind is raising hell in the rigging. We saw forty-one patients today and took in $59.00. It's a dark windy night and cold. Winter is in the air. We are almost into the Green Bay now where nothing can bother us very much. I have the saloon a little neater now, but I'll have it better arranged yet. Woke in Nipper's Harbor to have a fairly leisurely breakfast and start of work. It was pretty fast until lunch, which we took with people hanging over the fo'c'sle. This minister's son is the only special charity and he was certainly quick to put his wallet away when I said there would be no charge. In the afternoon I made a couple of shore calls. One was an unexplained high fever in a child. He didn't seem to have any tenderness in the belly and the story was not like appendicitis, but I'm scared of children. In any case, a conservative course seemed to be doing no harm. For the other case I had to go to the Bottom to the Pond which juts out below the harbor like the Pond at Norther Harbor. There we could see up the mountain. Down a scar in it a little stream of crystal cascaded. It was lovely indeed. We weren't through until 5:00 and we beat a very short run through clever sea and clearing sky to the wonderful Rogue's Harbor. There were rocks in the center of the entrance but you ease through a slit in the cliffs and are on a smooth pond. We tied up to a stage head with our anchor davit right in a kitchen window. The *Bonnie Nell* is very manageable in smooth water, but in anything rough she's like a bubble. There we saw only one patient and I speared a flounder, which I don't think Martin will cook for me. He doesn't think flounders are fit to eat. We entered Green Bay then and in the distance could see headland after headland a thousand feet high. We rounded a point and sneaked into Smith's Harbor, a long gouge in the shore, well protected. We pulled a couple of teeth and then put the saloon table up and declared a holiday because I wanted to do some carpentering. I made a rack for the rum bottles that we keep our medicines in. One wasn't quite empty yet so we spiked our cocoa. Had a pleasant time with the crew and Rita and now am making for bed rather determined not to do very much tomorrow—Sunday. It looks as if it were going to be fine and I want to get some sun.

September 1, '41. September morn was quiet in Smith's Harbor. We pulled a couple of teeth and the weather was civil for the first time this trip. We left early and went around the point to Burlington where we were rather busy. It too, like all the places on this rugged northern shore, is charming, snuggled in under the eight hummocks—Chip's Hill, Black Hill, and the Six White Hills all over a thousand feet. I had a long talk with a twenty-one-year-old son of the local merchant. He says his "brains are glued together." I was shocked at the ease with which his well-to-do father accepted my services for nothing. I took an acute dislike to him. We pulled out of there right after breakfast and went to Center Arm where Dalley says the tough Thomas' live, bandits, wreckers and what not. One of them was a little snotty. All we did was pull teeth. Then for a glorious hour down the southwest arm to Rattling Brook. The sun was definitely out, though the wind was cold and a bit of sea swept into the Green Bay even as far as this. This place is like a Scottish lake. We did a bit of work, though nothing like last year. The skipper got out his brush and painted up the ship a little. We walked down to the Rattling Brook, which tumbles off the plateau like Bridal Veil at Yosemite. I'm going up tomorrow to get a movie if the weather is anything at all.

September 3, '41. Yesterday we left Rattling Brook in dark raining weather and the wind behind us. We went deeper into the bay to King's Point. The rain balked my hope of getting up the brook for pictures. The falls opened up as we went down the run and you could see about 600 feet of the 800 which constitute the whole cataract. A woman was waiting on the dock when we warped into King's Point and we went from one to the next until 6:00. It rained like hell the whole time and they came dripping into the saloon until it was a mess. I was worn out and threatening all day to quit unless it stopped raining. We sent only one away after tea. A quiet evening at home. I wrote a few letters and we sat by the stove and listened to the radio. This morning the wind had risen and we bounded around a lot at the wharf. We had almost nothing to do here but this wind would make Jackson's Cove untenable. I scribbled off a few letters and went to mail them at the post office, an amazing structure—just like a country toilet—old dirty boards, just a lean-to thrown against the back of a house.

Right after dinner they left the wharf and went around a little point to anchor in a cove that is perfectly protected. I stayed on the wharf to cast off and followed in the punt. I heard them let out great quantities of anchor chain and even then it never touched bottom. I had to row a line ashore but we had a terrible time winning the anchor back. There was 90 feet of water twenty yards from shore. We finally made some arrangements but there were a worrisome few minutes. This afternoon just at tea the *Clyde* came. Lidge and I went down to get the moneybox and dental syringe. John and Stan sent notes. Captain Butcher had been looking for us all over the Green Bay. We went aboard and talked to him in his cabin. He said he had had a cup of tea with my sister in Lewisporte. Captain Butcher is a Twillingate man and one of my favorite people in the world. He's 64, gray, blue-eyed, and stocky. He went to work on the *Clyde* as a boy when she came to his bay from Scotland forty years ago. He's been captain for twenty-five years. He's part of the ship when he takes his wide stance on the bridge. He doesn't bother with charts and fancy navigation. He knows every rock and current on the coast. I remember talking to him on the bridge on a pitch-dark night in a roaring rain. I asked him if he was going to leave. "When the moon comes out," says he. In half an hour the darkness changed—perhaps the difference between tar and coal—and he took her out. He'll be talking to you on the bridge in a thick fog when for all you can see you might as well be in a cellar in Pittsburgh and he'll lean over to the speaking tube and say, "Port a wee bit." The *Clyde* herself, maybe 600 tons, looks like a yacht, sheer, clipper-bowed and graceful. There's a rakish slant to her mast and funnel. She's white topside, gilt trimmed and black hull. He handles her like a punt and takes her in among rocks that you can touch with your hand. Last winter during a poker game in my room, we heard a noise like the *Clyde*'s whistle. Captain Butcher started, then smiled and said, "That sounded like the *Clyde*—the day she blows and I'm not aboard is the day I die."

In the evening, I got rid of that box on the settee finally and made shelves for all the drugs. The place is still muddled but it's a start. I had more rum and cocoa tonight—that's very good stuff. Now to bed and I hear the wind blowing. Lidge says he's going to put another line ashore before we turn in. If the wind shifts much we'll be aground, but there's no real danger and that's his lookout, I suppose.

September 4, '41. Another rotten day. We woke in the bottom of Green Bay, our hook out with eighteen fathoms of irretrievable chain on it and a line to the shore as well. The wind still blew a gale and the air was full of rain spit. I don't suppose the sun will ever shine again. I would have gotten up as soon as Martin called me but he didn't put a fire in the saloon so I didn't stir until nearly 10:00. We couldn't look at the bay but I don't mind these days of forced inactivity. We kept swinging parallel to the shore and only twenty feet from it but the lead showed five to twelve fathoms—as close as that! Lidge and I walked around the bottom of the cove, fording the streams that make a large flat delta. After dinner we moved back to the wharf where we had to throw the mooring line six times before anybody caught it. They are lousy catchers. We thought we would try the bay. It was quiet enough below decks though the wind blew gales. Lidge said he was scared once or twice when the wind came in all directions. Great drifts of rain swept off the shore. The *Clyde* couldn't go to Tilt Cove because the wind circles down from that cliff and drives her against the wharf.

Jackson's Cove is not much of a place. We anchored inside the point and saw twenty patients in no time at all. That included a shore call on a nut. I hurried because Lidge was against spending the night there. The local people said it was a good place, but Lidge said they make their living from the ships that go aground. At 9:00, almost pitch dark, we crossed the bay. The wind fair took the paint off the deck and now we have the big hook out.

September 5, '41. It was a rough night over the ring of our anchor. The wind blew off the eight hummocks like "out of a pipe." I woke as I heard the men laboring at the windlass and with some reluctance shoved my pajamas into a pair of pants and unwashed, climbed on deck to help. A bit of wind was still at it and the current of the stream brought down a spume that might well have been slob ice. As I reached for the handle, I was hailed from a punt by a man who asked me to go ashore to see a swollen face. I knew it must be erysipelas and wanted to send some pills but I groaningly donned some clothes and grabbed the sulphathyasol. The patient had a swollen face and a sullen air. I gave him a quick one, two, three, and some pills. The charge was two dollars and a quarter. He hauled out a five and I took just two because I didn't want to fool around with change. He was unresponsive and thankless. I froze back towards the boat. It was weaving crazily around the harbor as if she were ducking torpedoes. The anchor had caught on the keel and they were trying to dislodge it. I had to do it for them by hand and scrambled aboard while they held the punt as steady as they could in the tide.

It was a clever trip to Green Bay Island and as we rounded it we did some fancy tossing with all the canvas on. We were in the lun then, but Martin took her so close to Brandis Rock that we caught the back lop and she jumped so that the skipper came on deck from his breakfast with a bound. Says he, "I don't believe it's necessary to go so handy to that rock." There was a big sea breaking in great long angry white and green whirlpools. Harry's Harbor was too tough for us to stay to the wharf. While we went around a corner to the harbor within a harbor, I tried to shave and cut the end of my nose. There we met Mr. Simmons. His daughter married the successful Redway and moved with him to Springdale when the herring trade failed. He died there and his last wish was that his wife should go to Ireland, his birthplace, to bring up their son. That she did and they were well off at first but had finally come to taking boarders. In one of the very few air raids on Ireland, her house has taken a direct hit. The son and six boys were killed but she had gone to the hospital the day before for some minor operation.

We did quite a business in children's teeth and scurried out around the point to Three Arms. We felt the greatly increased sea but it was short and we went deep into the cut, then through a tickle and down a long deep run to Southern Arm where we had good anchorage but no business. Mr. Yates' mill is here but he does only a bit of planing now because his boiler has been held to 60 pounds pressure. He probably didn't bribe the government boiler inspector enough, for the latter is a sonovabitch and a crook. Ted says so. He passed the hospital sterilizing boiler the day before it blew up. We had a quiet night. The wind is still north to northwest. The sky lifted slowly at 6:00 and now at midnight there are stars and moon.

This phosphorescent water is lovely in a dory on a dark night. The boat leaves a trail behind it of delicate white sparkling glimmer like a satin train of sequins in a dim night.

September 8, '41. The next day, namely Saturday, was a beaut, though proper cold. We had a lot of small ports to call at and coasted along easily enjoying ourselves. I woke to a magnificent clear crystal clever morning. I was dazzled as I poked my head out of the hatch, it was enough to make you cry—the blue overhead and the early morning light and the cliffs to our starboard as we went into Wild Bight. We had rounded a high point and were coming down on the lee side of it to enter this shallow scallop, which is a poor harbor. We spent a good part of the morning there. I didn't want to leave in a hurry because I was eager to clean the saloon. We scrubbed the dirty damned place and now it's beginning to look like a habitation for human beings. There used to be a mine here and old Boyd, 78, still hangs around the rotting wharfs of what was once a business. He busies himself in a vest and stiff collar by sawing wood. He was bemused entirely by my shorts and volunteered the information that the women were all away berry picking but I would scare them to death when they came back. I put on a coat and held the punt while the skipper painted the bow in a cold twilight. I forgot the lovely stop at Little Bay, shown on the sheet as Indian Bight. It was like being in a country strange to us as Bolivia would be—a straight deep indraft with seven fathoms right up to a sharp shingled beach. The hills look like slag piles, bare and loose. A tumbling stream cascaded off the slope to meander through a floodplain heavily turfed on which sheep and geese roamed. The houses were fenced and surrounded by lone groups of trees like western desert houses. We had a good time there seeing a few patients and painting.

By dark we made St. Patrick's and at the rotten wharf our chimney caught on fire and messed up all our new paint. We saw a few patients that night including a lady who began, "I may as well tell you, doctor, I'm a woman who has had five operations." We lay about the next morning doing very little and slowly made our way out of the bottom of the indraft to the perfect little Ward's Harbor, where wind was not enough to straighten out our grapple lines. The lovely day was gone. It was raining and cloudy again. I felt sorry for an old man— saw him for nothing. He turned out to be the owner of the Rambler Gold Mine, which he's trying to sell for $30,000. From there we wandered up the coast to Woodford Cove where an obliging gent yelled from the shore that no one was coming out to see us. Pleased, we went on for another hour around Cooper Island to dodge a reef. When we approached Little Bay Islands, I was below because it was cold and windy. I soon came on deck when I felt the short backlop that

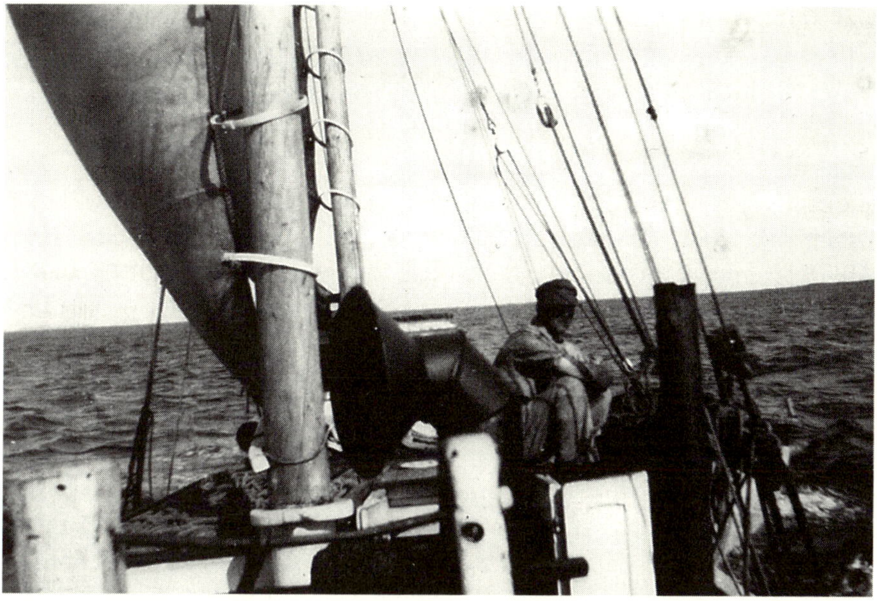

Martin, the "crew" on the *Bonnie Nell,* aft of the chimney. Author's photograph.

means rocks are near and I thought the skipper was trying to commit suicide. We were headed for a maelstrom of breaking seas. We coasted right through them into the perfect shelter of Little Bay Islands. We had hardly landed and pulled a few teeth for the swooning midwife when Jim Strong was aboard to invite me up for tea. Jim is an old friend of the hospital, but I didn't know him well. I went with misgivings but as in almost all such cases enjoyed myself very much. It has always been my experience that the Newfoundlander in his own home is a generous friendly and considerate host. I was aboard late with gifts of fish, maps, and meat. Today we ate the meat and it was a standard day of 39 patients and $37. I made a shore call on Uncle Dolph's mother-in-law, a fine, beautiful, spiritful, 85-year old Scotch woman with lots of cancer. I liked her very much. They paid me and gave me bread and butter. After our evening cocoa and chocolate cake that I bartered for two teeth, I listened to that 'Paul Revere' from Germany. I wish I could catch that bastard.

September 10, '41. Last night we received a wire from Stan telling us to resume his strep throat research in Lockport. We took off at the crack of dawn into the teeth of a northeaster. I stayed in the bunk and mentally followed the chart by the spurts of bad pitching and smoother water. It tested my bottle rack to the full as we went into Pilly Island Tickle and Long Tickle. I came on deck as we entered Seal Bay and got into a bit of a lun. To the skipper's surprise and my amusement, we found we had left Rita, our nurse, in Little Bay Islands. Her loving airman, home from Halifax on a furlough, had spent a fortune chasing her all over the bay on hired boats and finally had caught up with her in LBI. They all stayed ashore at Hillier's and had a time, but she had failed to tell us. We found Lockport, a fine landlocked harbor, and soon, after we anchored, I got shaved and dressed and followed an old crock ashore. He was far gone in beriberi, but scrabbled up over the rocks like a goat. At the first house I found all the children convalescing from bad throats. They had sent for the father to come home from the woods when the children were sick. He had caught it and was in bed with a terrific membrane on his tonsils. His sister, next door, had the worst throat I ever saw. It stank and was covered well up into the palate with a terrible, dirty membrane. Her uvula was a swollen little knob and she could get only a little whisper of air through. Her temperature was low, his was high. I was in doubt about diagnosis. It didn't behave like diphtheria, but the children, now well, had had nose bleeds and one was reported to have talked as if his palate were paralyzed. Some of them had vomited through their noses. The man who had died before Stan went to this place had dropped dead on the beach.

There had been a death in a nearby settlement. I followed a man over the hill for two miles through the rain to halloo for a boat across another tickle and wait for a decrepit old gent to go with him to a point of land with three families on it. I put them all under quarantine and saw the dead thirteen-year old girl. She had had such sickness often I was relieved to hear (that meant it couldn't be diphtheria) and was laid out pitifully, single blue wild flower in her rayon dress and pennies on her eyes. Rita arrived all of a sudden, scared, trembling, red in the face with Stan Hillier on the *Miss Labrador*. Her doughty pilot had hired still another boat, and a nice craft it was. I looked into the cabin where they were still at breakfast and was impressed to see a clean white tablecloth. It all looked very gemutlich. I set Rita to work on Ricka, our woman with the bad throat and by night we had her swallowing. In the evening we listened to the radio and the storm. I sent Hillier to Leading Tickle with a wire to the hospital for a microscope. This morning we were going to hang around and wait for Hillier to come back, but I got the bright idea that we ought to make a smear from the throat and take it to the Canadian army hospital at Botwood. We could get there in this weather. On every other trip I've carried a microscope but this time there wasn't a spare. I broke the glass on a picture of the Royal Family hanging in the wheelhouse. I took some of the stuff from Ricka's throat and made a smear on a jagged piece of glass.

Never again will I tell a layman that there is a medical emergency. It was no day to travel, but Lidge was determined to get me to Botwood to a microscope. He took the bit in his teeth and at 2:50 we left. I had an hour in the ashes while we punched to Leading Tickle. I took three stiff jolts of rum and sat on the floor trying to write a letter. We put our nose under a couple of lops and that frightened even Martin. I watched the Leading Tickle headland creep towards us to protect us, but I thought it would never do it. Into safety at Leading Tickle we stopped only ten minutes for a telegram to the hospital and off again, this time with canvas on, thank God, to hold us over. But the mountainous broadside lops really wet us. The skipper kept her into them well, but nothing could keep us off our beam. Soon we squared away with this one setting her backside on the following seas and scooting along like an old maid on a thunderbolt. We made Point Leamington in record time. In an hour we had a car bumping us over this execrable narrow road for twenty-three miles to Botwood. We were cold. A car caught up with us and they told us they had left a wire for us saying, "Come immediately" somewhere, they didn't remember where. We wondered about that all night but we were already On His Majesty's Service so we went to the hospital. We were received royally, the skipper and I, by Captain Levinsky, a mere youngster. He got out his microscope and stain and we spent a half-hour assuring ourselves that this was streptococcus and not diphtheria. I've always believed that dip smears gave me no trouble in diagnosis. He showed us about the one-floored "E" shaped hospital and it was done well. They're a little short on surgical equipment. A nursing sister from Prince Edward Island made us some coffee and toast and, seated in the little office with an electric heater to take the ice off, we had a tête-à-tête, which was fun. We were more than delighted with our reception. The twenty-three miles back took us an hour and twenty minutes. The wire turned out to have something to do with sending us antitoxin. Rumor here was that our patient had died though she was all right when we left, and no one could possibly have come down from Lockport.

September 11, '41. This day for the umpteenth in a row started with rain, but the wind was western and the sky a promise of better things. We decided to work Point Leamington, which we did. We saw eighteen patients and took in about eighteen dollars, finishing up at 4:00. We put our canvas on and pursued a course back to Leading Tickle. The water was some changed as we hit the familiar spots. There was quite a ground swell on. It was fun to review the trip down as we came around Northwest Rock and saw the light on the point where the sea had hit us so hard on the beam. We arrived at the wharf in a squall of wind and rain and were tied up only long enough to inquire at the post office. Evidently our wire had headed off the boat from Twillingate with the microscope and the diphtheria antitoxin. Back at Lockport we had tea and found things ashore much the same.

September 12, '41. This day dawned like a daisy—clear cold and bright. Someone came aboard pretty early so I sent the nurse ashore with him. I did a bit of washing, starting with handkerchiefs and going on through socks, sweater, and myself. I put on white pants and felt like a million dollars. I spent the day reading and writing. The skipper painted and Rita made a cake. A man was surprised when I told him that he was sick with a septic throat and couldn't run around town with the other boys even if they did have the same disease. Things ashore with Ricka are a little better. The irrigation cleaned a great hunk of membrane off the left tonsil with much bleeding. She's better but still in tough shape.

September 13, '41. We saw our patients this morning and accepted an offer of a few potatoes. We dug them ourselves because everybody's sick. I lay in the sun as we steamed around Leading Tickle, happy that the slough was coming off the other tonsil. We nudged our bow into a motley bunch of bullboats and nondescript motorboats. Few people came until after dinner because the usual mistaken or vicious rumors were abroad that we were going across the bay. I had to deny that I said Mr. Rowsel was dying, that the Hacketts had started it, and what not. Mr. Rowsel is Ricka's brother-in-law. The rest of the day was spent in examining patients and trying to get my sweater dry. I walked around the harbor to the justice of the peace to get my bill for $75 okayed. He was full of bromides—an apple a day and all the rest.

I couldn't get Martin to cook bacon for tea. He had heated the beans and it was too much of a problem to change pans. He won't wash the marmalade off the outside of the tin either. I wished we had someone on board I could order around. Rita is learning, though she does stand and stare while the blood runs down the patient's chin, or some woman dangles her baby down the hatch until it's blue in the face, or while I look for a light or a tongue stick. I have to tell her to wash the towels and the gloves. She is slow getting up and lets the patients talk and talk.

September 14, '41. This was a beautiful day. I woke before being called but Martin can't read my thoughts and would do as he pleased if he did. I got up in the cold with no fire, much surprised that I had slept, for the dogs were howling like the damned when I went to sleep and when I woke. Perhaps the precautionary veronal helped. Breakfast was a sad affair, no bread, the coffee cold, and the bacon all fat. I enjoyed it though and soon we were under steam back to Lockport. There we checked up on our throats. Mrs. Rowsel had gotten a bit better but she insisted on sleeping with her husband when I told her not to. She also wanted me to examine her son for bed-wetting and her husband for the gas, but I declined. Ricka was much better. We left through Dunier Tickle and around Seal Bay Head. I froze in shorts in the sun, which was hot, but the wind was bitter out of a profound blue north. The distribution of the ulnar nerve in my right arm got numb and white just as it did in Shoal Arm when I helped the skipper paint. We steamed into Beaumont North to find the whole population on the beach at an immersion ceremony of the Pentecostals. There was much hymn singing with 'h's dropped and added, which gives Scripture a peculiar twist. We watched the very chilly immersion from the boat. Across the harbor we could hear the preacher say, "You don't have to go over to the hospital boat. Belief will cure you."

September 15, '41. Belief must have cured them—we didn't do much there. We piddled along till noon. We got a wire telling us to come immediately to Jim's Cove—John Roberts was very sick. I had dinner at sea while we hurried through tickle after tickle cutting all the corners into Badger Bay. On Great Dunier Island we spied a lone, skinny gray horse and I felt very sorry for the poor thing for I know how companionable horses are. On Twillingate they congregate by the dozens on the mish. By 4:00 we were in Jim's Cove, populated entirely by Roberts all from the loins of the 90-year old crock who had sent for me. In spite of thousands of relatives and having been rich in his day, old John dwelt in a tiny shack with his blithe second wife, a mere 71, who is reported to have given his money to her children. The opening gun of old John was, "there's no charge for this, is there doctor?" I didn't tell him I planned to charge $30; after all we had brought four people and a gas-eating boat forty miles for more than a day. He was just old and rheumatic and adrift in his head. I went to the home of Stanley, his son, and there they gathered up $25. I sat in the dirty and fly-blown kitchen and watched the fourth generation—one Warrick some three years old having his afternoon nap. Like an old man he sat in the little high rocker, his chest covered by a torn sweater, across his tiny knees a coat, exposing his crossed black-nailed feet. His elbows rested on each arm symmetrically and his hands hung down. His head was thrown back in the mid-line and he was ticking it off like the just. We finished the town, having made a beautiful landing between an unloading schooner in the stream and a cluster of punts at the stagehead wharf. We turned on a dime and put our clear side in like a toy.

September 16, '41. I had planned to get up as soon as the engine started, but the pre-dawn was cold, rainy, and dark. I stayed abed even while we were going through fabulous Pretty Tickle. I had to get up though when I heard the engine skip the second time as the second tank ran out of gas. We made Lush's Bight on our emergency tank. I don't know what Martin does. The filthy fo'c'sle is full of dirty dishes, the saloon is dabbed out with a salt mop, mustard and jam pots are saved with a half inch of stuff in the bottom, our meals are poor, and the tanks empty. I had to leave a root in one seventeen-year old stoic after I loosened the wisdom behind and her twelve-year molar in the front. I made a shore call and an old cove talked me out of a dollar and I gave him fifty cents worth of codeine free. He had water on the knee. In the kitchen was a painting of Belle Isle, very local, where they had spent the winter. The son of a lighthouse keeper there did it and the wife said I was the only man she'd ever seen who looked like him. One old man, on whom I pulled a tooth, had worked on the *Grace Hickman*. That was something to be proud of, for she was the most beautiful three-master ever to leave the stocks of Newfoundland. Sheer as a bottle and a smooth 400 tons—fitted like a yacht—turnbuckles instead of lanyards—she made fourteen knots under canvas. She made one voyage to England in the last war and was torpedoed on her way home with salt. "It was a sin," the old man said with tears in his eyes.

Gladys Parsons, here, is famous for her canning. I got some canned strawberries. I saved the juice and added apricot juice, rum and alcohol. A Twillingate friend here on business, Henry Randall, came aboard and we had a party. We were going to play cards but we couldn't find any. We tried aboard the 86-ton big-bellied schooner beside us but they were shocked and said we wouldn't find any cards this side of the harbor. We planned to leave in the evening, but the northeaster breezed and it got thick. We drank instead. Randall was a riot. He sang and talked of his visits to the States and his argument with a subway turnstile and how a policeman gave him a nickel. I went to sleep unquietly.

September 17, '41. I woke when the engine refused to start and now it's noon and they've had the head off and found the cylinder full of seawater. It's frozen and God knows when we will get away. Then a wire came, asking us to hurry back to Lockport because Ricka was very sick. We are out of gas, tobacco, coal and what not—not a clean bit of linen and this racket is beginning to pall on me. What a day this turned out to be. They took the engine all apart again and swabbed the water out and wore out two batteries. At 6:00 they got it going but instead of going 'put put' and giving out smoke, it went 'foosh foosh' with a cloud of steam. Harry Randall came to dinner. I bought a jar of pickles when I couldn't get coffee in a dismal little shop. I dropped them into the fo'c'sle and they hit the 7/8 shotgun we are carrying back to have repaired for John Roberts and broke. I was going to salvage them but they are full of glass. Rita and I had a tea party. I had cooked breakfast and for once it was good. The eggs done properly and more bacon with the rind off than anyone could eat. Rita is the first person I ever met who didn't like bacon or canned roast beef. Just another one of her peculiarities.

We were ready to go at 6:30 and off we started on our two-hour run to Lockport. I went below after tea to try to read but the weather had me worried. I took a few drinks and followed the course carefully by my compass and the chart. I felt the bumps as we hit Badger Bay. I looked aloft and it was pitch dark. There were rain "dwys" and when we got to Seal Bay Head with the rocks just around it, I was petrified. You really couldn't see a goddam thing. Awhile back, I had seen the lights of Jim's Cove and suggested to the skipper that we put in. He said he'd love to but didn't know it well enough to try. I warned him to open Seal Bay wide before he turned in. My compass failed me. I found out later what it pointed at was not the magnetic pole but the cash box at the head of my bed. Nevertheless, I watched our eastward course waiting to detect our turn into the bay. But it didn't show a change of course. I heard the skipper yelling to Martin and went on deck. I expected open sea on our port and instead there was high looming land. I asked Lidge what it was and he said to my tremendous relief that it was the peninsula that makes Lockport Harbor or does the harbor being there make the peninsula? Well anyhow it was black. He told me to take the port quarter because he couldn't see. I warned him off the point and we made straight for the dark cliff and followed it in. I never had such respect for a man. He's God. He did anchor it too near the point and, in the rain, Martin rowed a line ashore to pull it away from the rocks. Rita and I went ashore to see our dying woman. Her throat had healed and her temperature normal. She was having "weak turns," a cough and was "stomach-sick." I gave her veronal and we had cocoa and went to bed after the tightest navigational spot I had ever been in. Not even considering the geography and the weather, I had listened to every turn of the engine for that failure I knew must be inevitable. It blew a gale all night but we scoffed at the groaning rigging.

September 18, '41. A good breakfast at 8:00 and soon ashore to see the sick. The nearer Rowsel family is in good shape and even Ricka is better—not dying as advertised. We scrounged some wood and some water and collected $10 from the brother David and were soon at sea. We have to abandon our trip and go home for a new engine or a new boat. Our engine only just caught and we were off in a cloud of steam for our five-hour journey. The skipper was afraid to stop in Leading Tickle. I wanted to send a telegram to the hospital saying we were coming home with a failing engine and not to let us drift too long. We hailed a man in a punt and threw him fifty cents and a message. We ignored the signals from the wharf.

September 19, '41. All went well yesterday. I kept the bottle busy and it was a clever voyage. A good-sized lop developed getting larger as we approached Long Point. We took turns getting shaved and neat. We sighted a boat coming out of Twillingate Harbor and thought it was sent to meet us, but it was making heavy weather and turned deep into the bay. Just as we got by Long Point the wind freshened seriously enough to make us take in our canvas. We heeled well over before we got it furled. The

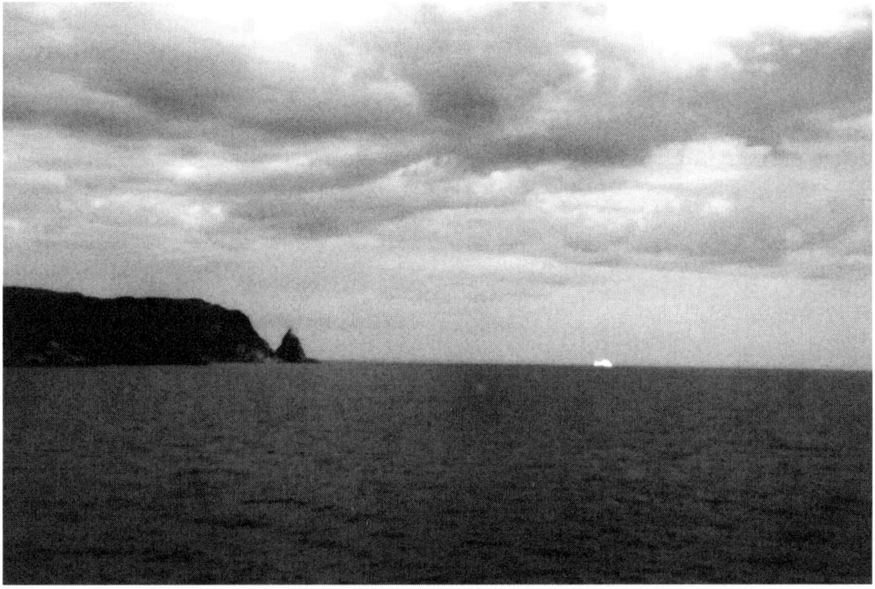

Mother Burke, a.k.a. Bishops Rock, Cape St. John, Newfoundland. Author's photograph..

wind by then was a fresh gale from the northwest. It was really blowing by the time we had dropped our little anchor well inside and pulled in the heavy mooring that has a 3000-pound anchor on it. The chain weighs ten pounds a link. No one has seen the anchor for years. It may well be rusted to crump. We all went below for a farewell drink, which discouraged the waiting John who gave up and returned to the hospital. Stan met us at the wharf in the station wagon that John had strangely bought. The greetings were warm and I was happy to feel that people were glad to see me. I had a tub and we finished off the rum in my room before a nice tea. They've been busy. John was sick in bed for two days and Betty is not well. Stan thinks she has an ulcer.

The wind breezed all night and by morning was a roaring northeaster. They couldn't work on the *Bonnie Nell* and I watched her all day, thinking she might go ashore. The waves go the full height of Paradise Head, and Carter's Head is a boiling cauldron. The harbor mouth is breaking right across and that is fourteen fathoms. This is the first time I have seen the waves go over the coastal wharf and breakwater. Stan went over to the wharf to watch the sea, and stones as big as his head were hurled onto the wharf. There are a few Labradormen anchored in the harbor, but they seem to be holding. One of them is very low in the water with its summer catch. The rain in the window frames gurgled like bilge all day. Jim Finney, one of the students, is staying here until November. That's a big help to us. I didn't operate today. I was loath to get back into that practice which gives me my morning qualms. John has been taking prostates out from below and having lots of success. Stan went to the Tilt today though Annette said she didn't care to fight rats. I gave them a dozen eggs.

September 21, '41. The lovely northeaster of Friday receded finally and left us with nondescript weather. The sun came out only a little today and the wind backed around to the west, but the sky to the northeast is bad and the wind is pulling around again to the quarter. Nobody bothered to tell me that the *Bonnie Nell* has been condemned and we won't voyage further in her until the engine is replaced. I think it will be difficult to operate in Hillier's boat, the *Miss Labrador*, but it's the best boat I can think of. While I am here, John and Stan and Jim are getting some time in at the Tilt. I've been in a stinking mood, helped neither by Benzedrine nor alcohol. I see no refuge but Luminal and bed. I don't know what is doing it. I shouldn't feel like this after three weeks away. I have the 'must get going' feeling—ulcer-like in my epigastrium. I'm unable to tell anyone about it and am surprised to find myself being pleasant. Talk does not come easy and I wonder how it will work out. I have some understanding for Chalian. He replaced me last year while I was away. Word came a week ago that he committed suicide. I wonder why he didn't crack up while he was still here if he had it in him. I want to go to the tropics now.

September 29, '41. Here is a whole week wasted except that perhaps I recovered a bit of my surgical confidence, never too good at best—an appendix with Jim and some adult tonsils. The supporting team say they prefer to have me do the tonsils, there is less noise and confusion. I helped the boss do a difficult tumor of the face that involved the facial nerve and the large artery.

Much of the week was spent in trying to get a boat to finish the bay trip. Finally the *Miss Labrador* was chartered, a nice two-cabined job, a little slow, with Herb Hillier at the throttle. It will be crowded and we may even come to doing the work ashore. I don't give a damn what happens, I will be so glad to get away from the hospital. Ever since I am back, and all tell me I have lost weight, I have a nausea, an apprehensive feeling in my stomach which sometimes makes me think I really am going to vomit. I feel about keeping this journal the same way that Wilson, who was with Scott at the South Pole, felt about Nansen's taking pictures of himself and a friend killing each others' dogs. It's introversion, and any introversion is bound to lead to self-consciousness of emotion, and that heaps up like images in a hall of mirrors until you don't know whether you are doing something for its effect on yourself or not. I have that sensation almost every time I weep. Tears in my eyes make me self-conscious and the emotion is dulled by wondering what I look like. Today I thought we would be leaving. John came into my bedroom to wake me. He sat down and chatted awhile. I'd had a bad night. I didn't sleep well, had delivered a baby at 3:00, and listened to the dogs as I turned and groaned. When I did fall asleep, it was to attend a convention in Bridgeport where the Earl of Connaught and a large, motorized series of connected stoves were featured. Each stove had a large roast of beef on it and there was much running up and down stairs. John finally got up to leave and asked me if I were ill.

After the operation he said he wanted to ask me a question. I assented and he asked how long I planned to stay, as Swanker was available and he would sign him up if I were leaving. Well I didn't know. I suppose I ought to make up my mind. All year I felt that Swanker was a competitor, and tonight I told John so. I said he should consider if he wants a man who won't do intern work, who will take his weekends regularly, and will want to operate. Perhaps I will get out and let him come. It would be a mild sort of punishment for them for their lack of appreciation of the factors that make me useful to this place—poor scared ineffectual that I am. Even Walter, the dentist, in the absence of his wife has taken to talking to me and telling me that I need self-assurance. I don't know and Christ, I think I'm going just a little crazy. I have to get out of this.

The wind today was strong from the west and Ted tied his boat to the crippled *Bonnie Nell.* As definite and sudden as the opening of a window, the wind hove in from the northeast with a great lop tossing the boats in the harbor and straightening their chains. Ted moved his after ramming the *Bonnie Nell* and really burying his head in spray.

October 1, '41. Yesterday I spent the whole twenty-four hours being on the point of leaving, but the wind was a gale from the west and southwest and the new skipper, Herb Hillier of Little Bay Islands, wouldn't budge. He's a man after my own heart and I don't think I have to worry with him. Stan was up all night on an OB case. He sent for Stella in the morning but before she could get there, the patient fooshed and there was no need. I didn't scrub. I found myself alone in the OPD all afternoon. John was in Friday's Bay and Stan made calls. A red-hot belly came in (white count 19,000). I wondered about waiting for John to come back, but Stan urged me to get it over with before John turned up. He thought it would be good to have John feel that we could take care of things. It was a good idea except that my evil fate pursued me. It was perhaps the toughest I've ever done. I had to rotate entirely the loose ascending colon and, pasted to the back of it, covered by a veil of thin adhesions, the appendix curled on itself and was ten inches long and way the hell up under the liver. The incision had to be enlarged. I started in the middle and went both ways. It took one and a half hours but came out intact with no bleeding. Saturday Stan and Annette went to the Tilt to put hot compresses on Stan's boil. I joined them for tea. Jim broached a bottle of rum just before I left. The bloody light doesn't work on the cycle and it wouldn't go into low. It backfired and took skin off my foot and cut my shoe. I had to give myself a tetanus shot.

John was disgusted with Hillier's reluctance to face the wind. He went down to the boat and practically ordered him out of the harbor. As we started out of the harbor, Hillier, unruffled, confided to me that as skipper of schooners he always moved on when the owners got mad even if he only went around the next point and anchored. We shied out through the back door, Burnt Island Tickle and over to Moreton's Harbor through Main Tickle. That kept Twillingate Island between us and the weather. This lovely, but poorly powered craft is a dream in rough water. I called at the Osmonds' and came back to the ship for a nap. About 4:00 the wind abated and we started across the bay to the fabulous Fortune Harbor, hidden among the crags. The rain poured down. I was prepared for something terrible as we crossed the run outside of Exploits and Black Island. I took some veronal and read Wilson's Antarctic book. I was delightfully surprised to feel so little movement. Northern Head was gruff and gray and it was good to find that narrow entrance to shelter. The boat was snug and nice. The eating quarters are comfortable. Meals are fun. The skipper's taciturn, overgrown boy of sixteen is the cook. It's hard to get a word out of him. After tea we had lots of talk. In the last war the skipper served on a 17,000-ton auxiliary cruiser that took four torpedoes aboard and sank in two minutes with loss of over a hundred. He then volunteered for minesweeping. I like him very much and am going to see that he gets the money for a new engine.

Sleeping is a little heads and tails aboard this one and it's no joke to stow our gear. Rita has a bunk in the narrow fo'c'sle, the two men sleep aft and I have a bed in the cabin. We eat, cook, and see patients in the same cabin. I will have to use my own bed for examining patients. We had our evening cocoa, the rain beating down on our roof and I am tired. The night will be pleasant, I think, in spite of a hard bunk. It was fun to be kicked out of the harbor. John must have had a good time throwing us out.

October 2, '41. After our worries and trials of yesterday, it was nice to have a quiet day in port. The halyards slapped on the main-mast all night and the wind blew a gale from the northwest. We saw twenty-four patients or so, including the delectable Mrs. Freeman Fowlow, who is a prime whatsis with her pains and her change of life and her introspection. Her poor old husband takes it on the chin. I was talking to him for quite a while before I found out who he was. I remembered him as a thin older man and I find him a fat young one. He has gained twenty-odd pounds since last we met. The clinical work was nothing special—the regular stuff, babies and teeth. The new priest was away. He was away the last time I was here. I'm afraid he doesn't have the missionary zeal of his predecessor, Father Casey, nor like that of Father Henry of Parry Sound in *Kabloona*. In the evening we had a couple of patients and went to Fowlow's until 2 A.M. for Auction 45 and a scoff (refreshments). Fowlow had scratched around to get a bit of beer and dandelion wine. We talked a lot and had a good time. Herb grew mellow and told us about his troubles as a purser on one of the Newfoundland steamers. He spoke particularly of the rough-spoken Brigus man, Captain Clark, who had his own methods of navigation, but couldn't make out an accident report without Herb. He moved the heavens to keep Herb on his ship. They put into a tiny harbor once for refuge. Herb's mother and father happened to live there and he hadn't seen them for two years. The crew didn't dare speak to the old man, but Herb with trembling says, "Captain, will you put the mail boat out for me," and explained why. The captain stepped on deck and bawled to the bo'sun to lower away. Herb asked how long he could stay. The Captain snapped, "Use your own judgment." Herb found his parents and they talked for hours with no mind to the weather. His brother suddenly noticed the fog had lifted. They got out a punt and went for the ship as fast as they could. The smoke was going straight up. He heard the whistle. As they rounded the bow, the anchor started up. As he stepped aboard, the captain snarled,

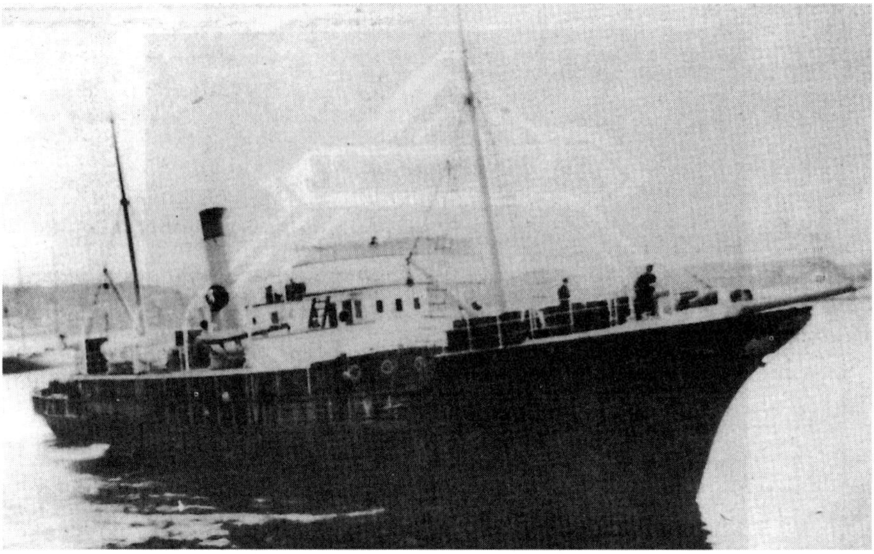

S.S. *Clyde,* life blood to Notre Dame Bay.

"Is that you, purser?" "Yes" weakly—he heard the bell for full speed ahead. His frightened crewmates told him he would be skinned. Herb went below, got cleaned up, and crept to the bridge. "I'm sorry, captain," he started, but didn't have a chance to say any more. Looking straight ahead at the lifting fog the captain said, "How are the old people? I knew you couldn't hear the whistle, or you would have been back sooner."

There were two old brothers, eighty-odd, living together. One unmarried, religious, and one a tough widower. After a heavy meal the gentle one said, "I must have a pee." The other said, "Great God, the likes of thee and I brought up on blubber and gurf—saying pee, when the finest lady in New York would say piss."

October 3, '41. The halyards hammered all night. Right after breakfast the skipper decided to go out and see what was to be done. I sent a wire saying we were off and fortified myself with ten grains of veronal. I went to the after cabin near the wheel. It was cheering when still in the narrows to hear Herb say we couldn't do anything, but not so cheering when he kept on. The sea was mountains, the wind was a cold northeast and we weren't in it yet, but my God, what a lop—end on end, squirms, screw-motions, reversed slides and pitches. It is amazing the number of dimensions in which a craft this size can operate. Herb kept on into it and I was in a panic. I got violently ill, not nauseated, but really in a vasomotor cyclone. Clear of the rocks and away from the backlop, I saw Herb with steel in his eyes brace himself to bring her around. Feeling all gone I held on with a merciful kind of void in me, while she broached. I remembered what the *Bonnie Nell* did when Lidge pulled her around. I waited but she spun around with never a murmur. She's a daisy in a broadside. I felt lovely as we skipped in with the lop on our tail. We fooled around all day and at 6:00, suddenly the skipper decided to try again. I never liked that word "try." I was not delighted. Out we went and down the straight front. It was a tumbly time, everything shifted. We cleared New Bay Head wide so as not to come in with the wind right on our beam. The *Clyde* passed us making heavy weather. Silver Buckle Island gave us shelter in the lovely red sunset. The sky cleared with the evening star vivid, and the moon only waiting for the sun to go. It presaged a good day. Tea was late at Cottle's Cove. I slept, of course, before dinner and after tea, being full of veronal, but I slept the night too, even though the halyards got to work again.

October 4, '41. A gale from the southwest and the rain had snow in it. A few patients came aboard and a solicitous character took me for a shore call. He saw us last night coming in and thought we had broken down, that's how slow this engine is. He put a Cape Ann oilskin on my head and tied it under my chin. The storm warnings on Gerald Doyle's program made the skipper anxious to get across New Bay. We left while I ate my dinner. That Rita cooked me three eggs, which leaves only three more and someone will have to go without his breakfast. It blew hard crossing New Bay. Leading Tickle seemed nice and quiet. The skipper was worried but past Thimble Head it was calm, so we went comfortably across Seal Bay and Badger Bay inside the rocks for Little Dunier accompanied by a coterie of gamboling porpoises. One was throwing himself clear of the water with abandon. One kept going right under the bow showing his white belly. Only once did I get a good view of his flat tail. Triton is a charming land-locked harbor. I fed a dog through the porthole—a can of salmon. The evening was quiet and the promised northwest storm has not broken. I dare say the halyards will start popping tomorrow. We don't care now. We can do everything but Wellman's Cove. A bad northwest wind will keep us out of Hall's Bay, but nothing can really worry us until we start home. God give us a decent passage, for I am sure my nerve is shot.

Having a lovely time this evening. The hated electric light gave out and I am writing and reading by lamps. The cabin is quiet, warm, and cozy. All have gone ashore, and I have a noggin of rum by my side and couldn't be happier.

October 5, '41. Not much to say about this day, shore calls for beriberi, strokes, and pre-natals. I pulled a few teeth and then kind of called things off. The wind was northeast and rather strong, but not the promised storm. Another quiet evening aboard with the lamps and everyone gone. I read *This Above All.* I was offended by the unnecessary familiarity. He has a good enough idea without introducing that extra stuff.

October 6, '41. A nice enough day. For a change the wind is easterly. There was no rain. Worked like hell all day. Didn't get dinner until 2:00. We stayed in Triton until 3:30. At the end I went up to Mrs. Jackie Thomas, the lady with the big smile who forges checks. She sent for me and said she couldn't pay. She has such pain in her chest that people have to stay with her all night. I did order her baby to the hospital, a little two-year-old holding on to the arm of her mother's chair like an old lady. She had an ulcer on her eye.

We steamed around the point to Brighton. The skipper showed me the place where Fudge, with a clear following moderate wind and a lovely afternoon, put a schooner ashore not five minutes out of harbor. He claimed that the wind had failed. Herb told me about his experience with a man named Smith. Smith asked him for a berth on Herb's 120-ton schooner. Herb went to see him. He was sleeping on the floor of his one room shack. His fourteen-year-old daughter kept house for him. He didn't even have any clothes. Herb fitted him out, down to underwear and gave him a job. They were leaving Little Bay Islands through the devilish tickle, when the wind sort of turned against them. He ordered Smith to man the motorboat because she was falling away on the rocks. He moved so slowly that Herb ran from the wheel and said hurry up. Smith stopped what he was doing and with the schooner drifting onto the point, looked Herb in the face and said he would never let any man, skipper or anyone else, talk to him like that. Herb canned him, putting back to the harbor to do so. We worked hard in Brighton, seeing many a screwball and didn't get tea till 9:00. I was especially irked by one woman who came aboard saying she had a weakness in her back, not a pain, but a weak feeling. It was not until I asked her that she admitted she was eight months pregnant. Another told a friend she had missed a period, but wasn't going to tell me unless I asked. Inasmuch as I was trying to be nice to her and not frighten her about TB, I could have nipped her. I put tea off to see another one because she wanted only one tooth out. When she got below, she said never mind about the tooth, she wanted to talk to me about an itch. When I mentioned sulfur, she said she wouldn't use that and started talking about her stomach. She was a dizzy one. I must look up her operation back at the hospital. I bet she had nothing wrong. We ordered two cakes and bought all the eggs in town and finished off the Teacher's Highland Cream before a very lovely tea. I was so tired I sort of snoozed all evening.

October 7, '41. Waited and waited in the cold north wind for that bloody cake, taking a scattered tooth out the while and finally getting off to Heads Harbor at 10:45. It was a quick run and we weren't there long. I made a shore call and reported to the hospital by wire. The trip to Pilley's Island was beautiful. Amidst the rich full verdure of the evergreen, the autumn frost brought out the fine yellows and bronzes of the hard woods. Little streaks of white birch showed through like the webbing in a worn hanging. The people were slow to arrive because of the rumor that we didn't work in the evenings.

October 8, '41. They didn't even come at a decent hour this morning. We finally were busy. I got an order off to the control office so there will be a drop of rum waiting for me in Twillingate. I was a little mystified by the resemblance of the postmistress here to the one in Nipper's Harbor. She turned out to be the same Mrs. Roberts. It turned cold and sleety before we got to Robert's Arm and the wind is breezing from the east. The teeth here seem to be in especially bad shape. Patients crowded all over the boat. In the crush, in the wheelhouse some dried fish got pushed up against the hot chimney and I blamed the terrible smell on the patients. Some time I must make a list of the things that Rita does that annoy me—her long hair all over the wash stand and all over the butter—her saying to the patients, "here's something to spit in,"—her not being able to get up in the morning.

October 12, '41. Sunday, Port Anson, Sunday Cove Island. Arrived here at 7 P.M. or a little after. Had quite a time tying on, for the lee space behind the government wharf was crowded. We had to move several motor boats and put our lines aboard an 80-ton schooner, a beauty with firm smooth woodwork and towering spars. We left Robert's Arm on a lovely brisk Tuesday morning with bright sun. It was no run at all down to Wolf Cove—on the chart, Springdale in ordinary society. I was looking forward to this stop because it would be a chance to see Edith Simms, now Mrs. Roy Manuel, wife of the constable. He was at the wharf and took me right up for a dinner of salt junk (beef). I had a good bed for once in the attic and was enjoying it at sixty miles per hour only to be called at 5 A.M. by a man who wanted me to go to Little Bay Island. His wife was about to have a baby, was spitting blood. I griped while the poor man went from house to house until he located Rita, who was sleeping ashore. I thought it might be a confinement and took along a catched-up outfit for such work. He had a fine boat and we drank coffee aboard as we watched the sun come up. With the full slanting light, Hall's Bay was lovely indeed and I was glad to have been gotten out. The sea was tremendous. The rocky entrance to Little Bay Island was disconcerting and I chain-smoked cigarettes as soon as I saw the breakers. They were so high I thought at first they were clouds in the sky. Black Rock was hidden and that doesn't happen once in years. The wind was off though, and the passage between the rocks was nothing to what I had expected. The patient is great with imminent child, but still had a tight cervix. There was a general slight swelling, but that had declined since she had gone to bed. Blood pressure was 195/90, heart sounded OK and she was not feverish. She was spitting bright red sputum. The right chest had tubular breathing at the base with coarse rales around it but no great flatness. The left chest had a few rales. There was considerable pain in what I thought was the right diaphragm. It didn't seem wise to get her into labor until we had fixed up the chest. She didn't seem awfully sick, but she was uncomfortable. I left about six dollars worth of sulfa and a little morphine with detailed instructions for its use. It's awfully hard to see patients just once and not know how they came out.

Coming back, the skipper's sister, here from Boston on vacation, said she knew me from the Massachusetts General Hospital. (I had spent the winter of 1934 at Harvard Medical School and had worked in surgery at the M.G.H.) She cooked us a good breakfast as we bowled along and I was never snugger or nicer in my life. I loved it and we were back at work in Springdale too soon. Edith had duck for dinner. She had started to kill her ducks because they were sick and lame. This was a well one, she assured me. The night ashore was comfortable. After breakfast the patients were waiting in scores. The *Northern Ranger* was called to Little Bay Islands because of trouble on the Portuguese ship I saw loading at Strong's. He and the magistrate went off in the face of a northeaster. I tried to work on board but it was no use. We rocked furiously and the rain was solid. I gave up about three after seeing Dr. Lidstone and having the pleasure of witnessing his extreme relief and gratitude when I gave him a clean bill of health. Edith came down about two and waited in the wheelhouse till I finished up. I put one man's tooth off till Sunday, but he said he won't come because he won't have teeth pulled on Sunday. The magistrate came back with Roy to dinner. He's a manic young man, who criticized his colleagues to me and talked till three in the morning. I objected to sleeping with him and I lost a cold poker hand for the big bed. He insisted I sleep in it all the same. He's younger than I. He had found that the trouble in Little Bay Islands was that some young fellows had opened a seal on a bonded keg and done some siphoning. The magistrate couldn't see why they should bother to bring in the full majesty of the law and why they couldn't fix up the seal and crack the boys over the behind.

Sunday morning after some mutton at Edith's, we were off to a late start. A powerful northwest wind with a rising glass blew us down the bay and a good thing it was because the magneto was bad and quitting.

October 13, '41. Up early because the schooner we were hitched to was leaving. They moved her out to the end of the wharf and put us on the inside. We saw about twenty during the day, reaching the 200 mark. Mrs. Reuben Goudy wanted all her teeth out and balked when I would take only four. She says she's tired of having teeth out by the two's and three's. I went aboard the schooner and she's a good one. The load of dried fish in the saloon didn't obscure its cleanliness and light. The fo'c'sle is large and clean. They wound in her anchor at great length pulling themselves well into the stream, then hooked up to a motorboat, for the wind had dropped to a draught. It's raining tonight but the glass is at the top, and I think we'll be able to get to Wellman's Cove and Paddock's Bight tomorrow and then it's through Leading Tickle at last on our way home. We sent a wire off today ordering a new Red Wing engine for *Miss Labrador.*

November 5, '41. Guy Fawkes' Day. Yesterday seemed quiet at first in the OPD. A car stopped at the door and then the bustle and scraping in the hall, which always means someone coming in on a stretcher. The bearers lifted an unconscious fifteen-year-old boy to the table. His neck was rigid with meningitis, his face pallid and his breathing slow, irregular, and gasping. "He's dying, Bessie, get him warm and give him caffeine as quickly as you can." Then I talked to his quiet, frightened mother about her family. "This is the only child I have left", she told me. "I had three little girls but they're all dead." I asked for details.

"One was just a baby—I smothered it."

My quizzled brow brought clarification. "I suppose I smothered it. It was sleeping in bed with me and when I woke up it was dead. The next girl died here in the hospital, paralyzed." I remember hearing about a strange paralysis case that had come in and died. It wasn't infantile—we never knew for sure what it was.

"And the other girl", I asked. "That was Marjorie—you remember Marjorie." I remembered Marjorie. I saw her here when I had been a student. The first two girls had died and the mother was doing all she could to keep her last little girl. Marjorie was four, two years older than we usually take in the Baby Clinic but her mother brought her every Wednesday. Marjorie had long bright red curls. She was husky and seemed well. She had a simple small cleft palate that interfered with her speech. Every Wednesday whoever was in the baby clinic would tell Mrs. Blake she ought to have it fixed while the baby was young. "It's my last little girl," she would say, "and I don't know what I would do if anything happened to her." We always explained that the cleft was so small that it would mean only a few whiffs of ether and about two stitches—much simpler than tonsils. She finally brought her in and the operation took only ten minutes, hardly a drop of blood and no trouble at all. But there was something wrong in all those children. That night after recovering perfectly without even vomiting from ether, Marjorie went into convulsions. John worked with her all night but in the morning she was dead. As we handed the baby wrapped in a blanket to the mother all we heard was "It's God's will."

Now here she was with her last child dying and her husband away to St. John's on a schooner. I helped move the boy into the plaster room and prayed hopelessly while I put a tube into his stomach and poured in sulphadiazine. He was too far gone to swallow. By teatime he was demanding to be allowed to go to the bathroom and this morning he was telling us he wanted to be in the ward with other people. His is the most miraculous cure I have ever witnessed and we will be only too pleased to move him out of the dying room.

November 14, '41. A boat got in from Leading Tickles this afternoon with three patients. They all had to be admitted—an OB, an infected hand, and a neglected burn on a small boy. The man with the hand told us that he had heard that Ricka Rowsell, our sore throat patient in Lockport, had died three weeks after we had been there on the *Bonnie Nell.* I don't understand that. She was almost entirely well when I left her.

November 21, '41. Sunday, and a quiet one, though there is promise of activity. An 'On His Majesty's Service' wire came today requesting that we investigate the sore throat epidemic in Lockport. It's no season to go to Lockport. It means crossing the bay around Long Point passing Northern Head and New Bay Head, crossing New Bay through Leading Tickles and around Thimble Head to Lockport in Seal Bay. Wynn agreed to send his motor boat. He has two good men aboard as crew. I guess it's logical that I go. It means my thirty-second birthday will be spent at sea. I had a feeling last fall that we hadn't heard the last of those throats. This time I will take a dozen petri dishes with culture medium and see if I can't find out what germ is giving them all this trouble.

November 22, '41. Happy Birthday I said to myself as I scrabbled around before daylight getting my stuff together for the journey. The weather looked gray and uncivil so we had to give up the pipe dream of making it in an easy one-stage sail. I don't think the men ever intended to go outside. Nobody wants to spend the whole winter frozen in Lockport. We pointed the motor yacht, *Dorothy*, into the shelter of the Bay and sneaked around behind Exploits and Black Island to drop our anchor in my favorite harbor—Norther Harbor. There is only one trouble with Norther Harbor, you aren't anywhere when you get there. Leaving the men with the boat, I pushed on the lone four miles through six inches of virgin snow to Fortune Harbor. I sought the hospitality of the parsonage but Father Hinchey was away. Fowlow provided a mug-up of tea and soup, which I disposed of while he routed out a pony and sled to take me across the peninsula to Issac Boone's in Cottle's Cove. I enjoyed the ride in the gloaming. This untouched part of the world has big trees and people seem to live on a little larger scale than on the wind burnt islands. The Boone's treated me well. I amused myself in the evening trying to spin some yarn. I wound up buying six pounds of homespun wool. "All in all," I thought as I crept into a good bed, "This is a more wholesome and less Checovian

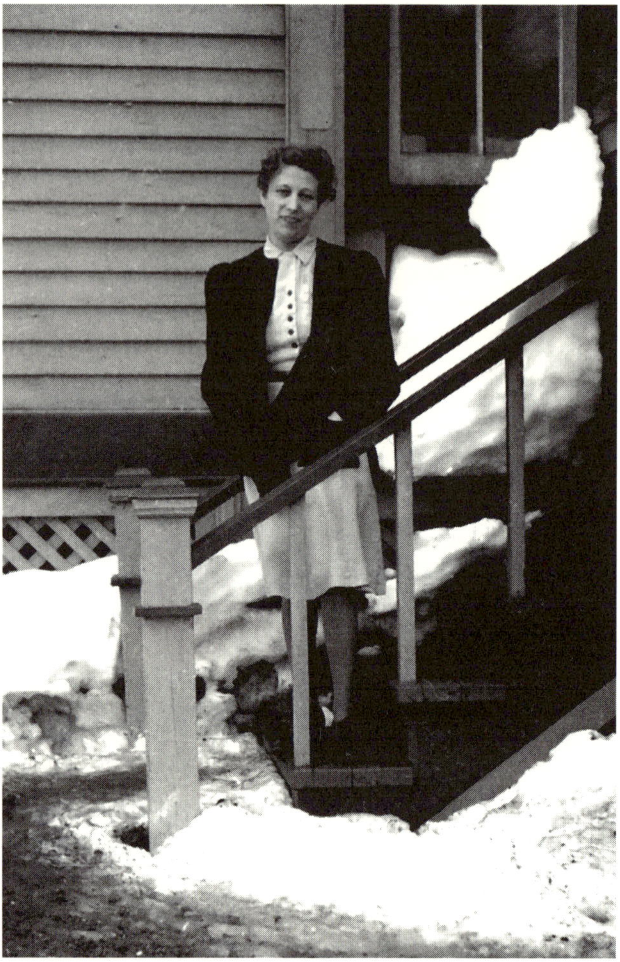

Stella Manuel of Twillingate, noble nurse, my mentor in tatting. Author's photograph..

birthday than my last—not a drink—not a fight—just good outdoor sport." I fell asleep before I could develop the theme.

November 23, '41. Things began to get interesting. In the morning Boone's two sons took me through Leading Tickles to the backside of Lockport. They improved the shining hour by making wide excursions to shoot six turrs during the trip. I trudged two miles across the neck and hailed a punt at the tickle. In no time I was in my old haunt, Lockport. There had been about twenty cases of bad throat during the past three weeks—one child had died. All the rest were well. It was hard to tell much from the descriptions but it sounded like the old business that Stan and I had been seeing here for the past four months. I did at least find that Ricka Rowell had recovered entirely from her throat. She had been caught in the rain in an open boat and died three days later. The throat might still have had something to do with it. Strep or Dip could have left a damaged heart.

I got out my twelve four-inch glass petri dishes with covers and made twelve smears from the throats of the most recently ill. To keep the cultures alive I put them under my shirt against my skin. Thus loaded I felt very fragile and pregnant as I retraced my steps. The Boone boys were impatiently watching the darkening November sky when I found them. No time was wasted on birds as we sped through Leading Tickles and faced the lop of New Bay to Cottle's Cove. My bed looked good to me. I have a faculty, after two nights in a place, of feeling as if I had always lived there. I even felt enough at home to try the parlor organ but the frost drove me back to the kitchen stove.

November 24, '41. The jaunt begins to be long. There were six patients waiting for me to get up this morning and they made me late in getting across the peninsula. At Fortune Harbor, after a cup of tea, Fowlow prevailed on the pony boy to take me to Norther Harbor. He was a little afraid of the deep snow on the unused trail. I reached the boat by late afternoon. Warrick, the mate, had had the luck to see a big lobster on the bottom when he inspected the mooring. He gaffed it (strictly against the law) and it was boiling when I arrived. It was so big that only the tail and claws would go into the pot. We sliced steaks off the tail and there was more than three could eat. The men were concerned about the rising wind and lowering sky. They wanted to get in the shelter of the islands before dark. We reached Exploits by dark. Things were looking bad enough to occasion a twenty-minute debate as to whether we ought to push on. Those twenty minutes I guess made the difference, for when we hit the weather we were sorry. It was only two miles to the two rocks known as Block Island. We crept into the narrow tickle and tied up to the shore. The bottom had dropped out of the glass and we can be glad we are here. It looks like a bleak Thanksgiving and these late November storms don't mind how long they stay. This hard wooden bench isn't much of a bed.

November 25, '41. THANKSGIVING. A day to count blessings. I count them as I sit in my overcoat on my bed. All I have to do is swing around and I am in bed. The wind has howled all day. The snow even now sifts through the ill-fitting hatch. The lack of fuel has reduced us to a few wet smoldering sticks. We foraged ashore for food this morning—there are only two houses here—and found nothing but candied orange peel. That topped off my Thanksgiving feast—tea with no milk or sugar—bread with no butter or jam—frozen sardines, granular and tasteless—dry old moldy rat cheese and then the orange peel. We tried playing Auction 45 but the deck is an inch thick with dampness and has seven cards missing. We have no tobacco. At least I remembered that the call bag has a bottle of Nembutal in it to soften my bed a little. We don't dare stick our bow out. Constant tapping of the barometer only made it go lower. The moaning of the storm means we won't get home tomorrow either. Oh Lord, how long?

November 29, '41. I am only just beginning to feel human. Thanksgiving Day, Friday, and Saturday, the three of us huddled in the cold cabin gazing blankly at the uncooperative barometer. We took turns tapping it every five minutes. Our larder grew no better and we scraped along on almost nothing. I finally threw the deck of cards overboard. The cold and hunger wasn't so bad if you kept full of Nembutal, two at bedtime and two first thing in the morning. Early Sunday morning it looked as if we wouldn't get out so I took two more and fell asleep. I awoke, surprised to find us moving. Ahead of us Twillingate shimmered in the clear winter sky in a new coat of snow.

These homecomings are sweet pleasure. We had been reported as leaving Exploits Wednesday night in a storm. No one had sighted us after that. I loved every one for the warm welcome. Our friend, Joe White, was here and my case of rum stood grandly in the middle of my living room floor. While it was being opened, I had the joy of a hot tub. Two drinks cemented our fraternity forever—John, Stan, Joe and Betty, Annette, and I. Dinner was gay while it lasted—I mean while I lasted. In the middle of the caribou course I rose unsteadily to my feet and excused myself—too much welcome—too much Nembutal—too much rum—too much excitement—too far to my bed. I didn't open an eye until this morning. All those culture plates I carried so carefully and warmed with my life's blood froze solid on the *Dorothy* and not a damn thing has grown on them. We weren't the only ones storm-bound. Wednesday night Captain Butcher had collapsed and become unconscious on the *Clyde* as she docked at Campbellton. His crew had put him in his bunk and rushed him towards Twillingate. Just outside of the Run the seas had taken the deck cargo over the side and she had to put back to Exploits. He got to the hospital Sunday morning and he is not going to live. He will never have to hear the *Clyde* blow and him not on it. The noble captain, unconscious, had still been part of the ship. At the worst of it he had roused enough to say, "Pretty rough, pretty rough for this one."

December 3, '41. Captain Butcher died last night and with him part of Twillingate. There are bright young graduates of navigation schools to take his place on the bridge, but the *Clyde* to many will never mean what she used to.

December 8, '41. What a day—a weird one which please God I shall never have to go through again. It started way last Friday when Malcom Simms and George Chaulker came to the Olds for tea. John suggested that I get my telegraph key and take a lesson in code from Simms and only to please him, I got it. Something was wrong with it and when I tried to fix it, John interfered with his notion of how the wires should go. In another ten minutes I'm certain that blood would have flowed. Just as Betty made peace with tea and brownies, the Slades yelled for another doctor. John argued a while because Doccy Wood had just been down there to see the fits, but when John found that Wood's car had broken down, he picked up Doccy Wood and went about 12:30. I read until they came back and then John and I settled the world's problems until 2:30. I was in bed exactly fifteen minutes when Hazel called me for an OB case in Indian Cove. I wrestled with the telephone, got Stevie and his horse out of bed and on a misty slippery night we started for Purcell's Harbor without knowing whether the road was open. The fog diapason warned me to bring my compass. I also took little David's sled in case I had to haul the OB bag. At Purcell's Harbor a boat was waiting for the quick punch across the tickle to Gauss', where I battled the whole night through urging Mrs. Gauss to push. I used intranasal pituitrin. By 7:30, a fine boy was screaming in the crib. Back at Purcell's Harbor, I put the bag on the sled and pulled like mad to Little Harbor where I telephoned Steve to come and get me and then walked all the way to the big hill before he hove into sight.

While I drew a tub, Swanker suddenly appeared. He had left Fogo and was on his way with Mrs. Swanker to the States. Their household goods were already in Lewisporte and they had reservations on the morrow's train. When Swanker heard that I was planning to take a holiday in the States the first of the year, he volunteered to stay at the hospital until I came back if I would go now. The idea was that I should take his reservations and leave within twenty-four hours. It would be a break for the hospital not to be shorthanded and it was a generous offer on Swanker's part. It meant a lot of rearranging for him. I stood with one foot in the tub and asked for an hour to think it over. Before I could get the other foot in, a rush OB call came from a patient I had promised to deliver down on the Arm. Bathless, I rounded up Stella and went on the call. While Stella watched the patient I sat by the kitchen stove pondering this going to the States. It was certainly best for the hospital to have three doctors, but did I want to go now? These were hectic times for the world. I wasn't eager to leave these people who are my friends. I liked our snug meals upstairs in the Olds' digs and in the Hardy's apartment. I would miss my friends in Twillingate and New World Island. The busy OPD didn't seem so bad. The ski runs with the dogs seemed only swift and smooth now, the slob didn't seem so deep, the sea not so rough. My patients all seemed reasonable grateful people who blessed your healing hand. Stella, handing me the brush and soap, stopped my reverie. For awhile there was no time for dreaming. At 3:00 back at the hospital, Joe White and John were in my room. I hadn't actually made up my mind but when I saw John's inquiring smile, I said, "O.K. I'll go now—be back in four weeks."

It was more fun to talk with Joe over a root of rum than to pack or take that bath. The tub was cold by now anyway. Tea was on us before I knew it and I had to play a return bout of poker so that Bert Pardy could get back the seven fifty I had won the last time. It was two-A.M. before any packing got started. At six, still tired, I scurried around to have breakfast and gather my stuff together and with papers still on my desk, clothes still in the laundry, I boarded Skipper Frank's *Little Grace* for the smoothest trip to Lewisporte I ever saw—like the glass. Lewisporte was gloomy, dark and wet. At the King George Hotel where I had always found sanctuary, a full-faced wench said there was no room. Manuel's Hotel, with which the hospital has always had a kind of feud, offered complete hospitality. Just before tea, a Canadian soldier reported the incredible rumor that Japan had bombed Manila. The next broadcast found a tense group around the radio—Pearl Harbor had been bombed too. I was in twelve minds about what to do. I went back to Skipper Frank's boat to talk with him and to think out my problem. I decided to go on. Skipper Frank offered to wake me for the 3:00 A.M. train. Mrs. Manuel offered to call me. The stationmaster offered to call me. I refused them all. The half-hour-warning whistle had never failed to wake me. Under the hotel window a switch engine shifted coal cars all night. A dozen times I got out of bed to check. Suddenly a strange man stuck his head in my door—"Are you leaving on the 3:00 o'clock train?" I nodded yes. "It's gone." He slammed the door. In the wet wind by the open window my lighter wouldn't ignite the lamp. Mr. March, the station agent, was surprised to see me in my coat and pajamas. Considerable burning of the wire to St. John's got permission for me to use the repair gang's speeder to catch the second section of the *Overland Limited.* Permission didn't come until 8:00 and, perched high on the speeder with my bag clutched in one hand, holding on to the center support with the other, we clanked along the twelve miles in the rain. There was a two-hour wait at the junction. Still we had no news and now on the train there is nothing but terrible rumor of eight cruisers sunk and God knows what. Olds wired me, "Advise immediate return, but do as you think best." I'm going on.

EPILOGUE

It was a thoughtful quiet ride cross-country. Rumor and speculation flourished on the lack of news. The Newfoundlanders and Canadians were excited, but of course could not feel as I did about the entry of my country into the war. To them it was a new ally and relief. Even though I felt we should have entered long ago, it was still a personal shock. The *Caribou* was crowded to the gunwales. We crossed the gulf convoyed by corvettes and for good reason. Eight of a twenty-eight-ship convoy had been sunk within the month in sight of Sydney Harbor. That wasn't my last crossing on the *Caribou*, but it's the one that stays in my mind. The blackout made us feel threatened. It must have been about 2:00 A.M. as I was getting myself a mug-up in the pantry off the darkened saloon, that I met the two young R. A. F. cadets. They were a little tight. One was singing. I'd never heard the song. They sang it for me waltzing together around the rocking saloon—"Bless them all—bless them all, the long and the short and the tall. You'll get no promotion this side of the ocean—bless them all, bless them all." The *Caribou* is on the bottom with her dead and somehow I know those happy flyers are gone too. The few words to draw the picture come hard.

Mother McKenzie in Sydney made me take a bath and put a boiled dinner in front of me. She gave me the details of the loss of the *Rodney* and the *Prince of Wales*. "I understand," she said, "I know that you can't eat. I'll give you a good cup of tea." She told me to go back to Newfoundland. I'm sure that it was through her offices that the railroad put me on an extra car that gave me a berth to Brunswick. At the border, I surrender my passport and with it my past. Newfoundland, I knew was a happy dream and I couldn't help wondering what Swanker would do with his half of the bargain. "Till I came back," I felt, might well be quite a while.

My Brooklyn draft board welcomed me. Who ever heard of Newfoundland? Three doctors for 30,000 people didn't make doctoring essential civilian occupation. My number would be called any minute, and where had I been and who the hell did I think I was. They didn't care if my name was Ickes. Where they got the idea my name was Ickes I don't know. I took it for granted that the chairman could read. I would fool them though. I rushed to Church Street to try for a commission in the Navy. Yes, the commander was in and would see me, lisped the yeoman. The navy office was empty and luxurious and quiet. An hour passed on a hard bench. More curly-haired lisping and "the commander would see me." After a half-hour, I allowed as how I would see the commander in hell. I went downstairs to the Army. There was no such nonsense there. Col. Lippold saw me right away and put the wheels in motion. He wasn't certain we could circumvent the eager draft board's intention to make me a private. He apparently had lost an occasional skirmish. Affidavits had to be collected. My diplomas and papers were in Twillingate. I rushed around to Governor's Island, the Central Draft Office, to my college, to my university, to Church Street, to Maine, to Madison Avenue. Like the Hound of Heaven, "I fled Him, down the nights and down the days; I fled Him, down the arches of the years."

The smallest comfort came from Governor's Island. They were certain my commission would come through. But they said, "For God's sake, send us a postcard every few days after you are inducted. We often get a commission for a draftee and then we can't find him. He's lost in some camp or other. We have had commissions kicking around for six months before we located the owner; I assured the captain I would write him every day. The race got hotter. I took my pre-induction exam and stood in my drawers all day with a thousand or so fellow New Yorkers. They lost the laboratory specimen. I lost the tag around my neck and had to wait till last to get my clothes back. There was some question of my passing the physical—blood pressure they said. I wasn't to worry. There would be an appeal for another exam. The day I was to take that, Valentines Day, as it happened, my commission came as a 1st Lieutenant, in an envelope with a bright red border. Various informants assured me that two weeks elapse before assignment to active duty. I believed them and while the draft board paged me in Grand Central Station, I grabbed a plane to Hollywood.

Three days later, in Santa Barbara, a much-forwarded telegram found me. It ordered me to report to duty at Governor's Island, New York, two days before. In this premonitory fashion, I started my army career—AWOL.

After fifty years, two of the star players are still on deck—
actually the deck of M.S. *Petite Forte*

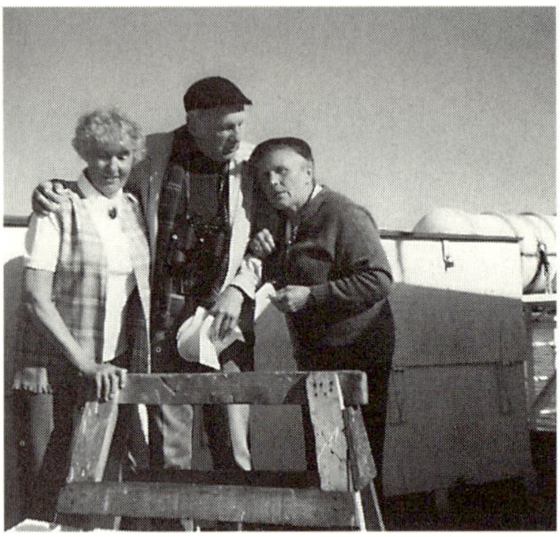

Left to right: Jesse Troake Drover R.N., Ecke, and Grace M. Sparks, twice an honorary doctor.

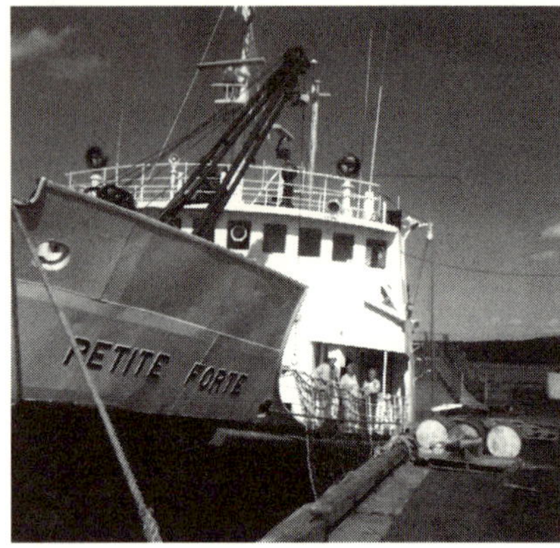

The ship.

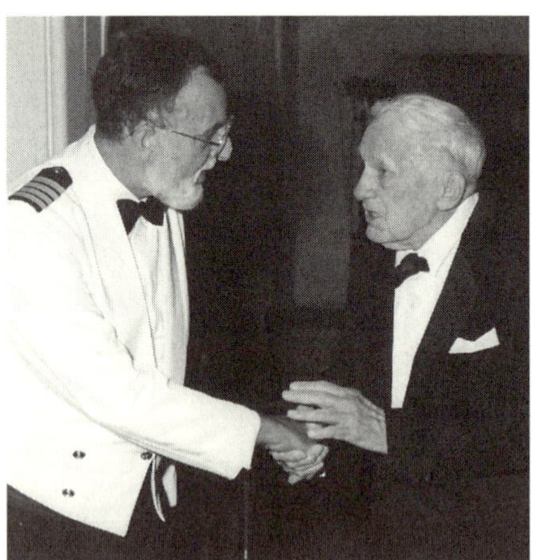

Ecke and friend
QE2 1998